TEACHER OF TH[E]
A Self Health Journey

by

SUZANNE LEWIS

An autobiographical story of healing during the decade of 1974–1984.

TEACHER OF THE HEART
A SELF HEALTH JOURNEY

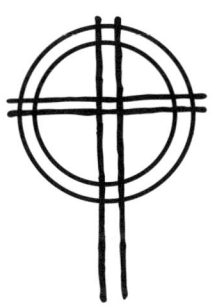

by
Suzanne Lewis

Cover Art by Cynthia Wearden
Photographs by Suzanne Lewis and friends

STAR ROSE PUBLISHING COMPANY
Boise, Idaho

Teacher of the Heart: A Self Health Journey. Copyright © 1997 by Suzanne Lewis. All rights reserved. Printed in the United States of America. No part of this book may be used or reproduced in any manner whatsoever without written permission except in the case of brief quotations embodied in critical articles and reviews. For information address STAR ROSE PUBLISHING COMPANY, Suzanne Lewis, 623 West Hays Street, Boise, Idaho 83702.

Original Book Design by Cynthia Wearden

SECOND EDITION

Lewis, Suzanne.
TEACHER OF THE HEART: A Self Health Journey / Suzanne Lewis. — 2nd edition
  Includes Index
  ISBN 1-887747-08-7
  Library of Congress Catalog Card Number 97–72310

1. Self Health/Help - Overcoming a life threatening brain disorder to becoming a healer.
2. Spiritual Healing/metaphysical 3. Autobiographical diary/journal of wholistic healing

DEDICATION

This book is dedicated to the Circle of Light and Life and to all my family, teachers and supportive co-hearts that have encouraged me to write my personal story of how I regained my vitality to live life healthily, filled with peace and joy inside and out. I thank each and every one of You for assisting me to show up with my heart, mind, spirit, emotions and body in better relations with all on this sweet Earth.

I especially want to thank my son, Nathan, for being my greatest teacher of patience and love. There is no coincidence that my first draft of *TEACHER OF THE HEART: A Self Health Journey* finally churned out of my trusty dinosaur of a computer one week after his graduation from high school. The book took twelve years to complete as did it take twelve years to assist my son to graduate from the public school system.

Through the years my son would say, "Mom, I think you need to go to the ocean or to the mountains and write." He knows how valuable a healing process it is for me to write, even when it meant going into isolation, leaving him to walk his own life. I am proud of both of us.

I also write to give great thanks to Mary Trail, who has often provided me the safe hermit's cottage by the ocean to write and the ongoing belief in this Journaling healing process. Gratitude floods over to Dr. Peggy Rowe whose own writing journey paralleled mine and propelled me to write even out of the 'structured education system' of recognition. Then I would like to recognize my soul brother, Garn Christensen for his ever present strength that reassured that my story was valuable. Lastly, great appreciation is sent to my soul sister, Cynthia Wearden, the artist who expressed a reflection of my journey through her interpretative creations.

Lorry Roberts, a long term friend and owner of Legendary Publishers, deserves respect and recognition for her advocacy of writing our stories for the sake of the women and the children and better relations in all aspects of life. For over five years she has consulted and shared important wisdom with me as the editing of this personal story unfolded. Thank you. I would like to also give deep gratitude to Carrie Chesnik, my editor, for honoring my unique writing style and choice of language and not structuring it to fit the typical accepted form.

Many others who appear in this book deserve great thanks. Our shared relations helped create the menu for my return to my self.

I thank you and We Meet as ONE.

DESIDERATA

GO PLACIDLY AMID THE NOISE and HASTE and

REMEMBER WHAT PEACE THERE MAY BE IN SILENCE.

AS FAR AS POSSIBLE WITHOUT SURRENDER
be on good terms with all persons. Speak the truth quietly and clearly; and listen to others, even the dull and ignorant; they too have their story. Avoid loud and aggressive persons, they are vexations to the spirit. If you compare yourself with others, you may become vain and bitter; for always there will be greater and lesser persons than yourself. Enjoy your achievements as well as your plans. Keep interested in your own career, however humble; it is a real possession in the changing fortunes of time. Exercise caution in your business affairs; for the world is full of trickery. But let this not blind you to what virtue there is; many persons strive for high ideals; and everywhere life is full of heroism.   Be yourself. Especially, do not feign affection. Neither by cynical about love; for in the face of all aridity and disenchantment it is perennial as the grass. Take kindly the counsel of the years, gracefully surrendering the things of youth. Nurture strength of spirit to shield you in sudden misfortune. But do not distress yourself with imaginings. Many fears are born of fatigue and loneliness. Beyond a wholesome discipline, be gentle with yourself.   You are a child of the universe, no less then the trees and the stars; you have a right to be here. And whether or not it is clear to you, no doubt the universe is unfolding as it should. Therefore, be at peace with God, whatever you conceive Him to be, and whatever our labors and aspirations, in the noisy confusion of life keep peace with your soul. With all its sham, drudgery and broken dreams it is still a beautiful world.   Be careful.   Strive to be HAPPY.

— FOUND IN OLD SAINT PAUL'S CHURCH, BALTIMORE
DATED 1692

DISCLAIMER

This book *TEACHER OF THE HEART: A Self Health Journey* is my perception of this 1974-1984 decade, its people, situations and political air.

There is a Zen story that come to me . . . Three people are walking down the street; all of them witness a real life situation where a person is striding along when all of a sudden the being slips on a banana peel and falls down into a mud puddle. One who watches the fall cries out in alarm; the second person observes the person falling and cracks up with nervous laughter, and the third person yells out "stupid person you should have been looking where you were going."

This book is my story told through my heart and mind. We each have our own sacred calling and life path we must walk. I have changed the names of the participants whose lives wove through mine so as to observe their rights to privacy. Most of my teachers are identified authentically, as they deserve this respect and honor. I am thankful that I trained with them personally rather than through books or videos. I was lucky to have lived during a time that they were accessible.

I told my story honestly. But, it was told through my eyes. Others have the right to their story or perspective.

PEACE TO ALL MY RELATIONS.

An associate of Suzanne's at Integrative Health Building, Bonnie Vestal, M.D., states:

"Suzanne is both a visionary and a wisdomkeeper, walking well ahead of her time in this complex and demanding world. Using the fundamental concept of remembered wellness, a powerful tool for restoring health, she weaves her story with simple elegance. Following her personal journey reminds us all that we must return to the heart before setting out on the path."

PERMISSIONS

Special thanks to Brooke Medicine Eagle for permission to quote extensively from *Buffalo Woman Comes Singing,* copyright 1991 by Ballantine Books. Thanks also to Kate Wolf for permission to quote her song *Medicine Wheel,* copyright 1982 by Another Sundown Publishing Company. Thanks to Dr. Richard Moss for permission to quote from a private workshop and author of the book *The I That is We Awakening to Higher Energies Through Unconditional Love,* copyright 1981 by Celestial Arts. Gratitude to Patti Weber Lightstone to print her add song I DREAMED A DREAM.

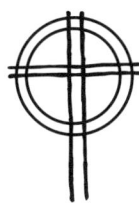

INTRODUCTION

My philosophical backbone of wholistic health is based on the short prose called *Desiderata*, found in an old Saint Paul's church in Baltimore dated 1692. At the beginning of each chapter a segment of this prose appears.

The knowledge I share has been gained or reclaimed during the last twenty years of my life. At the age of 24 I was diagnosed by Western Medicine to have an over-enlarged pituitary gland. The only way I became aware that the comptroller of the Endocrine system was 'out-of-order' was that my physical body began to change. I became taller, my body proportions grew. The chronic head pain (which I remember having since the third grade) was a constant companion in my life. The choices made in 1974 to heal my disorder wholistically have led me down and through a path of self health techniques, attitudes and cleansings that I now choose to call Wholistic Therapy. This body-mind-spirit-emotional relationship has developed into a way of living for me.

I contend that life is like a book. Collectively, I feel we share the same chapters, a person just opts to live the chapters at their own time line. What occurred in my life concerning a 'con' person happened at 32 years of age, whereas someone else may experience this same theme at 15 or 52.

My years as a health care practitioner have motivated me to share the vulnerabilities and the resultant strengths of these sometime painful and scarring life experiences, because I know I do not walk alone.

This decade from 1974-1984 took over twelve years to write. Upon rereading the early years there is a part of me that is embarrassed by the naivety and the broken spirit I share. The book travels an arduous journey as I learned to live life fully in peace rather than to continue as a broken, disbelieving, 'living dead' person. During the editing process I made the critical decision to leave my original journaled script and not rewrite impersonally, in my present day wise person language.

People have asked why it has taken so long to bring this book to fruition, my response is "It was the O. J. Simpson Trial travesty that demanded from my sense of justice to speak out for the battered and broken families of violence and to let go my own story of the consequence of abuse, especially when it affects children and subsequent long-term pain and suffering for all".

    If just one person can sense the similarities to their book of life and gain inspiration or choices to enhance their own well being, re-creating a healthier individual and family life styles; then the writing of this portion of my autobiographical journey has been worth it. The basic intention of this wounded healer's path is to assist more people to know that "Heaven on Earth is right now, right here" so let's get on with experiencing a wonderful way living on this sweet Earth in good relations with All The Family of Life.

CONTENTS

DEDICATION
DISCLAIMER
DESIDERATA
PERMISSIONS
INTRODUCTION

Chapter 1	TEACHER OF THE HEART: A Self Health Journey	
	ILLNESS ACKNOWLEDGED	1
Chapter 2	RAM DASS - BE HERE NOW	11
Chapter 3	YOGA - UNION	13
Chapter 4	CHILDHOOD REFLECTIONS	19
Chapter 5	THE FARM - 1975	23
Chapter 6	SHATTERED MARRIAGE	29
Chapter 7	PREPARATION FOR BIRTH - PRAYER FILLED REUNION	
	WITH GOD	35
Chapter 8	BIRTH OF SON - BIRTH OF SELF	39
Chapter 9	FEMALE/MOTHERING FRIENDSHIP	43
Chapter 10	DAILY HEALTH PRACTICES	45
Chapter 11	FEMALE ENERGY/EXTRA SENSORY PERCEPTION	53
Chapter 12	CULTIVATING SPIRITUALITY	57
Chapter 13	FAMILY PATTERNS - 1978	63
Chapter 14	EARTH CELEBRATION - TWO RAVENS AT TALL PINE	71
Chapter 15	1979 BOOK MAGIC	79
Chapter 16	SELF AND SELF WITH OTHERS	87
Chapter 17	TRANSFORMATIONAL ENERGY WORKSHOP	91
Chapter 18	BOOK MAGIC 1980	97
Chapter 19	SPIRITUAL EMERGENCY - 1980	103
Chapter 20	RIVER JOURNEY	107
Chapter 21	TRUE LOVE	113
Chapter 22	SAN FRANCISCO SURVIVAL SCHOOL APRIL - 1981	121
Chapter 23	HEALING THE SELF	125
Chapter 24	NEW AMERICAN MEDICINE SHOW - FALL 1981	141
Chapter 25	DECEMBER 1981	151
Chapter 26	EARTH MESSENGERS - 1982	155

Chapter 27	SPRING 1982	161
Chapter 28	WHITE BUFFALO CALF WOMAN TRAINING WITH BROOKE MEDICINE EAGLE	171
Chapter 29	THE FUTURIST - SETTING ONE'S INTENTIONS	179
Chapter 30	WHOLE PERSON - WHOLE PLANET	189
Chapter 31	THE LOST YEAR - 1983	197
Chapter 32	TRANSITIONS - 1984	209
	POSTSCRIPT	219
	LIFE SONG	221
	NATHAN'S WISH FOR THE WORLD	222
	REFERENCES	225
	ORDER FORM	231

PHOTOGRAPHS

Photo Title	page number
TEACHER	2
1968 MARRIAGE COMMITMENT	6
THE FARM	24
1976 PALENQUE, MEXICO	30
NOVEMBER 1976 BIRTHING OF SON	38
MOTHER AND SON	42
1978 FEMININE ENERGY WORKSHOP AT THE FARM	52
JULY 1978, TWO RAINBOWS EARTH GATHERING	59
"SUZI" AS A CHILD	62
"SUE" AS A TROUBLED TEEN	66
"SUE" IN HER TWENTIES RETURNING TO THE HIGH COUNTRY	69
1979, SUZANNE ON THE FARM	72
1979 TWO RAVENS FESTIVAL	76
TWO RAVENS FESTIVAL	77
1979 BOOK MAGIC OPENING	80
EXTENDED FAMILY'S CHILDREN	102
1980 EASTER ON THE FARM	106
1980 MIDDLEFORK OF THE SALMON RIVER TRIP	108
NAVIGATING WITH WILD RIVER	110
SUZANNE LETTING HER HEART ART OUT	117
COMPANION ON THE OCEAN — FIRST PHASE OF DR. MOSS'S PRESCRIPTION FOR HEALTH	119
1981 NORTHERN IDAHO HEALING CAMP FOR SUZANNE	126
SUZANNE LETTING GEOTHERMAL WATER HELP HEAL	142
BROOKE MEDICINE EAGLE	166
1982 TEEN SURVIVAL SCHOOL IN THE HIGH COUNTRY	188
1982 TWO RAVENS FESTIVAL	192, 193
1982 HOT AIR BALLOON AT THE FARM	199
NATURE HEALING SOJOURN	204
GRANDFATHER	210, 211
1984 HEALING SUZANNE	214
1984 SUZANNE AT THE OCEAN PRAYING FOR DIVINE GUIDANCE	217
1985 SUZANNE HAPPY WITH CHILDREN AND SUPPORTIVE FRIEND	220

TABLE OF INSERTS

	page number
CHAKRAS	14
ENDOCRINE SYSTEM	17
PRAYER OF SAINT FRANCIS	37
TRUE CREED'S SEVEN CONCEPTS	48
NEUROPHONE INFORMATION	101
ORIENTAL FIVE ELEMENT THEORY	130
FIRST CORINTHIANS, VERSE 12	133
FOOD-COMBINING CHART	134
HERBAL MANUAL	135
SPIRITUAL PERSPECTIVE from ALAN WATTS	147
1995 PUBLIC APOLOGY for VIET NAM by MCNAMARA	154
TWIN CHARACTERISTICS	163
MEDICINE WHEEL by KATE WOLF	164
WOMEN by CRAZY HORSE	176
SUPERBEINGS INFORMATION	180
HOW THE BODY REFLECTS THE MIND	185
HOW TO LOVE YOURSELF	187
THOMAS BANYACA'S INTERPRETATION of HOPI PROPHECIES	190
I DREAMED A DREAM by PATTI WEBER LIGHTSTONE	221
MY WISH FOR THE WORLD by NATHAN	222
ORDER FORM	231

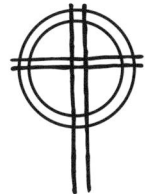

"GO PLACIDLY AMID THE NOISE and HASTE and REMEMBER WHAT PEACE THERE MAY BE IN SILENCE, AS FAR AS POSSIBLE WITHOUT SURRENDER BE ON GOOD TERMS WITH ALL PERSONS."

"TEACHER OF HEART: A Self Health Journal"

ILLNESS ACKNOWLEDGED

I have become known as a pioneer in the field of Wholistic Therapeutic Touch. How I wish that this success story could start in 1985 instead of 1974. It would be oh so easy to share my adventures with various cross cultural teachers that enriched my ability to be a ceremonial teacher of the Medicine Wheel and the Oriental Five Element Theory.

Numerous healing stories could be told regarding the decade of "hands on" therapeutic touch with a diverse clientele that willingly brought their personal dreams and pain to me to help each return to their authentic birth right of grace and trust to live fully with this sweet Earth. Quickly, an individual's effort to mend spilled over to their family with the recognition that "monkey see, monkey do." Ailments and structural imbalance easily are patterned into each and every family member, often totally unconsciously, sometimes even originating while in the womb. Over the past decade, my individual client healing work has spread to the mending of family's generational unhealthy traits.

I have taught one and two year-long Self Health and Wholistic Touch Apprenticeships for over a decade. My basic belief is that a Whole Person makes for a Whole Planet. Teachers, counselors, nurses, physical therapists, doctors and ordinary individuals have pursued studies with me to expand their own body-mind-spirit and emotional balance with enhanced validation of their own innate spiritual gifts of healing.

Coming from a generation which was trained to believe it was better to be "seen but not heard, and to smile pretty but say nothing," I have pursued training in diverse communication skill building from mediation, to conflict resolution within a Community setting and finally to family communication skills especially focused on the 'extended family' that now flourishes in our society. I perpetuate a circular, consensus approach to education not a hierarchial, antiquated mandating one.

I have gone one step further to acknowledge that these gained communication skills can be utilized to make peace not only with our external family and community but also with our internal family. My acute ability to read the body-mind is now recognized as leading edge self health technology. Though I never refers to myself as a 'healer' or 'medicine woman', the strength and integrity of my character is reflected in the

TEACHER

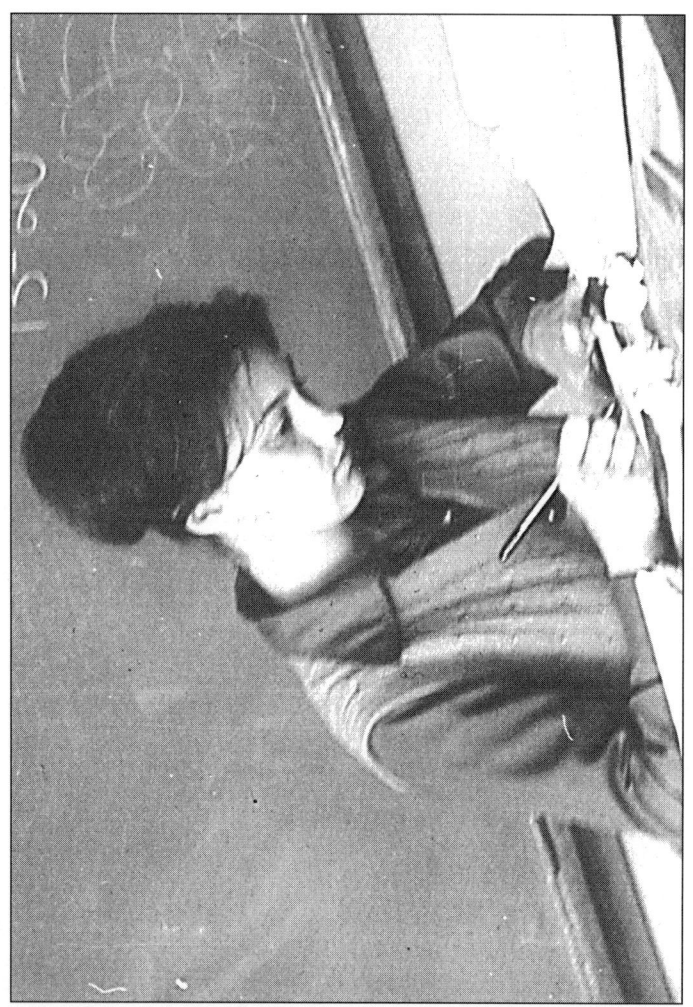

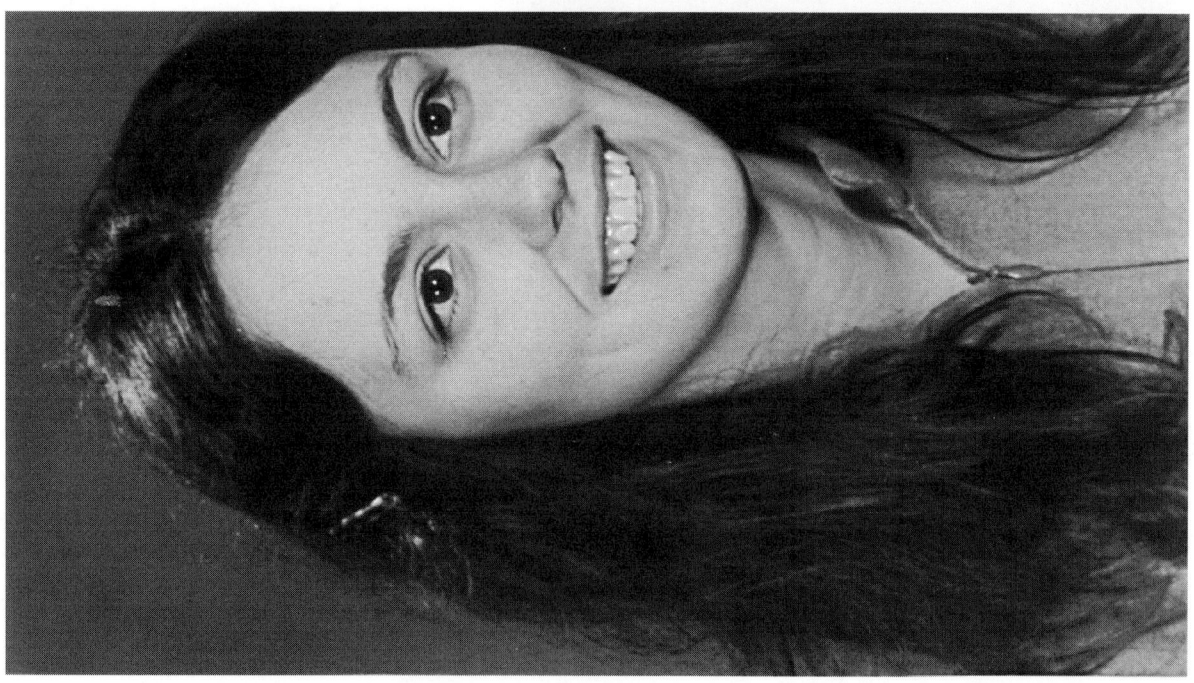

community touched and their renewed health and trust that this Earth and her family is a healthy, sustaining place to live.

One of my espousals is "most of society has been trained to believe that their mind is housed in the skull between one's ears." This is a fallacy, I believe. The mental capacity in the skull can lie and go unconscious especially regarding harmful, painful chapters in one's life. The body that rests below the skull houses one's honest history and trust. The body does not know how to lie. A trained touch technician can assist an individual to recognize an age and an emotional state that has created blocks in the person's ability (personality) to healthfully enjoy their moment to moment, day to day existence.

The most common questions I have been asked are "How did you get into this vocation? How did you know you were a healer?" This book is the true story of my reflections on the journey from a life threatening disorder to become a pioneer 'hands on' healer.

People have asked me why it has taken so long to bring this book to fruition. My response is "it was the O. J. Simpson trial travesty that demanded from my sense of justice to speak out for the battered and broken families of violence and to let go my own story of the consequence of abuse, especially when it affects children and subsequent long-term pain and suffering for all".

This very personal story begins in 1973 and continues into 1985. This decade of great inner and outer pain and suffering was an odyssey of exploring relations with myself, my blood and extended family, my contribution to my country and nature and most importantly coming home to my spiritual core.

When the editing process came for this story four years ago, I read for the first time the chapters put together. Immediately I felt great shame for how broken and "wimpy" that young twenty-four year old was. I was personally stunned at the undercurrent always present regarding male/female relationships. I was relieved that she didn't rule my current world and I pondered whether I should rewrite the script as a very mature, wise, forty plus year old. After much prayer and meditation, I decided to leave the script flavored authentically and allow you, the reader, the opportunity to be chagrined and hopefully elated with my growth of self and spirit through the decade of 1974 - 1985.

The clientele and students who have entered my world since 1984 have been mirrors to certain chapters in this book. By bringing the 'secrets out of the closet' healing begins. This does not mean we are to languish in the past. Rather, we are to recover broken personality parts, embrace and recognize them, forgiving ourselves for ever engaging in such misconceptions and let them go—telling ourselves, "don't go down that road again." I now can say to my clientele, I can identify with the 'yo-yo' relationship cycle it sounds to me you are in. Look in my book; see all those chapter with prose introduction reads "Be yourself. Especially do not feign affection..." those are my repeated search for a soul partner, my own 'yo-yo' relation.

What's important to know is that secrets kept hidden hurt everyone; if I can be a totem person to bring out some of my most awkward, embarrassing and deeply vulnerable sagas, others may benefit through simple mirroring identification.

The darkest, most unconscious times rest deep in the body and are often triggered by similar situations in our daily life. Incidents which are "the straw that breaks the camel's back" become the tools for retrieval of lost parts that deserve to be mended.

For me it is the sound of flesh being smacked that jerks my trigger totally involuntarily. Instantly my child self quivers and backs away. But, it is time to tell my story.

A long, long time ago on a faraway frontier, somewhere East of the moon and West of the sun, my young adult self began a long journey back to self and health. I noticed that my body was changing drastically and I could not control it. After nine months of exploratory medical research and study with an endocrinologist in Boise, Idaho, I was told the only thing left to do to help determine my health disorder was surgery. I had gone through an usual growth spurt at the age of 24. Not only did I grow taller but a persistent pain throbbed and seared behind my left eye.

The MRI (x-rays) reported an over-enlarged pituitary gland. At that time I did not even understand how this master gland functioned, let alone comprehend that it ruled the body's entire endocrine system, which includes the glandular secretor/regulator for the thyroid, hypothalamus, thymus, adrenals, sexual organ, thalamus, tonsils, and lymphatic system.

My body was drastically transforming and my mind could not get it to balance. No longer could I pretend that everything was perfect. For the first time, I decided to take charge of my life and health. Options to do exploratory surgery on the brain were totally unacceptable. The day the endocrinologist gave me the choice of cutting into the brain or not was the beginning of my deeply personal journey to self-health. Recent memories of the death of my beloved grandmother in the hospital and its system of machines, medicine and loss of personal dignity propelled me to walk out the doctor's office never to return.

At the same time, the rest of my world was exploding around me. My childhood sweetheart and savior from my blood family, Lion Heart, did not want to be monogamous any longer. He was in unconditional love, living in the Now and was magnetic and hot. We were going on five years of marriage, having married in our teens, and not only was I a wife but a teacher crusading and challenging the way young people were being educated.

After graduating from high school in 1967 during the height of the Vietnam tragedy (it was not named a war until after we were defeated) I was in a tremendous hurry to excel and gain an income. I graduated from college in 1970 with a degree in Mathematics and a Secondary Education teaching option. My teaching career began at a junior high where five teachers gave up their worst class so they could gain a prep period. Five classes to prepare daily plus handling the toughest, angriest teens imaginable created a mountain of stress for this twenty year old.

Besides the academic degree, little separated me from the students. I taught at the same junior high I had attended and at which my father had been the head physical education teacher and coach. I was the youngest teacher on staff at the toughest junior high in Boise. Many of my fellow teachers refused to acknowledge me as an equal. They thought of me as my father's child and their past student and thus continued to see me just as another student.

My participation in anti-war marches down our city's capital boulevard, dressed in mini-skirts and long, free flowing hair, actively protesting our involvement with Vietnam, did not help establish a good rapport with my school's principal, a retired military man. Luckily, the head of our city's math departments was a man whom I experienced mutual respect.

When I was an eighth grader, he was a fresh new teacher who volunteered to share a variety of philosophical pursuits after school for those students who wanted to communicate and understand life with a broader perspective. This special man gave me my lead to discover if I could find a better way to work with my mathematical students, especially the 'dead light bulbs' in the back of the room. I was fresh from the college regime and there was no way I could teach the 'same old way.' One of the reasons I had chosen to become a teacher was that during my high school years I was so disgusted with the quality of teachers I had that I was committed to share with students a more realistic, practical and heartfelt connection.

This doesn't mean that teaching agreed with me. During the first year of instructing mathematics and science, I suffered several stress-related disorders. At one point I started losing hair and actually developed bald spots that grew out as white hair. Jokingly, I have called these tufts of hair my stress barometer. The calmer I was the more likely the hair to be dark, the more challenged, the whiter the hair. Sometimes a strand of hair would be checkered, black-white, black-white.

The students were tough. The war was raging across the seas and war flaring in the classroom. Many youth would come to class stoned and angry, often camouflaging weapons. For many the greatest joy was breaking the teacher.

Transcendental Meditation was infiltrating the community in the early seventies, especially at the university from which I graduated. Knowing how vulnerable my mind was, I decided to be initiated into this Hindu mental calming process. I often said that during my last semester of college when I was getting a degree in Mathematics, my mind was shattered while participating in my last required math class, Abstract Algebra. It dealt with third and fourth dimensions of deliberation. That class, my senior year, was the only course in which I received a 'D'.

When I look back at my college education I can now find humor, though at the time it was so frustrating. I first started attending this junior college as a senior in high school. High School was a bore so I chose to challenge entrance requirements and was approved to attend while still in high school. During the next four years, my school grew with me. It became a four year college just as I need to go to upper division classes. By the fourth year it became an approved university. The Math Division brought in new teachers and new advanced courses and I found myself learning from novice instructors and brand new books.

My Abstract Algebra class with its fresh new teacher and book was the worse course I would ever take. It became very clear to me that a good teacher had to be a quality communicator. Advanced, complex math classes were like a foreign language. My last math instructor did not communicate well and I felt my mind literally frazzle with my over-achiever mentality. This class broke my perfection mode. I could not grasp any pattern or consistency. My brain went to overload and turned off.

A year later, dealing with social political changes, teaching aggressive, angry students, my health disorders were growing and consuming much more of my attention.

At the time my enlarged pituitary gland was diagnosed, my husband and I were considered the 'Golden Couple' in our peer group. My husband was a hero of sorts. He worked for the Boise International Fire Center and he and the crews he belonged to were renown for their heroic feats around fires. I called my husband and his male friends, the BIFC Boy's Club. They had little time for women. Their world was filled with their fiery escapades and machismo. When they would congregate around our home, I was to keep the quality food served but remain silent. If I did speak, I was mostly

1968 MARRIAGE COMMITTMENT

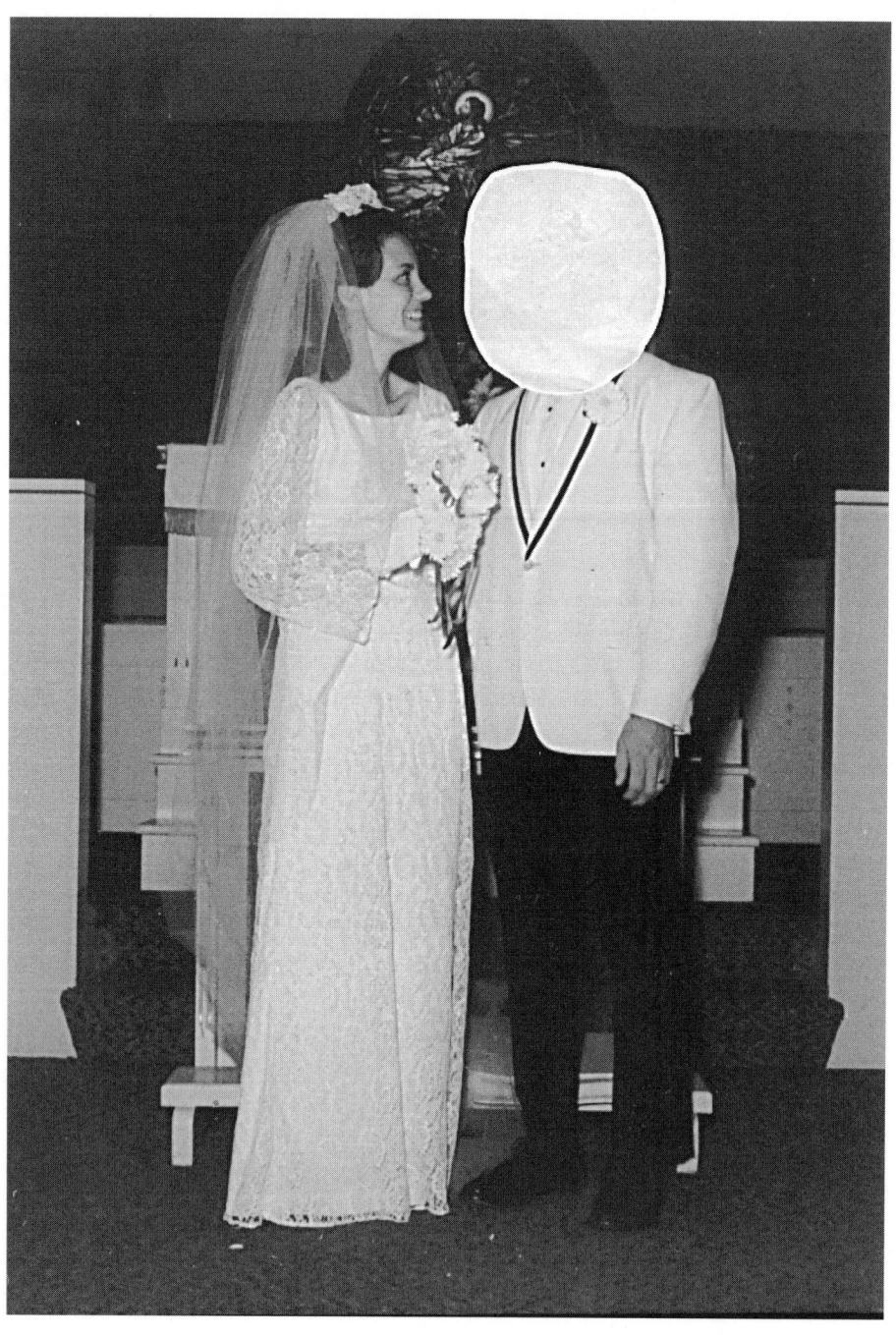

ignored or 'jived.' Being the brunt of people's humor, especially that of my blood family, was the story of my life. I was called naive or innocent. Much of their humor either went over my head or hurt.

Lion Heart and I were leaders. In our late teens, with the help of a wizard of a brother-in-law, we got involved in investing and rehabilitating real estate properties in Boise. One investment at a time, slowly but surely we built up a financial success, at least on paper.

When he was 22, my husband denounced the institution of monogamy and my world fell apart. As a teen I had searched for an understanding of religion and relationships. What was love? In my home I saw one form of love that had a repeated cycle of abuse and reconciliation. I refused to believe that my parents were examples of a caring, loving couple. Their love hurt.

In the Sixties, as I was going through high school, we were extremely peer conscious. There were 'in groups' and outcasts. I found it difficult to ever bring anyone over to my home for fear of what might occur and thus found myself a loner, separated often from all around me.

I started my dependency on Lion Heart at the age of fifteen. Girl friends took the back seat in my life. Most of my focus was on achieving good grades, learning how to keep up the living lie that surrounded my home and how to be in a relationship with a man.

As our marriage crumbled years later, it took on more and more of the qualities of the blood family I had left. Dishonesty, fear, verbal and emotional put downs, the endless cycles of shame and abuse defined the relationship. I knew if I could be just a little more sexy, or humorous, or prosperous our relationship would mend. It did not. In fact, Lion Heart coined his newly found focus on relationships as 'poly-monogamy' or 'love the one your with' in the now. My hero husband was confidant about his capacity to maintain an adequate love with his wife and still be in outside relationships. He had the ability and heart to love many, he said. After all he was a 'Leo', his lion nature had him out there leading, fiercely driven, to be independent while surrounded by his lair.

My response was to feel further devastation of my weak self esteem. Suicide seemed like an easy enough solution to end my stay in what seemed to be a miserly world.

It was at this same time, that I developed my first adult female friend. She was an art teacher at the junior high who gave me a copy of *Desiderata*. Slowly this piece of prose became my 'holy' reference. My woman friend did not stay long in my life, soon she moved to another state. I know her gift was to give me a point of spiritual reference for she had heard frequently my longing for rightness and moral structure in my life.

Guided by
DESIDERATA

GO PLACIDLY AMID THE NOISE and HASTE and REMEMBER WHAT PEACE THERE MAY BE IN SILENCE. AS FAR AS POSSIBLE WITHOUT surrender be on good terms with all persons. Speak the truth quietly and clearly; and listen to others, even the dull and ignorant; they too have their story. Avoid loud and aggressive persons, they are vexations to the spirit. If you compare yourself with others, you may become vain and bitter; for always there will be greater and lesser persons than yourself. Enjoy your achievements as well as your plans. Keep interested in your own career, however humble; it is a real possession in the changing fortunes of time. Exercise caution in your business affairs; for the world is full of trickery. But let this not blind you to what virtue there is; many persons strive for high ideals; and everywhere life is full of heroism. Be yourself. Especially, do not feign affection. Neither by cynical about love; for in the face of all aridity and disenchantment it is perennial as the grass. Take kindly the counsel of the years, gracefully surrendering the things of youth. Nurture strength of spirit to shield you in sudden misfortune. But do not distress yourself with imaginings. Many fears are born of fatigue and loneliness. Beyond a wholesome discipline, be gentle with yourself. You are a child of the universe, no less then the trees and the stars; you have a right to be here. And whether or not it is clear to you, no doubt the universe is unfolding as it should. Therefore, be at peace with GOD, whatever you conceive Him to be, and whatever our labors and aspirations, in the noisy confusion of life keep peace with your soul. With all its sham, drudgery and broken dreams it is still a beautiful world. Be careful. Strive to be HAPPY.

— FOUND IN OLD SAINT PAUL'S CHURCH, BALTIMORE
DATED 1692

As a young teen, I sought out various religious institutes trying to find a comprehension of GOD. I have learned that when 'one approaches the age of fourteen the dimension of soul starts growth—astral body forms, the motor starts to push one into spiritual action.'

I was raised without a formal religion in my home. I am a fifth generation Idahoan, whose great-great grandparents were pioneers brought over with the Church of Jesus Christ of Latter Day Saints. My roots go back to Wales and our Welch, Celtic blood. In junior high I became besieged with a hunger to understand God, and especially Jesus. I wanted to believe in something and I was intrigued by Jesus whether he was son of man or son of God.

I did not find a 'home' in any of the religious institutions I visited as a youth. As a freshman in Western Literature, a phenomenal teacher introduced me to the *EPIC OF GILGAMESH*. This knowledge that dated back a thousand of years before the time of Jesus disturbed my notion of there being only one son of God and that men and women were created in his image.

I learned about mythology and the power of the storyteller, the singer of history creating a story that is a common background for a multitude of religions which often starts with the unwritten word, but sung truths. Repeatedly I learned of Christ-like men with episodes of tragedy. Soul searching journeys into the desert and great floods commonly occurred. Individuals were called to mountain tops and retrieved doctrines often inscribed on stone tablets. I heard of a respect for the Earth her animals, plant, especially the trees, her waters, caves, stars and on and on.

My life was filled with complexities that did not conform with typical, normal everyday spiritual, physical or mental norms. My efforts to fit into the accepted social realm resulted in an illness that made my head ache and strain so badly that I could not think straight. Pain became my teacher.

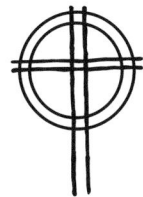

"SPEAK YOUR TRUTH QUIETLY AND CLEARLY; AND LISTEN TO OTHERS, EVEN THE DULL AND IGNORANT; THEY TOO HAVE THEIR STORY."

Ram Dass —BE HERE NOW

In the early seventies, Ram Dass was brought to Boise and he spoke about his book BE HERE NOW. It was quite revolutionary for my peers and myself. From high school forth many were trying to outwit the system to keep from getting drafted. Many got married, went to school, had babies, whatever to stay out of the Vietnam conflict.

To get in the present and enjoy each moment had not been an option. Meditation had been a natural lead in to quiet the mind. But many people dicovered that the attempts to get the mind quiet were great challenges. Now, Ram Dass further asked us to 'witness' our self, to watch our relationships, what we ate and how we thought.

He simplified people into two categories, those who watch others for their system of self worth and then the others who turn inward and get their accountability from a quality from within.

Part of what was drastically radical about Ram Dass was that in earlier times he was Dr. Richard Albert, who taught and did research with Timothy O'Leary at a renowned University setting, testing mind altering chemicals. His willingness to speak to altered states of consciousness shook the foundations of most conservatively raised Idahoans. He spoke in a language that was simple.

He described consciousness as being to the channels on a television; you can choose '2' or '12' or '27'. Just because one had not heard or recognized the various channels did not mean they did not exist. He encouraged us to still our busy, chattering mind and then to observe the option for greater peace. Ram Dass expressed the necessity of not judging any situation, to remove ourselves from the world of duality, right and wrong, asking us to shift to another realm of just going with the flow, not creating trauma.

Somehow his sitting cross legged with a beanie cap which had propellers swirling above his head added great humor to his intent to lighten our mental loads. The men in my life were sold on his message. Especially his recognition of drugs to assist in expanding one's consciousness.

The spring of my last year in college we decided to make a journey to the East coast and visit my husband's close friend. The man was a published scientific writer instructing and doing research at a university in North Carolina. This highly educated doctor's focus was on food additives and their effect on the body and total health.

Once there, I was plagued with my headaches and an upset system. I was unable to function let alone play. I remember holding my head up by the ocean's edge and then this doctor, concerned by the longevity of my pain, introduced me to an earth medicine called marijuana. Upon consuming some of this natural herb, it was as if my mind lightened, a part of me became less serious and I actually could play and be simple with the ocean.

Writing about my involvement with this earth herb is essential and honest. Yet at that time, and for years to come, it was another taboo that could not be discussed in open company or with the general public. It had a stereo-typing like venereal disease or worse. A movie came out in the fifties called *REEFER MADNESS* that portrayed tremendous exaggerations and distortions regarding the effect of this 'earth medicine'. My inner list of attitudes and family history abuse and societal prejudices was growing. Why alcohol and family battering was blindly condoned and consuming a natural herb was considered horrendously wrong made no sense. The chasm between my out-side public world and the inside private world was enlarging like the Grand Canyon.

How could I be here now and still recognize the drastic dualities in my life?

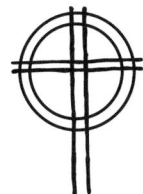

"BEYOND A WHOLESOME DISCIPLINE, BE GENTLE WITH YOURSELF.
YOU ARE A CHILD OF THE UNIVERSE,
NO LESS THAN THE TREES AND THE STARS."

Yoga — Union

My first yoga instructor, Jaye Ram Singh taught foot reflexology giving us a mapping of our total health through an understanding of neurological points on our feet. He started talking about life in terms of *Zen* and going with the flow. Where there is resistance, he asked us to let go. I did not understand then what he was sharing. Weekly we would study breathing, nutrition, yoga stretches, acupressure reflex points and guided imagery.

At the end of some series of exercises, this holy man, who wore a turban and was adorned in draping white clothes, would direct us through a multitude of different breathing techniques including short, puffing breath, alternate nostril breathing, deep three phase breathing and more. He put the greatest emphasis on not only how we inhaled but also on how we exhaled. Jaye Ram was assisting us to raise our vibration and balance.

He would have us get in a resting position and then proceeded to share a guided imagery exercise with us. He would suggest that we allow our minds to go on a make believe journey to a very peaceful place in nature. He would suggest we notice what we saw, what would come to us. I was often very uncomfortable with this process. When I would look from the inside with eyes closed I only saw darkness. I was ashamed to share this inability to visualize with anyone.

Jaye Ram was a strong advocate of conscious diet. He believed in macrobiotics, a dietary approach that relied on grains, live foods, careful preparation of the foods and no meats. He went on to proclaim that when an animal was being killed an adrenaline rush of fear goes through its body into its muscles. When humans consumed this fear hormone riddled meat, we had to digest destructive, aggressive disease creating matter.

The more peaceful our food chain, the easier it is to digest. Our personality becomes less aggressive and stressed. The interesting thing about having a disorder resting within the brain is that it mandates one look at the basic beliefs around the intensity with which one lives life. How much should I be in charge of my health? How much is determined by my mind? How much does it reflect my spirit and on and on. Being the intellectual I was, I soon learned if one part of the Endocrine System was out of balance, the rest would soon become affected whether it is the thyroid, thymus, adrenal, spleen and menses process, or the pituitary, the commander in charge of synchronized secretions and healthy emotional integrations.

As Jaye Ram continued training his Western indoctrinated students, we learned more and more about the chakra system, especially the Endocrine glands that were directed associated with each of the seven energy centers. In addition, we were informed that there were emotions, colors and sounds that connect with the chakra system.

CHAKRA - ENDOCRINE GLAND RELATIONSHIPS

CHAKRA	COLOR	ENDOCRINE	ELEMENT	TRAIT	LOCATION IN BODY
First	red	gonad	earth	stability	gonads/rectum
Second	orange	spleen	water	creativity	kidneys/female
Third	yellow	adrenal	fire	personal power	solar plexus
Fourth	green	thymus	air	open heart	lungs/heart
Fifth	blue	thyroid	ether	expression/manifestation	throat
Sixth	indigo	pituitary	mind	visualization	third eye
Seventh	violet	pineal	all there is	liberation/omniscience	crown

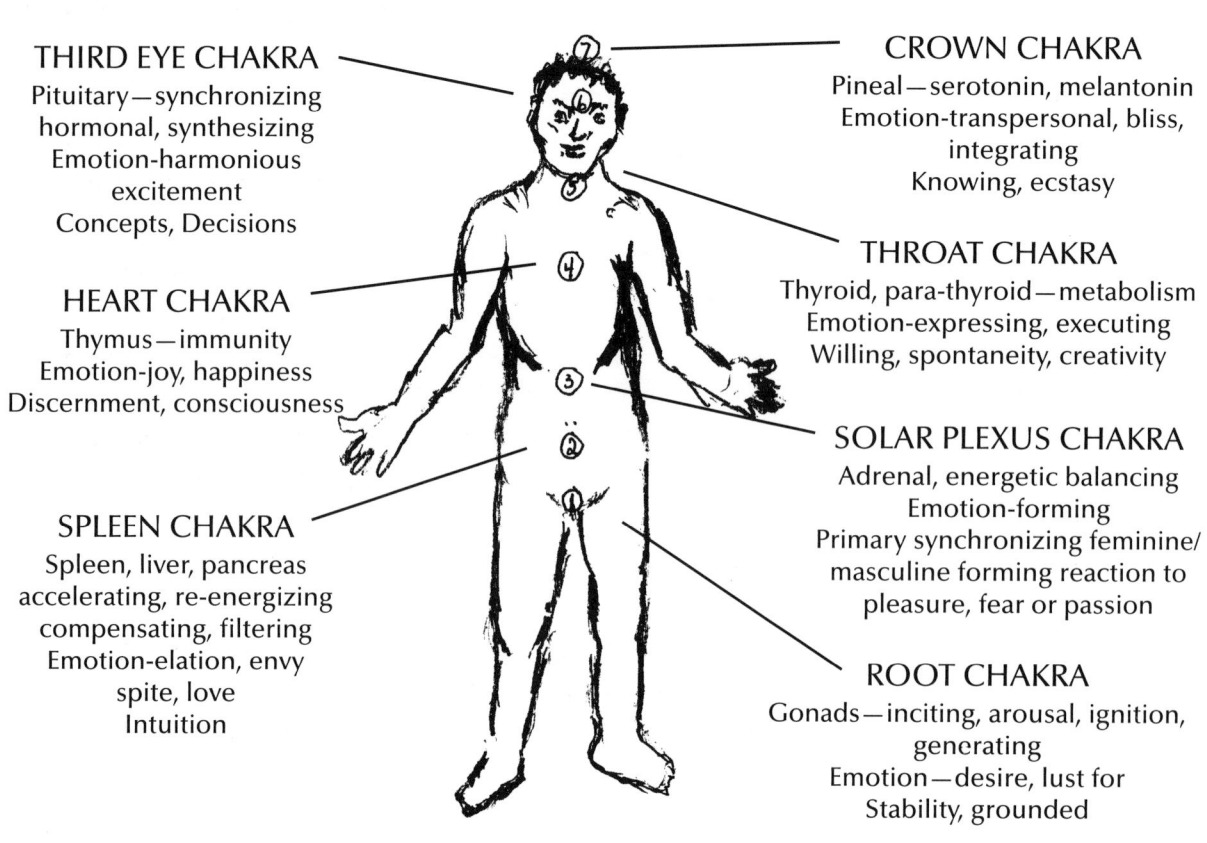

THIRD EYE CHAKRA
Pituitary—synchronizing hormonal, synthesizing
Emotion-harmonious excitement
Concepts, Decisions

HEART CHAKRA
Thymus—immunity
Emotion-joy, happiness
Discernment, consciousness

SPLEEN CHAKRA
Spleen, liver, pancreas accelerating, re-energizing compensating, filtering
Emotion-elation, envy spite, love
Intuition

CROWN CHAKRA
Pineal—serotonin, melantonin
Emotion-transpersonal, bliss, integrating
Knowing, ecstasy

THROAT CHAKRA
Thyroid, para-thyroid—metabolism
Emotion-expressing, executing
Willing, spontaneity, creativity

SOLAR PLEXUS CHAKRA
Adrenal, energetic balancing
Emotion-forming
Primary synchronizing feminine/masculine forming reaction to pleasure, fear or passion

ROOT CHAKRA
Gonads—inciting, arousal, ignition, generating
Emotion—desire, lust for
Stability, grounded

Jaye Ram was considered a celibate monk. Why did he preach celibacy? He emphasized that the men be non-orgasmic, to not let their semen flow. They would lose their kundalini energy, life force; he proclaimed. The second center, our passion and sexual center also housed the 'hara' or kundalini energy. Kundalini is often called 'chi' or 'ki' represent life force.

He made a symbolic connection to the spiraling energy on a physician staff- medicine of well being. The second chakra between the pubic bone and the belly button is not only the region of our sexual organs but our kidneys and bladder. Jaye Ram contended that a man was to breathe through the hara and by consciously bringing the breath up to the heart one could not only be charged but could access a deep meditative, 'zen-full' state of being. When one practiced celibacy he inferred, an individual had a greater opportunity for higher consciousness. The mundane ordinary life would be elevated.

Giving up meat was one tough challenge, but giving up sexual intimacy was devastating for me. Even worse, Lion Heart would not even discuss his view of intimacy. He was so focused on raising his kundalini, walking as God, he willingly ended our sexual exchanges. Plus it allowed him to be around more women, helping them get out of their ruts. He was a lion hearted man and he could love many and had nothing to worry about. It would not diminish our capacity to be in love, he reinforced.

It was really hard on me. He was around me less and others more. He contended quality time together was far more important than quantity time. The bottom line, too, was he was not going to worry. My problems were for me to elevate, not him. It was clear to him the he was getting high, a guru himself.

The tools I had been developing, meditation, witnessing and breathing slowly were showing me that I was an actress on a stage. I adjusted my personality to be the school teacher, to be the golden couple, to be the hurt daughter and to be a wife. No where had I learned to be just me. The witness part of me begged to be just ONE consistent being. I did not know how. I became more and more conscious of my lying. I called them white lies, just to make the story a little grander, richer embellishments to keep other's interest.

I really could not tell the truth simply. All my remembered life seemed to be untrue. Being raised in a battering, alcohol riddled home taught me to never let anyone outside the home know truly what my life was like. Truth was not good enough. *Desiderata* would speak to me:

"BEYOND A WHOLESOME DISCIPLINE, BE GENTLE WITH YOURSELF.
YOU ARE A CHILD OF THE UNIVERSE,
NO LESS THAN THE TREES AND THE STARS: YOU HAVE A RIGHT TO BE HERE.

AND WHETHER OR NOT IT IS CLEAR TO YOU, NO DOUBT THE
UNIVERSE IS UNFOLDING AS IT SHOULD.
THEREFORE BE AT PEACE WITH GOD, WHATEVER YOU CONCEIVE HIM TO BE,
AND WHATEVER YOUR LABORS AND ASPIRATIONS,
IN THE NOISY CONFUSION OF LIFE KEEP PEACE WITH YOUR SOUL"

I found continual solace in working with my yard and its multitude of roses and in quilting. My grandmother had been an avid quilter as was my mother-in-law. Quilting was a way to get in touch with feelings, storytelling and history for me.) In 1973-4, I felt like I was Humpty Dumpty, fallen and broken in so many pieces that there was no hope to put me back together again. Nixon and the Watergate scandal, the way Vietnam veterans were poorly received when brought back to the United States, my personal health, my marriage, my self image, my total lack of involvement with my blood family . . .all parts of my world felt broken. The book *1984* by George Orwell predicted the deterioration of the world as we knew it. It sure fit my interpretation of this earth life and slowly I became a 'doomsayer'

In Boise at the same time, major stands of trees were being destroyed in the name of bigger road systems. My quiet dead end street was widened and many precious roses from my front yard were eradicated in order to create a wider entrance a new city park at the end of our street.

ENDOCRINE SYSTEM

ADRENAL
The adrenals are the glands that help us deal with stress, mineral balances, and inflammation. They release adrenaline into the body to increase activity and energy. They may be overworked theses days in response to stress, caffeine, nicotine, and sugar. Adrenal glandular is suggested for people who experience fatigue, stress, environmental sensitivities or allergies, infections, and hypoglycemia. The symptoms that come from low blood sugar are probably more related to adrenal than to pancreas, and supporting the adrenals with freeze-dried adrenal at 50-100 mg. twice daily, along with stress-supporting nutrients, such as the B vitamins, vitamins C and A, and zinc, may be helpful

PANCREAS
Pancreas is used mainly to support digestion by providing extra digestive enzymes. Lipases, proteases, and amylases are found in the pancreas gland. Taking digestive enzymes 30-60 mg. after meals often helps us to better utilize the meal's nutrition, especially for people whose digestion has been weakened by emotional stress, chemical irritants, or poor eating habits. There are those who suggest that pancreatic insufficiency is at the heart of aging and much disease, including allergies, weight problems, arthritis and other inflammatory problems, gastrointestinal problems and cancer. Pancreatic support is important in cancer programs and the use of porkderived pancreas for therapy is currently under investigation.

THYMUS
The thymus is important to immunological activity. It contains the active hormone thymosin, which stimulates T lymphocyte (T cell) production and activity. T cells help the body defend itself against infection. Our thymus gland tends to weaken with age, and this may affect our defense system. If we experience fatigue, recurrent infections, or measurable immune deficiency, intake of oral thymus gland may be helpful. This is not well researched, but it most likely won't cause any problems. Injected thymus has been definitely shown to stimulate immune activity.

THYROID
Thyroid weakness can be cause by lack of iodine or too little protein in the diet and probably by emotional stress and blocked creativity as well. In such cases, thyroid glandular may helpful in supporting the gland to work better. Nutrients that contain thyroid tissue and hormone precursors, such as iodine and tyrosine, seem to be helpful. Thyroid glandular has been used for fatigue and to support immune function.

OTHER GLANDS
In brain (Pituitary & hypothalmus—endorphins), heart, lung, stomach, duodenum, testicular, ovarian, spleen, liver

(Dr. Haas, *STAYING HEALTHY WITH NUTRITION.* pg. 57)

METABOLISM OF PROTEINS—FROM INGESTION TO THE LIVER

MOUTH — Protein intake (long amino acid chains), Hydrochloric Acid, Pepsin and Proteases (enzymes) split peptide bonds between amino acid chains—turning them into long chain polypeptides.

STOMACH — Pancreatic enzyme Trypsin turns
PANCREAS — long chain polypeptides into
DUODENUM — shorter chain polypeptides,
tripeptide (3 amino acids) and dipeptide (2 amino acids).

SMALL INTESTINE — Amino Peptidases and Dipeptidases turn polypeptides, tripeptide and dipeptide into single amino acids, which are actively transported through the wall of the intestines into the bloodstream and then via the portal vein to the Liver,

LIVER — the principal site of Protein metabolism

PROTEINS — The Amino Acids
Proteins are complex molecules comprised of a combination of 22 naturally occurring amino acids . . . Essential amino acids are those our body cannot synthesize on its own and which we must acquire through our diet. These eight are isoleucine, leucine, lysine, methionine, phenylalanine, threonine, tryptophan and valine. Arginine and histidine are considered semi-essential in that they are essential for children and may be needed in increased growth demand states such as pregnancy. There are 12 non-essential amino acid, which the body produces to build the proteins for muscles and hair and important molecules (hemoglobin, enzymes, and antibodies) and hormones (thyroid and insulin).

AMINO ACIDS COMMONLY USED IN CLINICAL PRACTICE
(*STAYING HEALTHY THROUGH THE SEASONS* by Dr. Haas, pg.41)

Amino Acid	Uses
L-tryptophan	Sleep, anxiety
L-lysine	Herpes simplex treatment/prevention
DL-phenylalanine	Pain
L-carnitine	Weight loss, cardiovascular disease
L-arginine/L-ornithine	bodybuilding
L-taurine	depression, convulsions
L-cysteine	antioxidant, detoxifier
L-tyrosine	depression

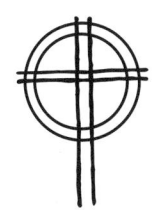

"AS FAR AS POSSIBLE WITHOUT SURRENDER BE ON GOOD TERMS WITH ALL PERSONS. SPEAK YOUR TRUTH QUIETLY AND CLEARLY; AND LISTEN TO OTHERS, EVEN THE DULL AND IGNORANT. THEY TOO HAVE THEIR STORY.   AVOID LOUD AND AGGRESSIVE PERSONS, THEY ARE VEXATIONS TO THE SPIRIT."

CHILDHOOD REFLECTIONS

From grade school forth, it was very important for me to be politically active. I can remember the admiration I felt for President Eisenhower and then how much I envied the Vice President's daughters. They were perfect. I also followed the Kennedy family when I was in junior high as if they were the hope of an image of what the American family could truly stand for.   All too quickly that fairy tale image shattered, first with the assassination and then by the ghastly rumoring of infidelity

Religion and politics are the two areas in my blood family that are open invitation to fiery, outspoken, loud arguing. Since my political beliefs put me in the minority of one in my family, I was severely chastised and belittled for my youthful political alliances. Even today I know not to speak about my political stands with my blood family.

The Viet Nam tragedy accelerated during the Kennedy presidency. I felt the confusion between the church and state and money and morals. Why were we really over there? Always I imagined these people and families being eradicated in their own homeland in the name of God with the influence of money.

I knew we, the USA, wanted what their lands and natural resources yielded, though we were told we were trying to stop the engulfing march of Communism. The natives got in our way so we killed them and bombed them with terrible defoliants. What I could sense was hurt. Hurt for the people's whose homes, lands and families that were being destroyed and maimed by our soldiers who were instructed to raid and kill an enemy who often was not dressed in army fatigues and who looked like ordinary grandmothers and children. In addition, that foreign land was cesspool of drugs and sexual exploits that many a young soldier succumbed to.

I could not determine who were the bad guys and who were the good guys. I just wanted us out of there. I was in the minority and I was not proud of my country.

In the mid-seventies, Nixon and the whole Watergate scandal filled me with political disgust and the ominous state of my physical health consumed my energy. Something deep inside of me yelled to get 'back to the land'. For the next year another couple and I scanned Idaho and the Northwest for a safer, saner, healthier place to live a simpler life.

We idealized about living a life that we were meant to, not one that was forced upon us by an industrialized, post World War II generation. With my crumbling marriage, I knew I had to leave the city in order to find a mental peace to encourage my whole health. My husband was willing to go along with my migration from the city. Divorce was not an option in my mind. I was very old fashioned. When I exchanged my marriage vows I truly committed to be married for life. I was putting up with it, but I was going to live somewhere that would be easier for my well being.

In the fall of 1974, the couple with whom we had looked for land with, introduced us to the option of going to an Encounter Group in order to help us know ourselves and each other better. Simultaneously, we had discovered some land with a rustic cabin in the mountains just above Boise along side a gentle stream. We quickly decided to set in motion purchasing this property.

What was so significant about this potential neighborhood was an interesting elderly couple who lived close to the cabin. Upon getting acquainted with this wizardlike couple, the grandmotherly gardener shared privately her connection with the earth and its elementals. Never had anyone, except in books like *WIND IN THE WILLOWS* and *WATER BABIES* which I devoured as a young child, spoken to me about the elemental and fairy world. This wise crone knew of it largely because of her own Welch and Celtic upbringing and with sparkling eyes told of wonderful things. A certain mystical quality surrounded this potential homesite. We decided to put down earnest money on the mountain cabin. I was ecstatic. It was close enough that I could still teach in the city and come home to the murmuring waters and singing winds

Meanwhile, we also committed to attend the three day encounter group facilitated by Mr. C. This tall, burly Viking-looking counselor introduced us to techniques of communication that helped to bring to the surface our fears, inadequacies and trust issues. It was the first time in my life that I tried to be honest in a group setting. The weekend experience was a safe enough center where masks fell away and we had options to trust and love ourselves and others like I'd always hoped for, but had never known. I experienced the 'hot seat', blind trust walks, singing, stretched perceptions of time and heart-felt hugs from both men and women with shy willingness.

That same weekend the facilitator, upon hearing about our quest to find a piece of land to live life more fully and closer with nature, suggested that we come down to his home territory, the Magic Valley and check out a remote and yet promising eighty acre farm. He said it was a natural setting for a planned community effort.

The next weekend many of us went down to Mr. C.'s home and then out to the farm. I must admit that just as soon as I walked on this rambling, rough eighty acre farm I felt to the depths of my soul the land was blessed by God. The only existing farm house had its doors wide open so that cows could meander through and pheasants could nest in broken light fixtures. Somehow the magic of the encounter group experience of the raw responsive nature calling to us brought nine individuals together. Within a month's time, we were buying this wild and woolly farm overlooking the Snake River Canyon.

Our closest neighbors were a quarter of a mile away and the nearest town was ten miles away. The Mennonites, who are quite prominent in the Magic Valley, had been share-farmers on this land. We formed a corporation and bought the farm, calling it Milepost #195 Inc. Nine people were in the corporation, three married couples and two single men and one single woman. The two single men were my husband's closest friends from the BIFC Boy's Club and the woman was the girl friend of Mr. C., who professed to not be supportive of monogamous relationships

In order to buy into the farm, my husband and I had to liquidate our possessions. Repeatedly I affirmed I wanted to be happy, healthy and holy. Physical possessions and niceties were not making me well. I knew I had to get to the land.

I felt all the dishonor in our country, the maiming of nature all about Boise, the electric energy fields of all the city's people and neighbors and I yearned for space and health. When we created the farm, idealism flourished. In the city I had everything any successful, middle class achiever could desire and I still was sick and sad.

The focus of my attention was the caring for the elemental aspects of nature, air, water, earth and us, knowing if we were out of balance in any facet of life, it would reflect an imbalance in all our existence with the Earth and beyond. Outside health reflects inside health. If we could just make one small statement/picture of a group of peoples, living with the land, healthy and spirit-filled, then our efforts would magnify outward and help balance all of what was happening away from our farm. Micro - macro consciousness. All the people and all the Earth are ONE. Our mind just keeps us separate.

Our coming together as a community was our chance to live what we innately believed was possible for people and the land. The verse from *Desiderata* would speak:

"YOU ARE A CHILD OF THE UNIVERSE, NO LESS
THAN THE TREES AND THE STARS;
YOU HAVE A RIGHT TO BE HERE.
AND WHETHER OR NOT IT IS CLEAR TO YOU,
NO DOUBT THE UNIVERSE IS UNFOLDING AS IT SHOULD"

It took me over nine months to leave Boise and get to the farm. Few could understand why we were ending a very profitable, successful real estate business in our state's capital city. My parents were disgusted that I would leave the world of teaching as it was well known how effectively I taught. In fact, by this time I had coauthored individualized math programs for grades 1 - 8. Repeatedly, my dad would say 'don't burn all your bridges.' All I knew was that I was sickened by the state of the world as I saw it. I felt the weight of our injustices within my mind and in my heart, literally. I was beginning to know that until I found that placidity and peace in the noise and haste of life, I wouldn't know happiness, holiness or health.

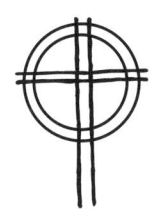

*"ENJOY YOUR ACHIEVEMENTS AS WELL AS YOUR PLANS;
KEEP INTERESTED IN YOUR OWN CAREER, HOWEVER HUMBLE;
IT IS A REAL POSSESSION IN THE CHANGING FORTUNES OF TIME"*

THE FARM — 1975

Our farm, Milepost #195, Inc., could only be located by the mile marker a half mile away from a dead end, inside the eighty acre parcel of 'God graced land'. Within a mile, a steep, tumbling river flowed through lava boulders and fish spawning beds to the Snake River floor commonly known as Magic Valley. We were drenched with wonderful sunrises over the canyon's edge to the East and a wide splendid view of the sunsets to the West over the desert bluff bordering our farm. A stream, lined with craggy Russian Olive trees, meandered through our farm.

Immediately we named our land an 'animal and bird reserve'. It was not uncommon to see and hear thousands of bird in migration overhead and in our trees and fields. Each year we would raise crops just for the wild life, sometimes not on purpose. We immediately aimed at growing organic 'people food'. Blue corn, garlic, black beans, lentils and alfalfa seeds were the focus of our attempted organic fields.

The alfalfa seeds were intended to be sprouted, making them rich with chlorophyll. A sprouted simple food that heals one's blood system. What an idealistic approach to the food chain. We knew our intentions but we were ignorant of the machinery needed or the labor intensive demands to have a successful harvest.

The locals snickered about us and our ideals. Lentils, they asked why lentils? And, Blue Corn, just because the Hopi Indians declared the deep, indigo blue kernels as sacred, inviting peace to the holder and the lands. Why were we choosing to not grow the field corn that the 'Jolly Green Giant' Company could quickly mash into canned cream corn or better yet, store the mashed corn in troughs and let it ferment and stink so that it could become cattle fodder.

Then there was the acre of garlic. Few outside of our farm community recognized this medicinal, ancient food. The English knew and did continue honor the essence and values of certain flowers, herbs and especially garlic. We Westerners were pretty ignorant unless a wise elder brought the healing knowledge from the old country.

THE FARM

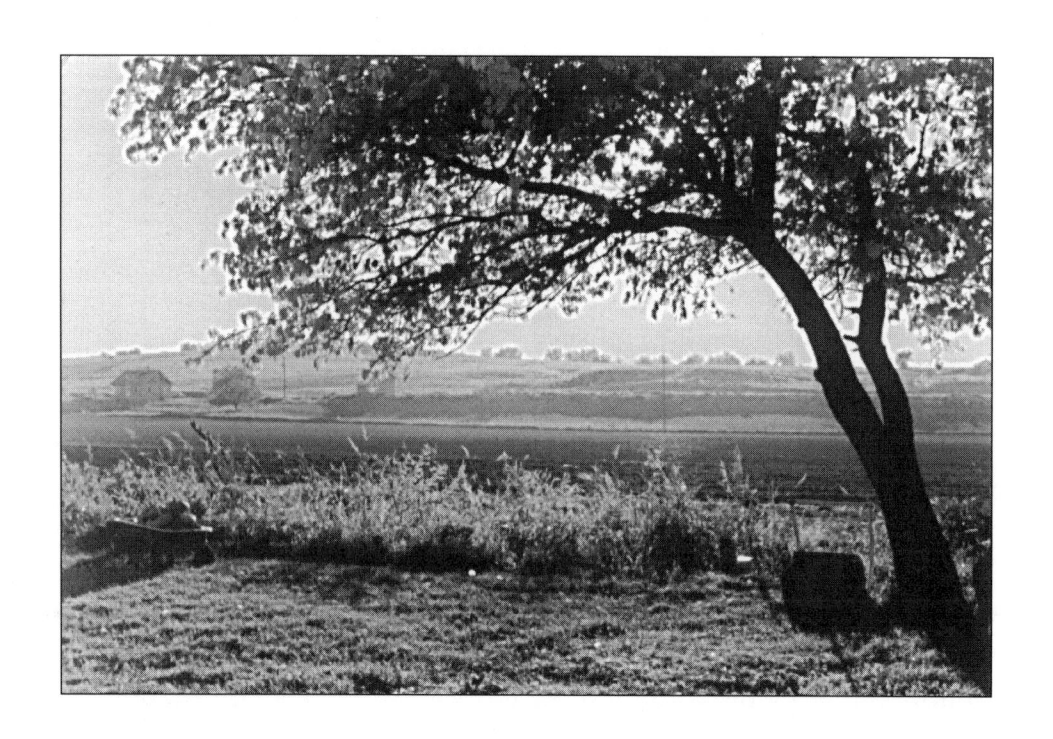

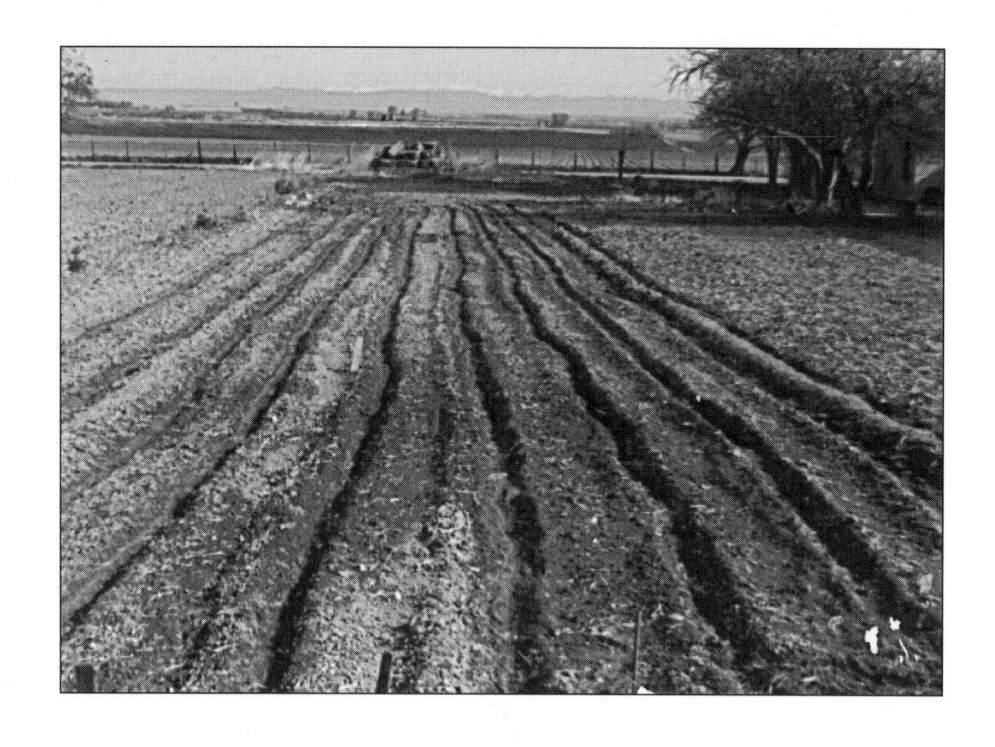

Garlic was a crop that also helped purify the blood, a definite agent to diminish impurities that perpetuate disease.

Since we were part of the forerunners of alternative organic fertilization (fish emulsion) to deadly man made chemicals, our crops were labor intensive, specialty crops. The locals scrutinized us and predicted failure. Since I was a fifth generation Idahoan from farm stock, I probably had the most knowledge of the land, and that wasn't much. We kept the Mennonites on until one member of the farm was trained and educated enough to become the responsible farmer for our field crops.

During the first few years my major focus was establishing a new home. I could count on one hand the number of times I'd moved in my entire life. Being stable and secure was important. I was one of the last ones to settle on the farm in it's solitary, dilapidated farm house. Upon my arrival in June, I found four other owners were already established in this new home, a home that had plastic for windows, no running water, no indoor bathroom, no kitchen and no privacy.

Ah, but we were idealists, we could live it. We could achieve that place of beginning again each day, unconditional love and being willing to work and work hard. It was quite a shock to find myself in relation with more than just a husband, but two other men and two woman.

One of the major reasons I chose to join the farm's communal setting was I wanted to change my belief system. I never wanted to put 'all my eggs in one basket' again. Focusing all nurturing and loving on just my mate had broken my heart and value system. I now wanted to develop an expanded family relationship, so that I would never be dependant on one person or allow all my sense of worth and quality intimate communication to be restricted to just one other mate. Since thoughts of divorce seemed impossible, choosing to come to the farm afforded me a chance to participate in a larger loving and caring family, yet still be conventionally married.

Since the intensity of living in a small space was so great, the land all around us became my 'salve' for sanity. I worked close to the earth, turning soils badly abused and weakened. Almost immediately, I started getting feedback from my new family that I was being unnecessarily chastised and verbally abused by my mate. One male, whom I had once called the 'Biggest Male Chauvinist of the World' finally took me aside and spoke to the worth and beauty he saw in me. He coached me to stand up for my self. I found though, that when I built up enough courage to speak, that the tremoring and fear would quake through me and my spoken words would be jumbled, ass-backwards and poorly expressed.

By this time we were calling the farm the 'crazy farm'. It felt like we were in this institution that droves of people came by to observe. Many of our friends from Boise and beyond came by just to get a feel for how it was going with this reality we were attempting to create. We'd hear how it was their dream too, but for one reason or another others chose to stay 'in the system.' Locals, though, hardly gave us the time of day. I knew I was angry at the world when I left Boise, but the reception of this small community incensed me. Here I was native born, with roots less than 150 miles away and it still did not make me accepted in this rural farm community.

In trying to attend to my head pain, absent menstrual cycles and surging mental stress plus my other physical concerns, I was forced to order books by mail. Twin Falls, the closest town only had a religious bookstore. Since my departure from Boise, I often questioned my sanity or rather my craziness. Movies like *ONE FLEW OVER THE CUCKOO'S NEST*, with Jack Nicholson's impressive acting, haunted me.

At one point my much loved friend, the renown researcher from the East coast, the doctor who had introduced me to 'marijuana as a medicine', was institutionalized because he `was not making sense' to his wife and others. I was really scared. I understood what he was communicating and fear shook me that I could be the next person institutionalized. I was watchful for someone `out there' to come and put me away.

Also the movie *ORDINARY PEOPLE,* exposing the insane way our society would hide from honest feelings and communication and thus perpetuate suicidal tendencies for sensitive people, helped me see the lying script I was raised with. Then the movie *STEPFORD WIVES,* further congratulated me that I was an individual not willing to just be a robot women filling the space for chauvinistic men. I knew I could not accept being 'brain dead'. Upon observing Jane Fonda in the movie *COMING HOME* and seeing her recognize that her boring, unconnected marriage was destroying her aliveness, I too registered how I had escaped the realness of my marriage through daydreaming beyond the moment out to space. I'd put my attention anywhere but the present moment. The script of this movie also brought home the tragedy of the Vietnam era. All of us were affected.

Slowly I started to read Jane Robert's *THE NATURE OF PERSONAL REALITY* and found her languaging of our multi-dimensional self to be very intriguing. As Jane Roberts explained, "Each natural element had its own key system that interlocked with others forming channels through which consciousness could flow from one kind of life to another. A person understood herself to be a separate entity, but one that was connected to all of nature. An over development of the ego would break down that knowing of *Oneness."* I was hungry for this wisdom, though I could only digest small bites at a time.

A Native American myth is that of White Buffalo Woman, which expanded this knowing by stating "initially language had nothing to do with words and in deed language emerged when man had lost a portion of his love, forgotten some of his identification with nature so that he no longer understood its' voice to be his also."

"In many contemplative tradition, it is readily acknowledged that association with an enlightened teacher is one of the most important and effective means of advancement on a spiritual path . . . many great spiritual teachers—especially those from Hindu, Sufi, Zen, and Tibetan Buddhist lineages—have maintained a life-long connection with their own teachers..." (*THE JOURNAL OF TRANSPERSONAL PSYCHOLOGY,* Vol 24, Number 1, 1992)   Even though at this time many Western intellectual circles ridiculed gurus and viewed those who associated with them as naive and immature, many people, including we at our group farm, continued to pursue the age-old tradition of spiritual apprenticeship.

Ram Dass and Jaye Ram Singh both preached the culturally sanctioned rites of passage of discipleship under a spiritual guide. The traditional saying goes 'When the student/disciple is ready the teacher/guru appears.' This willingness to trust someone as a teacher to engage in the process of inner transformation hopefully to gain some degree of illumination, if not complete enlightenment, was desired by many of us at the farm. I was leery of gurus since many thought my husband to be one.

When Jane Robert's book appeared, I was thrilled. Here a woman was 'channeling' a spirit guide called 'Seth' and spoke in such a manner that some of the dense, critical, dark parts of my brain actually were lightening. I noticed that up to now all my guru's and teachers had been males. I needed the feminine influence. I had been practicing Transcendental Meditation for four years, and was intrigued by the various dimensions I experienced while in this deep, restful state, plus my dream world seemed increasingly active. I seemed to be enjoying my time spent out of daily reality more and more. It fed my essence, my soul. At a retreat away from the farm I met a new teacher. He was a tall, philosophical, gentle man and appeared to be a close friend to my encounter group facilitator, now farm member. Up to this time my husband had encouraged me to find another partner to occupy some of my sensual, love needs. Here was my first viable candidate who happened to have access into some of the deep, vulnerable, feeling parts of my soul.

Since I was still morally bound by the marriage ceremony I committed to, I could not allow myself to be sexual with this man unless I first legally divorced my husband. Now I had this special potential lover, plus both of the men on the farm who were my husband's best friends, all encouraging me to finally take a healthy stand for myself. I was glowing and excited.

It wasn't until I would no longer meet the physical, sexual demands from Lion Heart, that I knew I was seriously capable of ending my nine year marriage. Funny how he forgot his aim for an elevated rate of kundalini energy when it appeared that another might meet my sexual passions.

Strangely, things became more and more intense for all at our small farm home. We were approaching winter, and one by one the other community members chose to leave the farm for the winter season, mostly because it was so cold and tough to exist in that skeletal, rough farmhouse. I too was leaving after many terrorizing rages directed at me by my husband. I came home after a journey and found my husband with a gun to his head. He said he was playing Russian roulette, the chamber was just partially loaded. Life without me left him without worth, he told me. He proceeded to break and destroy my treasures in this home and then he put the gun to his head and pulled the trigger.

What blew was my mind/heart. I collapsed hysterically to the floor. As synchronizity has it, our encounter group facilitator and farm member, Mr. C. walked through the door. He saw the situation and took my hand and asked me to leave with him. So I got up and walked out the door with Mr. C. telling my husband, former guru, 'go ahead and try again'. As we walked away from the house, no sounds were heard.

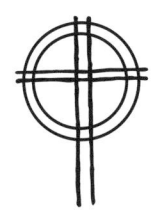

*"...AVOID LOUD AND AGGRESSIVE PERSONS,
THEY ARE VEXATIONS TO THE SPIRIT..."*

SHATTERED MARRIAGE

During the next few days I could not stop the inner chatter that I had caused my husband to go over the edge and he really did care for me, I was at fault for not knowing it. Being the 'Golden Couple' and all the social pressure that came with our success had stressedour relationship.

My husband convinced me that we needed to leave the farm and go on a long shared goal of a journey to South America. Within a week we were packed and gone. I did not let me dear other man friend know that I was giving my husband another chance. In a way the potential of a loving relationship with another disappeared out of my fragile mental reality.

We left our car in Arizona and proceeded to enter Mexico via the train system. I was aghast at the standard of living, the grime and lack of respect for women. I did not feel safe and thus clung to Lion Heart. For a few days he was willing to be protective. Then his patience ran out and he wanted his individual freedom. His anthem of self independence was renewed.

The second week on our journey, Lion Heart abandoned me in central Mexico after another fight over my insecurities. I checked into a hotel and began making arrangements to return to the states. Within a few days he returned, apologizing. We agreed that we both deserved this vacation, but would have to rearrange our relationship form. From that point on we vowed to be friends through the trip and upon returning to Idaho would finish up our divorce process.

Basically he needed more female attention than I was able to provide. So we traveled South, and I continued to draw attention from the men who called me 'mucho grande; big woman. This did little for my self confidence. For a while I thought it was my size that attracted the flirtation and pinches. I soon discovered that many Mexican men's goal was to 'screw a white American woman'. Once again I heard I was not special.

1976 PALENQUE, MEXICO

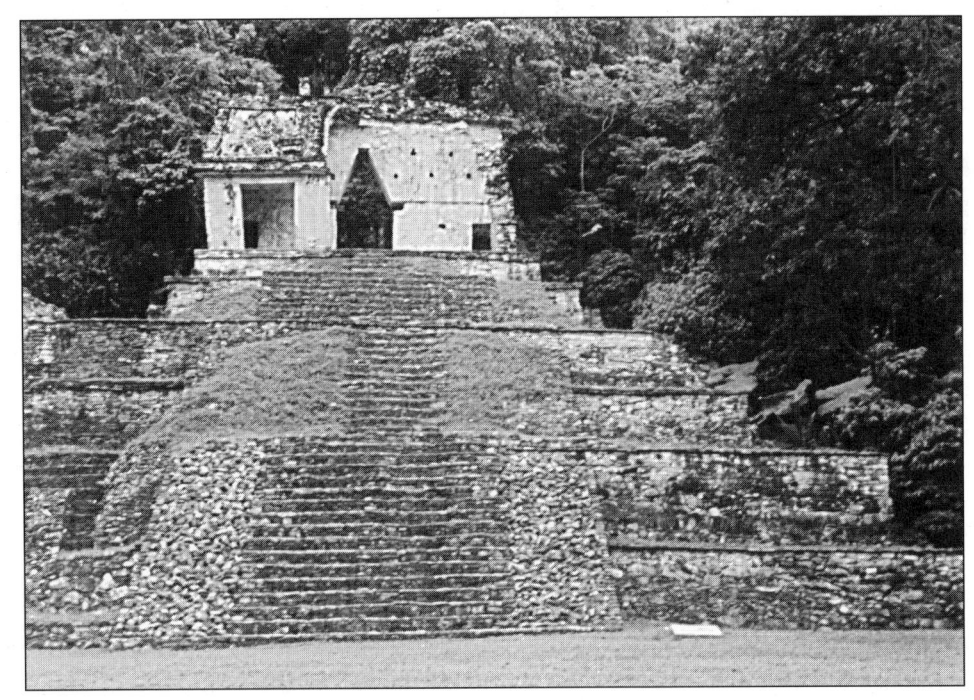

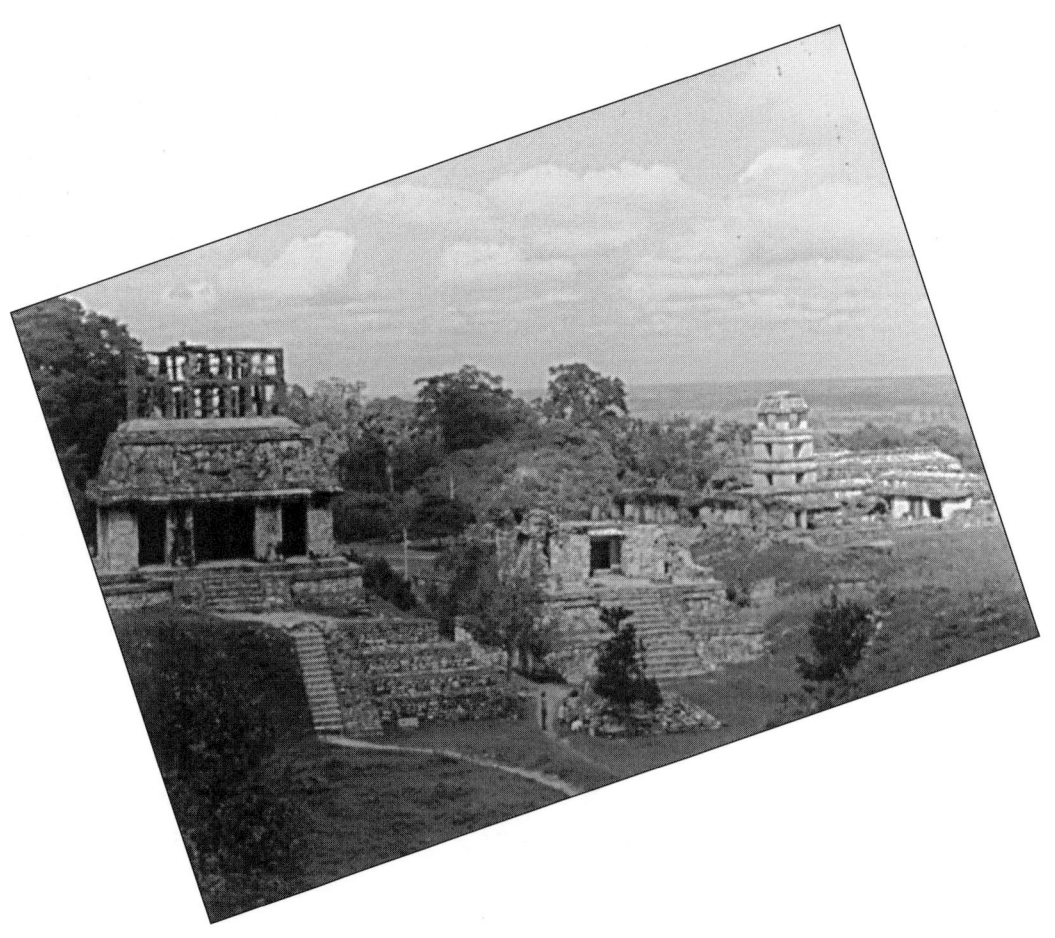

The oldest Mayan ruins in Palenque stole my heart and soul. I was so intrigued with their skyward focus, their space men, their sun, moon and star pyramids. It was the mystery of the civilization which just disappeared that grabbed my fantasy mind. The whole area felt mystical.

When we journeyed further into the Yucatan peninsula, I was disappointed with the various Aztec ruins. The Aztec were much more war like and practiced human sacrifice. I was uncomfortable there and wanted to quickly move on. We finally arrived at the Caribbean Ocean front and decided to stay put for a week or two near Tulum. The warm sun and glorious turquoise waters were so welcoming.

Almost immediately my husband discovered another available woman from Canada and struck up a relationship. I began seething and I felt hate for him. Luckily there was another single woman who liked me. Finally, I had a companion to walk the beach front and to talk with. When she left I decided to return to Palenque which so intrigued me I was dreaming about it. My husband and his girlfriend followed me. I was bitter and unhappy.

The bus ride was long and upon arriving back in Palenque, the motel proprietor put us all in one room, much to my chagrin. Immediately, Lion Heart wanted to go visit the cow pastures for he had heard there were magical blue hallucinogenic mushroom growing. So out he went.

Hours later he returned and while showering he started yelling in outrage. We learned that he was covered with ticks from his waist down. In Southern Mexico, the ticks were much smaller than the ones I was familiar with in the United States. My husband soon pleaded for help to pinch them off him. I told him to suffer. His girlfriend hid her head under a blanket. After an hour of his growing pain, I broke down and began to help remove, tick by tick, his infested genitals and other body parts. One aspect of me would have preferred to just let him die, but he was quick to remind me that I owed him one.

On a high mountain trek a year or so back he had caught me just as I leaped across a gorge and missed the handhold on the embankment. He had saved my life and I owed him one—even though he was the one who demanded I jump. For hours I proceeded to remove the tiny ticks from him. It was the goriest, bloodiest, ugliest task I had ever been asked to do.

When I finally finished the process, all I knew was that I needed a drink. I walked down to the corner liquor dispenser. A huge, five story tall, fiery, red full moon filled the horizon. This surreal setting, I bought a small bottle of tequila and returned to the motel room. I proceeded to pour each of us a drink. I clearly remember telling the other two to be happy with each other, that I was fine and my husband and I were through. I observed, curiously detached as I slowly entered a different consciousness or rather unconsciousness.

The next morning I was back and miserably sick. My mate's girlfriend decided she needed to leave and did so. There was a Catholic Church up on a knoll that drew me in to pray. A crucified Christ bled at the altar. Much of me felt bloodied and needed a transformation.

Within the next week we flew high into the mountains, preparing to enter Guatemala. Earthquakes rattled and shook the mountainsides while various public transportation dropped into cracks and lakes. We had to have special vaccinations to enter the country. From the time of the vaccination on I became ill.

Imagine riding in a squatty van, elbow to elbow, knees pressed hard against one's chest, with the local natives stoically sitting not seeing us or the chickens that squawked and pooped overhead. Often we were the only Americans and the only woman aboard. Bathroom stops did not occur when the illness racked through me. There were no bathroom facilities.

Though part of me loved the remote experience, I could not handle the embarrassment of dropping my pants at those quick release stops and having all the men in the bus stare and chuckle as I eliminated, which I had to do often. I was not feeling well at all.

Enough was enough, I decided I was going home. My husband wanted to go on to Costa Rica but I was miserable. I had to head north, not further south. Again my mate followed. The trek home took two solid weeks. I had a dream that I had a baby. Then a second dream showed me returning to the pyramids with a fourteen year old boy, a young man that traveled freely in the world. Neither made any sense to me. I knew I was sterile, unable to bear children.

Throughout the ten years of being married I yearned deeply to have a child. For seven years I practiced no birth control. Because of my pituitary mysfunctioning and faulty menstrual system I thought I was unable to conceive a child. Plus my husband did not want to be responsible for raising a youngster. He wanted his freedom. It was a constant sore point in our marriage. Often I would dream of a long table filled with loved children. I would be serving wonderful meals.

Finally we arrived back in the States. Spring was slowly beginning to blossom and other members of our farm family returned to the land. My husband quickly began an intimate relationship with another woman on the farm. Since I was going for a divorce what did it matter?

I still did not feel well. Even though it was not unusual for me not to have menses, it finally dawned on me that I may be 'with child'. Upon sharing my condition with Lion Heart, he immediately suggested that I consider getting an abortion; after all, we had not been sexual for months and months. He was not the father of it, he stated. In fact, he elaborated that the night I had drunk the tequila in the ancient Mayan town, I had left the motel room. He was sure I had ended up screwing some Chicano. It wasn't his concern. He knew it was not his child. Abort It.

There was no way I could end the life of this growing baby within, especially since it was one of my most fervent prayers to have a child. No part of me could accept that I had abandoned my morals and just screwed a stranger. I declared immaculate conception and that the baby indwelling was the gift from the gods of Palenque.

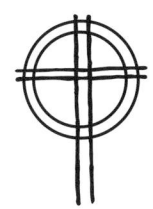

> "NURTURE STRENGTH OF SPIRIT TO SHIELD YOU IN SUDDEN MISFORTUNE. BUT DO NOT DISTRESS YOURSELF WITH IMAGININGS.
> MANY FEARS ARE BORN OF FATIGUE AND LONELINESS."

PREPARING FOR BIRTH - PRAYER FILLED REUNION WITH GOD

I was pregnant, filled with hatred towards my husband, alienated from my blood family, and living on an eighty acre farm with five other people. I was in a house with minimal electricity, no running water or bathroom and heated solely with wood. I learned directly about living off the land, much like my Welch ancestors a hundred year before in the same Southeastern part of Idaho.

Only one couple from the farm corporation had children. The others had consciously chosen not to have a family. It was the consensus that anyone over twenty-five and had not decided to have kids by then, probably never would. I had often dreamed of a long table filled with children. It was a deep hurt in my marriage that my husband didn't want children. Lion Heart's goals were focused on lots of money and maximum freedom. He aspired to being retired by the age of thirty.

At this time, being pregnant, I was not strong enough to follow through with a divorce. It was a cultural 'no-no' to be a single mother. We clarified that as soon as I birthed the baby, I would proceed to complete our divorce. Somehow I kindled enough energy to insist we build an addition to our rough house. That spring and summer we created an addition to the ramshackle farm house a kitchen and bathroom equipped with electricity and running water. A greenhouse was attached to the kitchen affording freedom to be out of doors during the endless windy spring and fall seasons.

I was asserting myself. Being pregnant made me very demanding. I knew I needed a way to wash and cook. The purist way of cooking on a wood stove had lost its romantic tones. I wanted to wash clothes and body, other than in a bucket.

Idealistically, I planted an acre garden and all of the farm members put in an acre of seedling pine trees. Little did I know about soil quality or water conservation. It was very frustrating fighting back the weeds and watching the poor yield from the great quantity of hard labor.

Our group coagulated around an encounter group, initiated regular meetings on Sunday meetings to discuss "what was happening at the farm". Our communications leader, Mr. C., often facilitated these sharings. Nothing was sacred or left hidden. Though married, he did not believe in monogamy. I learned that one of the nine members of our farm group was one of his mistresses. We had started out with three married couples and three single people, two men and one woman.

Soon the nine of us were divided into two factions, the "wimps" and the "assholes". I was a "wimp"! The married couples became totally a non-monogamous group. I did not want to recognize that I was the only idealistic, monogamous, marriage committed member of our farm.   I was nicknamed an 'airy fairy'.

Towards the end of the summer when I was six months pregnant, Lion Heart informed me that he and another female member of the farm had decided to take an extended journey to India together. She would be leaving her husband behind.

Troubles flared on the farm. No amount of communication could ease the anger that raged in me. The other woman was a childhood friend of mine. I was deeply wounded at her insensitivity towards another female friend, especially one who was pregnant.

Only one of the single men actually lived on the farm at this time and he was a golden, long haired, environmental activist, government helicopter foreman. He worked for the U.S. government in crisis situation and was gone much of the summer months. By the fall of 1976, I found myself completely alone on the farm. Twice daily I would walk the mile long path around the farm singing, crying and praying for guidance. My strong maternal instincts had me tune into my womb and pray continually for a healthy, happy and holy child.

A deep honesty roared through me. I had no time for 'bull shit or jive'. I felt as if I had driven all the others farm members off the land. All the talk of being in unconditional love, beginning again each moment of life with everyone one met, didn't fit me. I just knew love didn't mean hurting another for selfish reasons.

My attempts to be healthy during my pregnancy were kindled by a very sensitive inner system. I truly credit this period with the cognitive understanding of "you are what you eat". Any time that I would indulge in greasy foods or poor choices of protein, I would be instantly ill. Not only could I sense the growth of my "gift from God" within but I learned better how to honor myself.

Daily as the sun rose and set, I would be embraced by the most panoramic, majestic of beauty that would lighten even my darkest moments.   As I planted my feet I would sing a mantra, a spiritual verse or song of affirmation, filled with holy tones. Over and over again I would pray for the birth of a healthy, happy and holy baby. My constant focus was on the 'well-being' of this unborn child which helped balance the angry, mental part of my brain.   Even though I was challenged by the concept of God, I still prayed to him. All my life I had prayed, especially during my toughest times. It was my salve against mental torture.

With the rapid disintegration of my belief in human man at this time in my life, I was beginning to recognize that God, father in heaven, and earth father was too jumbled together in my mind. I was angry at my own father, and at the next man who had come into my life, Lion Heart. I was beginning to pray to the Earth Mother. I did not know how, but she was sending me messages that I could strongly sense through my body. The unspoken mystery about our relationship with nature, the Earth, moved through me.

If I didn't pay attention, it felt like something would die. If I put direct, loving focus on some aspect of the plant kingdom, it would flourish and so would I. If I was in need of a boost, a bird would swoop close and drop a feather. I was receiving a lot more from the earth than from any outside person. One particular night as I strode along on my walk, my mind was screaming at the way my relationship with my husband was going. I couldn't believe I was going to bear this child alone, with no caring support and that I was going to proceed with the divorce that was currently on hold until after the birth of my child.

To be a divorced, single parent was a sin as far as I was concerned. I wanted to know how not to be angry at God for the course my life had taken. I fervently asked for a sign that I could not miss. As the golden peach hues of sunset streaked across the waters beside my path, I felt a jolting bolt come up through my body and a glow of intense golden white, showering light come down through my head and shoulders. My spine crawled and the hair on my body stood on end. I felt a connection with grace that soothed me deeply and without a doubt I knew that God had taken root in my soul. Many times a day from that point forth I would test my relationship with Grace. I'd get quiet, prayer-like and ask that the "Lord, make me an instrument of your peace." If I was truly centered with at-one-ness, the rush would spread up and down and across my body. If I was in distraction and casually requesting alignment nothing would happen. It would become a barometer that I still use today.

I would refer to the *PRAYER OF SAINT FRANCIS:*

"Lord, make me an instrument of Your Peace.
Where there is hatred let me sow love.
Where there is injury, pardon.
Where there is despair, hope.
Where there is darkness, light and where there
    is sadness, joy.
Divine Master, grant that I may not so much
    seek to be consoled, as to console;
To be understood,
    as to understand;
To be loved, as to love;
For it is in giving that we receive—
It is in pardoning that we are pardoned;
And it is in dying that we are born to eternal life."

My heart was broken, my mind shattered, but my spiritual connection became a constant grounding wire. I felt the rush of recognition, that I was not alone; spirit embraced me.

NOVEMBER 1976, BIRTHING OF SON

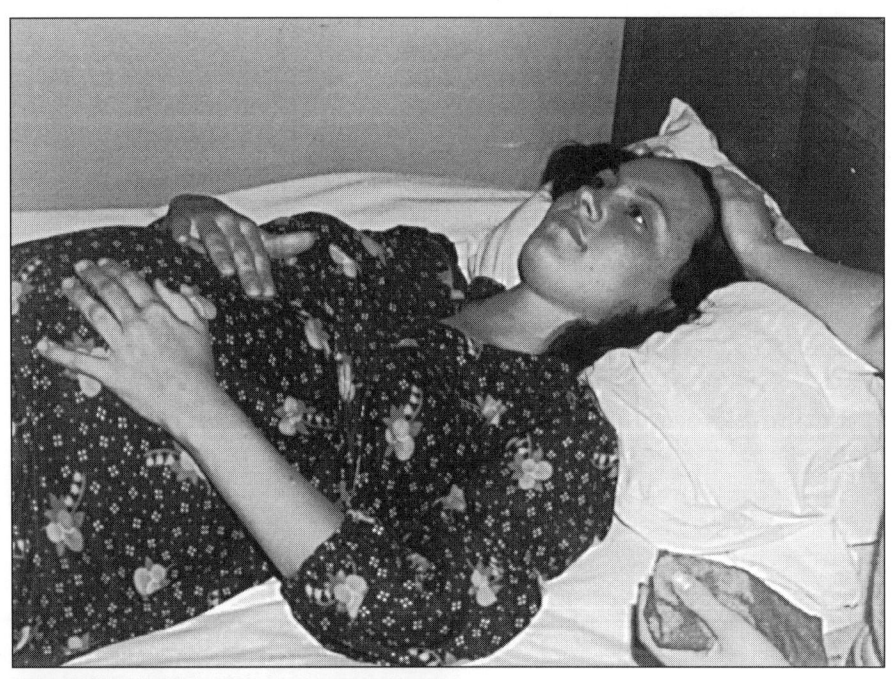

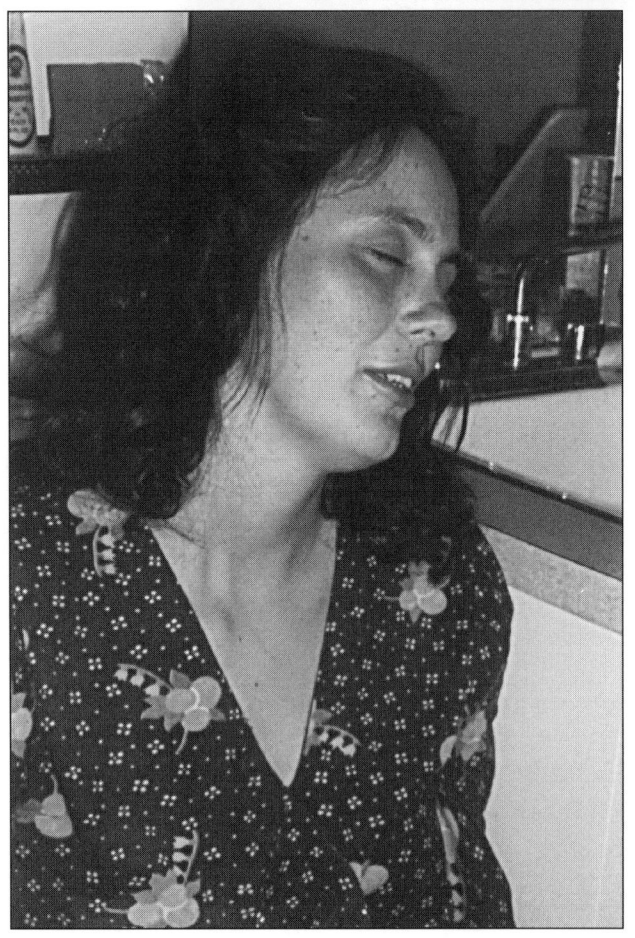

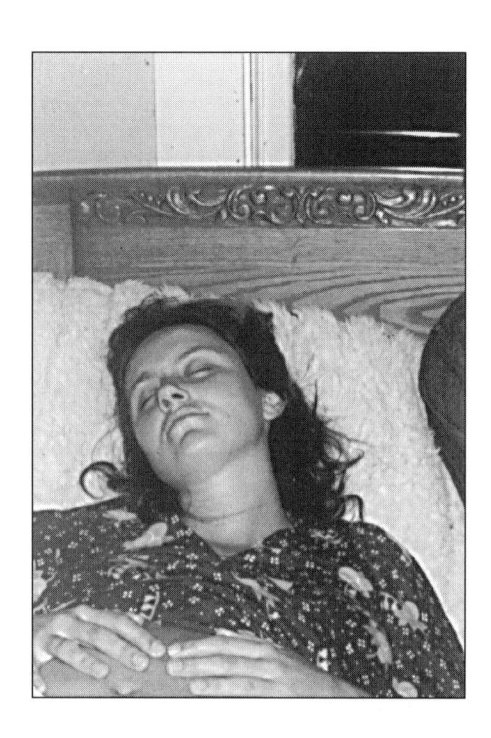

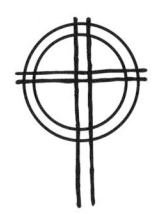

"BEYOND A WHOLESOME DISCIPLINE , BE GENTLE WITH YOUR SELF."

BIRTH OF SON - BIRTH OF SELF - 1976

During our marriage my mate worked diligently to help me overcome my fear of the dark by hiding from me and jumping out of nowhere 'to scare the life from me'. His intentions were to train me to react to unknown situations or beings by staying cool and collected. He also tried to break my pattern of avoiding being hit about the face. As a child, my face was hit often. Any time I was 'smart mouthed' or in the wrong place as a child, I would be slapped.

Lion Heart hated the way I involuntarily recoiled or jerked when a hand would approach my face. For years he pretended he was going to hit me in order to train me to not respond. My life was often a startling set of unforeseen tests of my neutrality to potential abuse.

During the long days awaiting the birth of my child, I listened and reviewed how responsive to nature I had become. Giving birth was something I alone was responsible for so I decided to do a natural childbirth, in contrast to the common drug administered birth procedures.

The doctor whom I chose to assist me lived 150 miles away and he and his wife had a private home clinic. As I educated myself about childbirth, I became very "cocky". I believed I could birth this baby by myself if necessary, so strong was I in my belief in the naturalness of woman giving birth.

As I prepared myself, I practiced deep breathing, a breath that rolled from my navel up through my stomach and all the way up to my heart. I also trained myself to experience a point of focus until I could alter my state of consciousness to lessen my sensitivity to my physical body.

In the fall, the golden haired hero, was the first to return to the farm. As a single man, he watched me closely, especially as I nestled deeper into a protected cocoon readying for the birth. The last month of pregnancy, I prayed to deliver early. It seemed that each day I gained another pound. I felt gargantuan and humongous—Amazon like. My husband and his lady friend arrived back at the farm shortly before my delivery date. He was surprised that I didn't expect his return.

Much to my chagrin, I went two weeks over my due date. When I finally went into serious labor, I could barely sit, let alone drive the 150 miles to my doctor. Contractions began on a Friday morning. I soaked down at Miracle Hot Springs and the contractions kept getting closer. I danced inwardly with my labor. Barely was I aware that my house was filled with my 'husband', his girlfriend, a dear lady friend and three other men.

Midnight approached and I was in the transitional stage (next to the time one pushes the baby out) and was in minute or less contractions for the next nine hours. All I could do was focus on a crack on my bedroom ceiling and pray. With each internal strain, I prayed for the health of the baby. After twenty-four hours, my birth attendant decided something was awry and demanded I go to the local hospital, which was about twenty miles away.

In the van ride to the hospital, I wanted to push the baby out. Instead my companions yelled at me not to push. Upon arriving at the hospital, I was whisked immediately upstairs. The doctor on duty was delivering another baby. I had a serious complication, a 'placenta previa.' The intensity of labor was great for both me and the baby. In a normal setting, I would have had no choice but go through a C section to save both our lives.

A strength came through me that helped me be very clear about not receiving any medications. The old-time doctor performed a quick alternative cut and my son popped into the world. I would not let the nurses take him away. Since I had not been officially registered into the hospital, they had no authority over me. Twenty minutes after the birth, I left the hospital with my special 'gift from God'.

My mate was gone within a few days of my son's birth. He and most of the farm crew went up to Canada for a major Earth conference. When my son was less than a week old, I traveled to my doctor 150 miles away to have our health checked out. Since I had never had the measles, the doctor insisted on giving me a measles inoculation.

Within a few days of receiving my shot, I came down with all the symptoms of the disorder. Feverish, alone in an unheated home at the end of November, I cried in pain as I held this pure new soul in my arms. I was so alone. No one was there to help me or my son stay warm. Yet some deep strength continued to surface and we both survived.

Upon regaining my health, I began a practice of giving my son a total massage daily. I was so sorry that he had such a painful, arduous birth, and part of me knew we both could have died. I recognized my son's poor head had suffered. One of my friends had gifted me with an infant massage book called *LOVING HANDS* which beautifully illustrated an East Indian woman's techniques of baby massage.

The previous summer I had the good fortune of training with Swami Gitananda and his main wife in breath and yoga practices. I was drawn to the East Indian health practices.

Partly I was motivated to work with my son because I knew that he had been in my birth canal way too long. I just knew that he had endured undo cranial pressure. What began as an awkward exploration of a bulbous little body, grew daily in a respectful awe of the muscular, skeletal development of someone I loved deeply. I was particularly fascinated by the cranial bones and the relaxation that would result in my child when they would be touched.

The other practice I did daily was to swim in a wonderful natural hot springs close by our farm called Miracle Hot Springs. Early each morning we would travel several miles down river from our home and swim. It became a 'family' experience. There were regular elderly, retired men that became grandfathers to my son. I was especially relieved that he was receiving doting attention by grandparent people since my own blood family and I were still quite distant.

It took me a full year to complete my divorce. Amazingly, Lion Heart's best male friend became the 'sunshine of my life'. Daily he would validate my unique worth. My struggle for recognition with the BIFC Boy's Club worked. He was a Yoga instructor and a vegetarian. Also he was an outspoken advocate for protecting the Earth, especially Idaho. The author Edward Abby was a hero to him and inspired him to protect this wonderful earth.

This political activist created a T-shirt which read "Idaho It's Not For Sale'. He encouraged me to speak my own thoughts and just not parrot my husband and father's philosophies. He felt that no one deserved to be treated so minimizing as I was with Lion Heart.

Of the three single people on the farm, one was the mistress to our encounter group leader and the other two were my ex's best friends from the BIFC Boy's Club, that I had considered women haters and male chauvinists. By the time my divorce rolled around, both of Lion Heart's best friends stood beside me and supported my actions for freedom and personal worth. A guru-God Junior had fallen from his throne because his ego got in the way of humanitarian equality.

MOTHER and SON

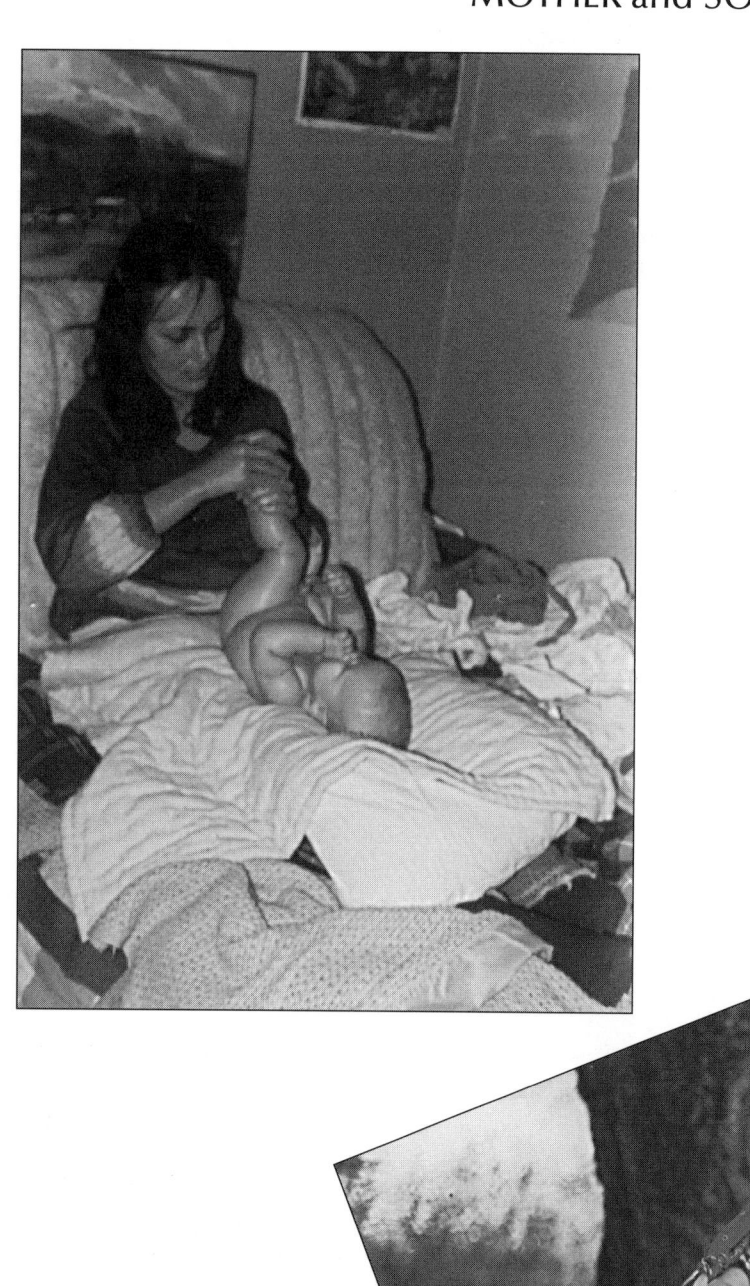

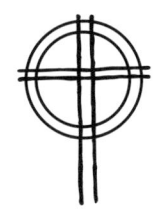

"BE YOURSELF. ESPECIALLY DO NOT FEIGN AFFECTION."

FEMALE/MOTHERING FRIENDSHIP

One day when my son was just a few months old, there was a knock at my door and a friend of a friend asked if he could come in. He had some special acquaintances that he would like to introduce to me. In came a pixy-like, long blond haired, smiling woman with a charming bubbling two year old daughter. The woman was pregnant with her second child and was lonely for female friendship.

She became the first friend in my life who loved children. Also, her husband and she radiated a strong, fun-loving marriage. I was so pleased to finally have family-oriented friends enter my life. The only problem was that she lived fifty plus miles away in a remote town, so we did not get to see each other regularly.

On one of our shared visits, my friends who were jewelers, brought some clients by the farm on their way to the local hot springs. Invited to come along, I gladly traveled to the warm water soaking oasis.

My friends' clients had a baby in arms like I did. As the conversation came around to age, skills, first child, we were to discover that our babies were exactly the same age, born only fourteen hours apart. What even became more fascinating was the fact that this couple also lived in a remote location in Idaho and had researched birth alternatives and had chosen the same home birth clinic and physician as I had, and we both described our offspring as 'gifts from God'.

If I had followed through with my initial birth plans, my son would have been born at the same home clinic as their son. But since I was so uncomfortable, being two weeks overdue, I had opted to stay home and do it myself. After all, I had thought it was a natural woman's process.

I explored what it was that brought them to my jeweler friends. I was told that the wife had ordered a red catlinite ceremonial pipe for her husband as a Christmas present and was picking it up. Questioning the significance of the pipe, I was informed that the husband, True Creed, was a Sioux trained medicine person and the pipe would be used in medicinal earth ceremonies and healing processes. From my youth, a part of me had fantasized about Sacajawea and the way of Native Americans. Because my last name is Lewis and famous wilderness explorers Lewis and Clark had journeyed through Idaho with the help of this Indian maiden, I felt an unexplainable closeness.

The almost white haired medicine person, was a 'far cry' away from my the idealized image of a Indian teacher but he oozed the sense of a wise elder person. Another intense male entered my life.

The wife of the "twin-like" baby was from the same city that I was though several years younger. She had attended the same schools I had. Things were a little eerie,

43

too much synchronism for comfort. Little did I know that I was creating my dreamed of `extended family'.

My personal health took a sharp turn for the worse at the time of my divorce when my son was one year old. My greatest fear was that my ex-husband would come and take my child and disappear. During the last months before the legal divorce I was constantly challenged to not collapse from the intense feelings we had for each other.

Lion Heart seemed to feel that there was no need to divorce. Life could just keep going as it was and that was fine. I knew that there were not enough shreds of respect left in me. The constant reminders of how much of my life had been spent with him and his family stirred deep sadness. How could I not love some part of this person who had protected me from my blood family and then introduced me into a surrogate family . Twelve years of relationship was a lot to end.

On Thanksgiving my soon to be ex came to take my son to his blood family dinner. Twenty-four hours passed and he did not return. Finally one of the men from the farm went with me to Boise to retrieve my baby. Since I was still actively nursing him, I was painfully engorged. When we finally rendezvoused with Lion Heart, he was at his parent's home. With my arms stretched out to hold my child, he quickly pivoted putting the boy child in my male friend's arm. Twirling, he calculatingly punched me squarely in the face.

I crumpled on the floor. My 6'4" friend helped me up, baby in one arm, me on the other and we went out to his car. No words came from us, while Lion Heart's mother screamed and fluttered about. My head reeled with wrenching pain and my heart collapsed in confusion. My in-laws wailed and said they were so sorry. Why would he do such a thing?

I went to my parents' home. Where else does one turn but back to our blood relatives when time get really tough? My mind was filled with static and pain. Ten years had passed since I had entered my family home. The home-coming was less than welcoming. Noticing the wounded face, my family shrugged. Slaps in the face were pretty typical happenings. It got one's point across. Within hours I left to return to the farm.

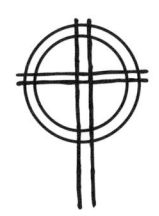

"NEITHER BE CYNICAL ABOUT LOVE; FOR IN THE FACE OF ALL ARIDITY AND DISENCHANTMENT IT IS PERENNIAL AS THE GRASS."

DAILY HEALTH PRACTICES

Back on the farm, winter deepened. I was currently sharing a home with two men, two women, and one young child. Occasionally my ex-husband would return to the farm from one of his various escapades with no advance notice.

> BE HERE NOW
> LOVE IS ALL THERE IS
> STAY IN THE MOMENT
> LIFE IS A LIVING ORGASM (Ram Dass)
> LOVE THE ONE YOU'RE WITH

These were some of the guidelines for those of us living on the farm. The vegetarian teacher's famous epistle was "a stiff mind yields a stiff body". He contended the only difference between old age and youth was stiffness. Daily we would do yoga movements and breathing exercises. We ate simply. We would consume foods and juices that were grown locally and organically. More and more attention was put into understanding how to combine foods, and attending to chewing our food and loving each of the steps to maintaining health.

Daily, I tried to begin again without registering anger at another or holding on to grudges or pre-judgements. It was difficult. I was understanding the importance of picturing the life I wished to live rather than being a broken record of the type of existence I wanted to leave behind. Stepping into the greatest potential called for every inch of effort to creatively live it in the now. The witness in me was quick to catch when I was negative or scornful.

At night, I would record in my journal the events of the day. Since junior high the diary or journal had often been my best confidential friend. When it was unsafe to share my thoughts with any other, the intimate writing tool became my agent for communication.

Journaling also could haunt me especially when I would notice a constant repeated complaint or confusion. From thirteen years old on I was consistently asking 'What was love?' Why does caring mean hurting? Why aren't people fair?' Why do I get hit and hurt?'

Currently the dialoguing was about becoming lighter, more spiritual, spirit-filled. I wanted to turn things over to God and trust life was unfolding at just the right time line and way. Relationships continued to be a undercurrent theme in my journals. After my divorce I had vowed to never marry again. I did not believe in that institution any longer.

Yet the ongoing life I was sharing with the men at the farm stretched my understanding of caring and loving.

In the fall many from the farm attended a conference at the YWCA in Boise focused on *Alternative Communities in the Northwest.* Throughout the past year, different members of our farm had traveled to organized planned communities throughout the United States. Hungrily we searched for well developed smoothly functioning communities. We did not want to 're-invent the wheel'. We welcomed the opportunity to participate in this conference.

Our group was intrigued by the people who attended. It was fascinating to be introduced to Sun Bear and Wabun, Two Rainbows Affiliates, True Creed and others like our farm group.

Most of the folks we met shared their experiences about relationships, philosophy and life practices such as food, exercises, diet, meditations and circles. It became clear that we were all experiential—not one except maybe *The Farm* in Tennessee had a long term, successful community history and reference book.

Sun Bear spoke clearly of his 'Medicine Society' which consisted of a group of people who shared a common 'vision'. Attaining a Vision is not something simple. A tribal leader or recognized medicine person usually receives the message of 'blueprint' after years of training.

The medicine person may be a chosen person this life time and are willing to sacrifice for the good of their tribe. When receiving a group message, the follow through models the trust, honor and commitment of those who can hear and understand the message delivered. Sun Bear's physical presence commanded respect. He was a man capable of disappearing in a blink and then being so physical he felt like a bull ready to charge.

The 'Bear Tribe', he related, was an example of a multi-racial medicine society composed of people who wanted to understand, then teach others about the coming earth changes, especially how to prepare for the upcoming upheaval on this sweet Earth. The Bear Tribe was "also trying to build a true love relationship with their brothers and sisters in the group, and to avoid being negative, violent or possessive." (Wabun, *WOMAN OF THE DAWN,* pg. 22)

His willingness to speak to a new form of rainbow relationship between man and woman, Earth and Sky, attracted me. Sun Bear spoke with such tender compassion for the Earth. He called it the Mother. Endearingly, he implored us to wake up. Sadly he knew the white immigrant had not been reared with this respectful exchange with the Earth.

The Mother was being torn up. The Sacred Mountain where all life began was being destroyed. Sarcasm for the white man's arrogance came through. The Earth could wipe out the two legged with a simple burp.

White man wants to own everything. He's taken the land from the Red People not knowing they don't claim to own the land but believe that they are part of a family, the earth family where everything is related. Nothing is taken for granted, ceremony and thanksgiving are extremely important. The Maker of All Things represents everything. He implored us to pray for and with the Earth. He implored us to listen and be respectful.

That was a theme of our Milepost #195 Farm group, too. The book *1984* and *HOW TO SURVIVE THE UPCOMING EARTH DISASTER* had influenced our group's decision to leave the professional, city life and to return to the earth. I know we were focused on growing healthy, organic people food and establishing sounder neighborhood consciousness. We wanted to model another way of living these short remaining years on earth. We were prepared for major earth disruptions in the upcoming eighties.

I watched with intense interest this woman called Wabun that seemed to walk beside Sun Bear. All my teachers to date had been men and I was hungry for a woman teacher. So it was at this time that I joined my first woman's circle facilitated by Wabun. For four days she shared Earth Mother language, expansion of our strength, our rightful purpose and sacred step dancing. I can still see her in the basement of the "Y" pulling the drapes, locking the door, lighting the candles, sharing the smudge, calling the directions, and speaking prayerful thanksgiving.

In 1977 it was illegal for Native Americans to share their natural spirituality. Shortly thereafter in 1978 the white man's laws changed to allow Native Americans to practice some of their ancient spiritual ways. Much of what she offered, I had never heard spoken before.

The 'Step Dance' evoked involuntary remembering inside my mind and within my heart. I knew that these women and I shared something from long, long ago. Without a doubt I connected with a spiritual lineage that had been persecuted and killed. I was almost in a daze after the dance when we looked in each other's tear-filled eyes, speaking hesitantly of what we now knew. Wabun made us vow to never use this new/old knowledge inappropriately. My inner memory was of being burned at the stake. It was so real I could still smell the smoke and the flesh. I felt horrendous pain and a raw fear of being found out. I heard each of the other women in the circle quietly with intensity describe a common 'past-life' experience. A part of me could not believe what I was witnessing.

Nothing like this had ever occurred in my life before. What did that life which found me 'judged bad—a witch' have to do with me in the seventies? Would I have to revisit this lifetime being in the public's judgmental eyes—getting terrorized and then maimed and killed?

Whew, I prayed not.

A day before the last dance, Wabun stopped me in the hall. Having watched me among the "men" in my life, she intensely related "Grow up! Quit kissing ass!   Be in your power, woman power!" Being hit by a 'mack' truck couldn't have impressed me more.   I was intimidated, yet I heard something.

During this last ceremonial lineage step circle, when Wabun stepped us into remembering our inheritance of who we truly were, each of us went back to another group experience, the dawning of the sisterhood based on integrity. Relating to the good Mother Earth was rekindled in me.   Being burned at the stake meant one was named a witch. And as everyone I knew would tell you, being a witch was bad. Now all of a sudden this term was being redefined as a caring person who nurtured children and the earth. Believe me, I was not going to talk to anyone outside of that intimate circle about my step dance gift from Wabun.

I loved finding out more about the *Two Rainbow* group**,** sponsored by True Creed and his wife. Just the name created a deeper bond with our farm group. One of the greatest natural gifts at our farm was the veranda which afforded stunning views of tremendous single and double rainbows plus stupendously color washed sunrises and sunsets.

We wanted to work and play with the Earth, not use her up and spit her out. The Two Rainbow people had a goal of facilitating their first Summer Festival in the high country in the Sawtooths where they were inspired to buy land. Their whole group stood behind a seven phase doctrine that True Creed had received in communion with St. German and Merlin. These spiritual connections rang so true for him, that his whole life pivoted around the following truths:

> One   Sun
> Two   Shoe
> Three   Tree
> Four   Door
> Five   Dive
> Six   Sticks fire
> Seven Heaven

True Creed explained the above simple ways with the following explanation:

"These seven survivial concepts re not only useful in an emergency survival situation, but also valuable in working through many problems in daily life. The first two of these concepts have been discussed; Honesty and Personal Responsibility For Your Life. I discovered the high level of interest given these concepts while training Army personnel. The first of these concepts is Honesty (Sun). All too often we will not admit we have a problem or we try to cover up the problem with a lie.

The worse lies are the lies we tell ourselves. The sooner we acknowledge we have a problem, the sooner corrective action can be accomplished. To do otherwise wastes precious time and energy. This concept has a strong bearing on all our lives. We all feel we are honest but, in reality, we often create illusions and rationalizations which are not in harmony with what we know to be truth. Sometimes we live our lives by another person's value system or expectations, yet all the while carry resentment, guilt or a feeling of helplessness.

Even socially accepted "white lies" do nothing but postpone what must be confronted and ultimately dealt with. The result is that we waste energy and undermine our self confidence. Without honesty, there is no foundation upon which to build a solid life. Be as honest with yourself as you can and let that honesty permeate all aspects of life. You will be amazed at how problems will be solved and eventually disappear.

The second concept is that you are Personally Responsible For The Life Which You Create (Shoes). No one is responsible for the conduct of your life but you. We tend to give our individual power to others or institutions in exchange for promised security. This is an illusion. True security comes from discovering one's own abilities and strengths. You must live your own life and take full personal responsibility for it.

The third concept is the acknowledgement and realization that Your Truths and Strengths Come From A Universal Power (Tree) accessible to all of us. Your concept of this power is your own decision. Many call it GOD. Without exception, I have never met a person who went through an intense survival experience or severe life and death problem who did not acknowledge or rediscover that source of help and comfort. That power is real. Recognize this truth and call freely upon the source.

    The fourth concept is Prayer (Door). We must communicate in our acknowledgement and giving thanks for our individual abilities, strengths and opportunities. There is an old saying the Army, "There are no atheists in foxholes". In a survival situation, you may find yourself really alone for the first time. You will experience an overwhelming need and urge to communicate with this source of power, giving thanks for what you have and asking for what you need and hope to achieve.

    The fifth concept is to be still and Listen To Your Inner Voice (Dive). In other words, you should sit, be still and think. In a stressful or panic situation, the most important task you must accomplish is gaining self control. Sit down on the ground and breathe deeply and slowly. Allow your mind to clear and your body to calm. Listen to your thoughts and they will give you the answers required. In a more relaxed and calm frame of mind, it will become much easier to make clear evaluations of your problems and sound judgements needed to take the most appropriate actions.

    The sixth concept is to Live In The Present (Sticks to make fire). Worrying about past mistakes, bad predicaments or anticipating problems in the future can be a tremendous waste of energy. It can also weaken the focus and concentration necessary to deal with the present situation. This concept is particularly relevant in a survival situation or emergency. Live in the present and take care of today. It conserves energy and survival depends on the conservation of energy.

    The last of these seven survival concepts is to Be Positive (Heaven) in your thoughts, feelings and actions. Approach life with a positive attitude and attend to any task with which you are confronted, striving for excellence and doing the best job possible. Be positive; it will get you through some rough times.

    There is a Native American Indian proverb that states, "The Great Spirit will never give us more than we are equipped to deal with". I am sure we all feel sometimes we have more problems than we can handle; however, remember you can make it. It's a matter of how and what you think and do."

    This code of received ethics and True Creed's desire to celebrate with the Earth stirred our farm group to commit to work together with them. In fact, the weekend community workshop brought forth the knowing that there just was not one light center on the earth. There was not one perfect right community or leader. Each community where there was a union of respect for Earth/Mother and Sky/ Father with the two legged beings; participating in a rainbow bridge with above and below was a light center. Our over-all goal became to connect the light centers, thus lighting up the entire world. There was no place on this earth that did not deserve to be an acknowledged light center.In particular our Farm and True Creed's group committed to work together to assist the farm with its' organic labor intensive crops and the Two Rainbows Spiritual Earth Gatherings. Our sense of community consciousness was expanding.

I knew I wanted to share this collection of communication with my home community. I asked many of the presenters of this conference if they would be willing to come to our farm the next summer to share their insights and talents in our part of the state. I especially wanted to further pursue the right brain stuff, the feminine. I saw too many women walking around with feminine exteriors and masculine dominated interiors.

I was discovering that I knew next to nothing of what was being spoken about the right side of the brain. All too well, I was familiar with the left side, the logical, analytical, systematic, competitive, masculine side of me—the math major—the super do gooder!

The right hemisphere related to the intuitive, sensing, feeling, artistic, freeing feminine side of one's personality process. My left side was so strained, and it was the source of the constant head pain I felt behind my left eye.

The next step in my healing ('that which makes one well') process was opening up the right side of my brain. And if work was life and life was work, I had to put more playful, light, spirited sensing activities into my reality. For the summer of 1978 I planned a *Feminine Energy Workshop* at the farm.

While practicing to be perfect, I was raising a two year old intense child. He was a child whose rumbling chuckles could seduce a room to tearful laughter and whose loud rages could all but break windows with forceful intensity.

When the warmer weather hit the farm, everyone left our tiny rough farm house to move outdoors. Whether to alternatively live in a trailer, tipi or truck, they left the house.

My son was a handful and each one living on The Farm had not chosen to have a child or "caretake" a young one. This child was a pain in the rear for the farm family.

Even though I was divorced from my son's father, Lion Heart was a legitimate shareholder of our Milepost #195 farm corporation, so my ex had free reign to come and go on our eighty acre parcel of earth. As the time for the Feminine Energy Workshop approached, I was clear that I did not want his participation, nor that of his current companion.

One of the features of the farm was regular communication workouts, usually facilitated by our own therapist member. Angry, spark-filled releasing came out as we tried to re-establish safe boundaries and freedom so that I did not have to include those who might disturb my conference project. I did not buckle under the pressure to forgive Lion Heart and his current love, also a member of the farm and invite them to participate. This was quite a coup for one of "wimps" of the farm.

One of the reasons I had left the city was that I was extremely sensitive to all the vibes of my neighbors and community. I was a sponge that was absorbing unwanted dense energy. I could feel someone's thoughts, especially if they were negative. My ex and I during many of his summers away from our home would practice telepathy and sensing into each other. We consciously made notes of when we would either dream of the other, or if our thoughts would be dominated on the other. We had been pretty tuned in to the other being or presence. Now I was establishing that the vibes I felt with my ex and the 'other woman' were damaging to the peace and clarity I wanted to maintain.

One of my strongest allies was another new mother. She and her husband at the last minute had chosen not to buy into the farm but had maintained involvement. In her late thirties, this glorious South African adopted a new born boy. It was a wonderful event as she and her husband had longed for children and were down to the wire age wise to adopt a child. They had only one week's notice before receiving their son.

We shared the new mother's wonders together as her son was only two months younger than mine. This lady's heart was large and caring.

Two nights before the Feminine Energy Workshop, this loving, spirit-filled friend was critically injured in a front-end car accident. She curled her body instinctively around her precious young son, taking the impact on herself, crushing her skull and spine. Her husband was also injured but the boy child was not hurt.
　　I wanted to cancel the Feminine Energy Worship as I was totally stunned and sickened by this tragedy. It was impossible to stop the event at the midnight hour. The course of my life was altered. How could I be responsible when my soul was intensely sad and stretched?

1978 FEMININE ENERGY WORKSHOP AT THE FARM

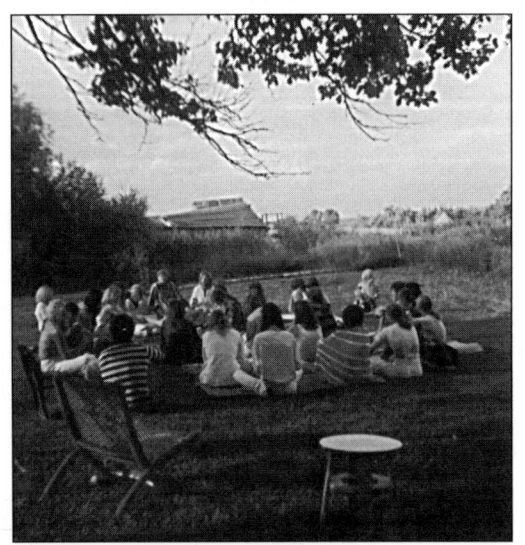

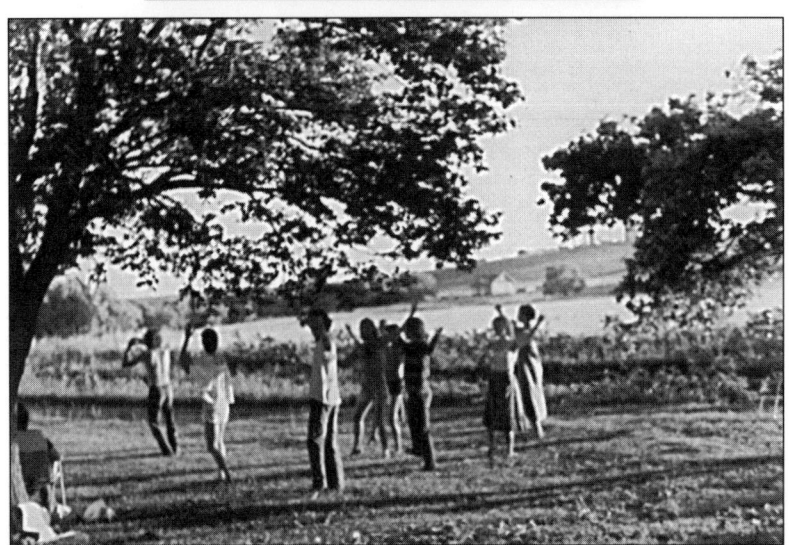

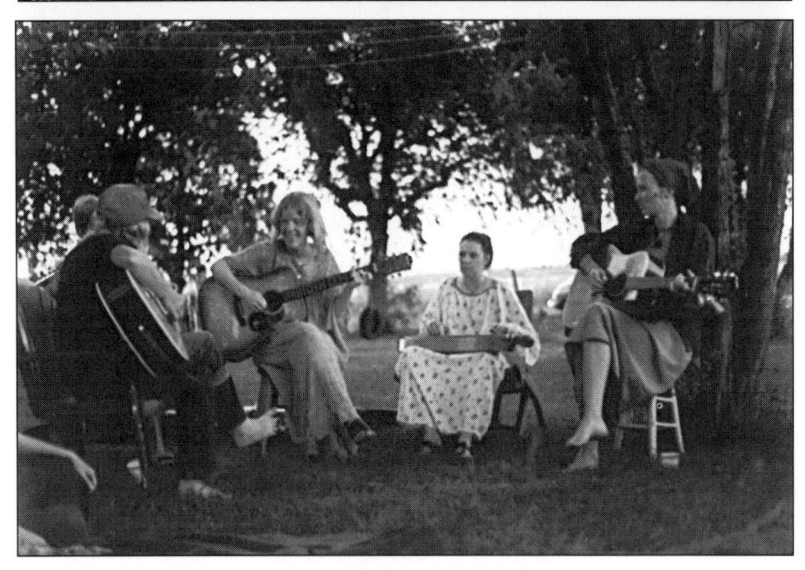

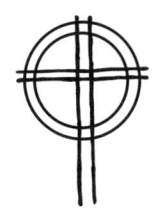

*"NURTURE STRENGTH OF SPIRIT TO SHIELD YOU IN SUDDEN MISFORTUNE. BUT DO NOT DISTRESS YOURSELF WITH IMAGININGS.
MANY FEARS ARE BORN OF FATIGUE AND LONELINESS."*

FEMININE ENERGY - EXTRA SENSORY PERCEPTION

Fifty people showed up at the farm while many of us were deeply grieving our friend who was in a coma close to death. There were psychologists, teachers, and various community members committed to participate in this three day event.
We began the morning with yoga, tai chi and meditations. Interwoven through the various workshops, songs were sung and the harmony of sacred chanting. Because our emotions running close to the surface with our lady friend's car accident, the intensity of the weekend heightened with each event.

Linda O'Hare, a talented seer and clairvoyant, guided the majority of us in a past life regression. For many, it was a first time to experience the slip into a mysterious journey back in to another time period when we had walked together. As a group we went back in our spirit and soul's history. There was not enough time allotted for individuals to share their experience when we came back to the here and now. What we sensed, saw or experienced was kept private. For some, nothing but darkness occurred. I know for myself I was stunned that I returned to the time of Christ. I was aware only of his feet and the path he walked, and of tears.

Many sought me out privately, in safe secluded places, to share that they, too, went back to the time with Christ. It was awesome to even consider this as part of my soul's experience, let alone language it with someone else. Coming to clarify myself and others as a tribe that had chosen to reincarnate together felt right but I could not find a comfortable spot to rest in my rational mind.

Without a doubt though, I now knew myself to be a 'Living Disciple of God's Son'. I was relieved. It felt like my spiritual seeking was providing some substance I could believe and truly be. From that moment forth I did not flounder again about how to live my days. I had gained faith in the Great Teacher and his words and teachings filled me.

Towards the end of the workshop, we were doing a special group healing prayer circle, directing loving thoughts to our critically injured friend. Three times she had all but died, and she laid in a faraway hospital, comatose. We prayed for her to be care taken and to pass through the limbo of living dead. Hands connected, eyes closed, hearts united, we sent our intentions.

As the tears flowed, she appeared to some of us, in her lovely green Easter ceremonial dress, imparting to us that she was okay. I remember seeing/sensing her and having my hair stand on end, I literally was lifted off the ground by the strength of the energy of the exchange. Pretty amazing! The encounter was so eerie, somewhat like an "out-of-body" feeling. Various others in the circle experienced different forms of exchange with this woman.

Western Medicine brought her back to life three different times. I don't feel our prayer group interfered with her death process, but the medical world did. She ended up a living vegetable, kept alive for another decade. This experience taught me to be very clear before praying for another's well-being or course of life. My dear friend truly became one of my most meaningful teachers. Any time I would start feeling sorry for myself because of how bad I felt, I'd think of her and know I had to lighten up.

Our extended family expanded. I became one of her son's surrogate mothers. My son and I got to spend lots of time around an individual that could only spasm and cry.

At the Feminine Energy Workshop, I participated in my first official "sweat" with the white Sioux Medicine Man, True Creed. Previously, I had been introduced to the sweat lodge in a rather informal manner. We had gleaned the worth of this natural cleansing, healing process from various books and real experience. We called this eclectic, natural ceremony, Farm Sweats.

I immediately felt a deep respect for this medicine person. As we walked over to the fire pit next to the sweat lodge, nestled into the curve of our creek, protected by Russian Olive trees, I asked; "What is your philosophy on monogamy, marriage, and committed relationships?" He said, "Number one, I don't believe in monogamy. Any honest man would have to answer the same," he stated. "Love the one you're with." True Creed said, "that any time two people connect on the sexual realm, they have to be responsible for creating a child. God was a trickster, and no matter what form of protection a couple my take, a sacred new being could be created. That potential offspring is one's first consideration before becoming intimate or sexual with another!"

He inferred that even if a couple thought they were taking adequate prevention to not conceive, if the Maker, God intended creation of a special new being, it could occur. To be sure that one was willing to be meshed for life with a potential co-parent was essential before being sexual.

I listened very thoughtfully since relationships with men seemed to be one of the weakest suites in my life. At this point in my life, I was physically intimate with two men. Two males whose different range of perceptions and talents filled me more than I had ever known while married. Yet neither one of them was monogamous nor even wanted to be committed. Recently divorced, freshly single, I had vowed never to marry again. I was curious and this man was willing and safe to talk to.

In the lodge, True Creed prayerfully called to all the relatives on this good earth. The manner in which he shared was through what the indigenous people call the Medicine Wheel, a symbolic life expression mapped within a sacred circle. The wheel expresses one's physical (earth), mental (air), emotional (water), and spiritual (fire) aspects of being. The wheel was described like a clock of life, East/Birth, South/youth and family, West/lineage spirit, and North/crone or elder; each of the main quadrants represented a direction through animal representative, plant life, seasons of the year, stages of a life, instruments, and on and on.

He offered so much and I loved how the Medicine Wheel reflected all of the outside of self, nature, as a mirror for all the inside of a self, the personal being. True Creed expounded that the power of prayer throughout this sacred ceremony was essential. Also, the manner of reference in the lodge reflected the locality a tribe was raised in. A Northwest Indian would language his symbolic world differently from an Indian raised on the plains. The study of the Medicine Wheel is a lifetime of work and contemplation. This was a memory making workshop, an episode in my life that would teach me much through the course of time.

I was introduced to tai chi, an oriental dance like exercise movement that has a story of nature and her animals and elements expressed through it. By coordinating stance, hand movement, breath, focus and prayer, one can bring a sense of balance to self and the world we live in. The terms yin and yang were introduced again, giving me another way of looking at female and male energy.

Our own East Indian advocate and yoga instructor shared the postures called the Salute to the Sun to the group each morning. I gradually was learning to love knowing about my internal organ systems, the muscular support system and how through an exercise program I could assist my body's health. In the past both my father and ex-husband had used ridicule and criticism to push me to make my body as beautiful as it could be. I never felt in the past even a semblance of being attractive with the body I had.

For this mother whose left hip was so trained to jet up and out to support a hefty little boy, I was struck by the awkwardness and unsteadiness of my system. I was a klutz, who deserved another way to 'caretake' herself.

Another highlight of the Feminine Energy weekend came through a teacher called Tara Nelson who shared sound and color therapy with us. She came up from California and was introducing us to what seemed to be the leading edge of self health techniques. She wove the concept of chakras, the seven energy centers in our body that respond to specific colors, emotion, endocrine gland, and sound. She clarified these vibrational regions in terms and tones that had previously seemed like Greek when I had trained earlier with my yoga instructor in Boise.

Tara, with her flaming red hair was like the sun beaming out warmth and joy as her small frame drenched us with intense tonal vibrations. I was moved by what I felt inside, but it was very difficult for me to verbalize what I was experiencing.

At the closing ceremony Tara, knowing that I was in dire need of a throat chakra healing (I was characterized as a workhorse, famous for my ability to help behind the scenes to make other leaders, teachers, men succeed) asked if I would be willing to experience a group healing procedure. Work I could do, but speak out I could not. I would open my mouth to express myself and words would scramble, I'd stutter and squeak. The more effort I would put to getting something stated, the worse my delivery would be. I'd choke, gasp and become humiliated.

With no time to run away, I hesitantly entered the center of the large circle of participants. She had a dear male friend hold my feet and a kind woman friend cradle my head and she then asked all in the circle to tonal with her as she prayed for God, the Maker, to come through and assist in releasing whatever blocked my throat.

I was asked to become a hollow flute receiving, allowing myself to be tuned. The vibration created by all the participants set me to trembling. Shivers made my hair stand on end. With eyes closed colors splashed in my inner sight. The touch of her hand on my energy centers, was like electrical currents plugged into an intense source. At times I felt like I was inside a huge ringing bell. I vibrated. As she worked above and below my throat center, tears came to the surface and rippled non-stop down my cheeks.

I perceived the intensity of staring into the bright glowing sun. My insides were stretching.   I was a glowing light. I knew I was being deeply touched by light and grace.
When the experience was completed, I was changed. Never in my life had I received so much love and blessings.

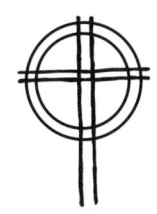

"THEREFORE, BE AT PEACE WITH GOD, WHATEVER YOU CONCEIVE HIM TO BE, AND WHATEVER YOUR LABORS AND ASPIRATIONS, IN THE NOISY CONFUSION OF LIFE KEEP PEACE WITH YOUR SOUL..."

CULTIVATING SPIRITUALITY

After the Feminine Energy Workshop, my focus on healing intensified especially as it related to Jesus and his influence as an example teacher/healer. I truly began to believe that what he could do, I could do and even more.

From the age of twelve I sought out various religious institutes trying to find and understand God. I Often referred to God as 'IT'. I sincerely yearned to know Him. Even though I am a fifth generation Idahoan whose great-great grandparents were original pioneers in Idaho in the mid 1800. A lineage that was brought over with the L.D.S. missionaries from Wales where my deep roots mingled with Celtic natural spiritual wisdom. A blood line filled with instinctive understanding of the Earth, her elements and all Her beauties and expressions. The church wanted bodies to claim land for there religious domain.

By the seventh grade, my deep thoughts were dominated by a hunger to understand God and especially his son, Jesus. I wanted to believe in something and I was keenly intrigued by Jesus — was he a human man or a God man?

Repeatedly I read of Christ-like men who experienced episodes of tragedy, a voluptuous flood, great learning that came from mountain tops often inscribed in stone, and a respect for the earth, her animals, plants, especially the trees and her waters, caves and inhabitants. Plus, in all these hero's stories there would be conflict about the physical yearning for comfort and passion with a woman and the ultimate test of staying on there spiritual path.

Often a spokesperson would arrive giving the wake-up call to the two legged to remember their Earth commitment of integrity, honor, peace, trust and good relations.

For years I had read every book I could get my hands on that would give another insight to Christ, the teacher; Christ the man. I was so curious how he could create miracles and feed the masses and with an ongoing intent and prayer. He could reach out and touch the sick healing those with the greatest belief. Now it all made sense all those years of wondering. I felt Christ's presence in me as a much loved family member and outstanding teacher.

One of the main virtues of The Farm was to set an example of how neighborhoods could exist peacefully and healthfully. We were affected to our moral backbone by Vietnam, Religion, Nixon and Watergate. Quickly we learned that until peace and health are found within, there couldn't be a real peace in the Earth world outside our own community and self.

Seeing the strife on the farm, many of the farm family decided to travel to Oregon two weeks after the Feminine Energy Workshop. I had been hearing about this remote, annual Fourth of July week-long Rainbow Earth Gathering and knew I was to attend. Significantly I chose to hire a Mennonite family in neighborhood to be the caretaker of my son, while I traveled alone to the depths of Oregon. This would be the second time my son was away from me. He was now 20 months old.

Arriving at the trail head, I packed all my stuff for staying a week on my back and stepped on a well worn steep, forest trail that lead to a meadow a mile away. As I walked slowly down the path, I immediately received smiling greetings from each person traversing the path. There were obvious stages or stratums of life being shared as I descended. I noticed some sweat lodges, people sitting in meditation, people dancing in circles, a huge kitchen and food storage, a fire pit and ragged looking 'survivors'.

Almost immediately the rains began to pour down, and I had to make a quick decision on where to pitch my tipi tent. I bounded up to a Northern mountain side. Pitching the tent in the downpour was a challenge. Once inside the tent, I was overwhelmed with what I had gotten myself into. This was the first time since my son's birth that I had been completely alone, yet strangely enough, I was not afraid.

Nestled on my steep eagle's perch, I began to watch the community get setup for the thousands of people to live cooperatively. They exuded a healthy, non-toxic relationship with this beautiful high country river valley. The rains ceased, and the neighborhood of those who inhabited the precariously, pitched tents on the mountain side appeared in the sunshine. We discovered that we were a bunch of 'lone wolves' from Montana, Idaho and Washington. We were in need of space and freedom from the crowds below. An example of human nature expressed unintentionally with the Earth nature.

The most exciting gift I experienced that week came from circle dancing with hundreds of people. We had a Sufi Master who interpreted dance through story telling and we would be guided on how to do the movements. The sequence of dances wove us into a deep trance-like state. Sufi dancing has your whole body/mind involved in movement, sound, and eye contact with an inner circulating circle. One can quit being mental and can become more loving, accepting and simply being.

The windows of our souls, our eyes, mirrored deep "unjudgemental love", and we exchanged `vows' and commitments to be God-like. The great number of participants, we created circles within circles within circles. It was joyful and wonderful. This participatory event anchored into my knowing what tremendous energetic power comes through people who form a connected hand-to-hand circle, praying and moving simultaneously. It reverberates and spirals inwardly and then outwardly. A natural high that when celebrated out of doors, the family of nature participates in the ascending harmonious feelings. I loved this sharing and enthusiasm. There were many options to purify, whether through fasting, sweating, meditation, prayer, community service, or circle dancing. After the third day there I felt pretty `blissed' out. This was all natural as no drugs were involved, at least that I knew of.

I returned from a sweat lodge, to my amazement, two small-gnome like people came skipping, hand-in-hand towards me. These tiny, fairy-like beings, dressed in green and brown were three feet off the ground. Gasping, my hair standing on end, jaw dropping, I watched them disappear just when I could have reached out to touch them. Spinning around, I bumped into several others (like me) gaping in the direction that the

JULY 1978, TWO RAINBOWS EARTH GATHERING

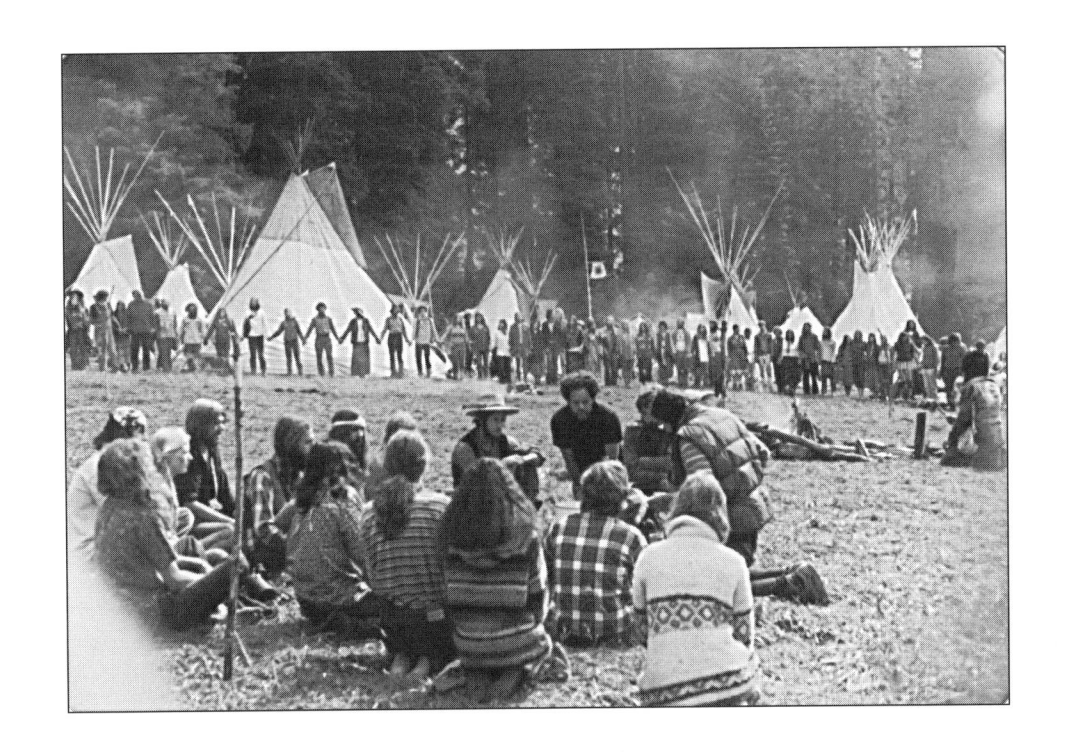

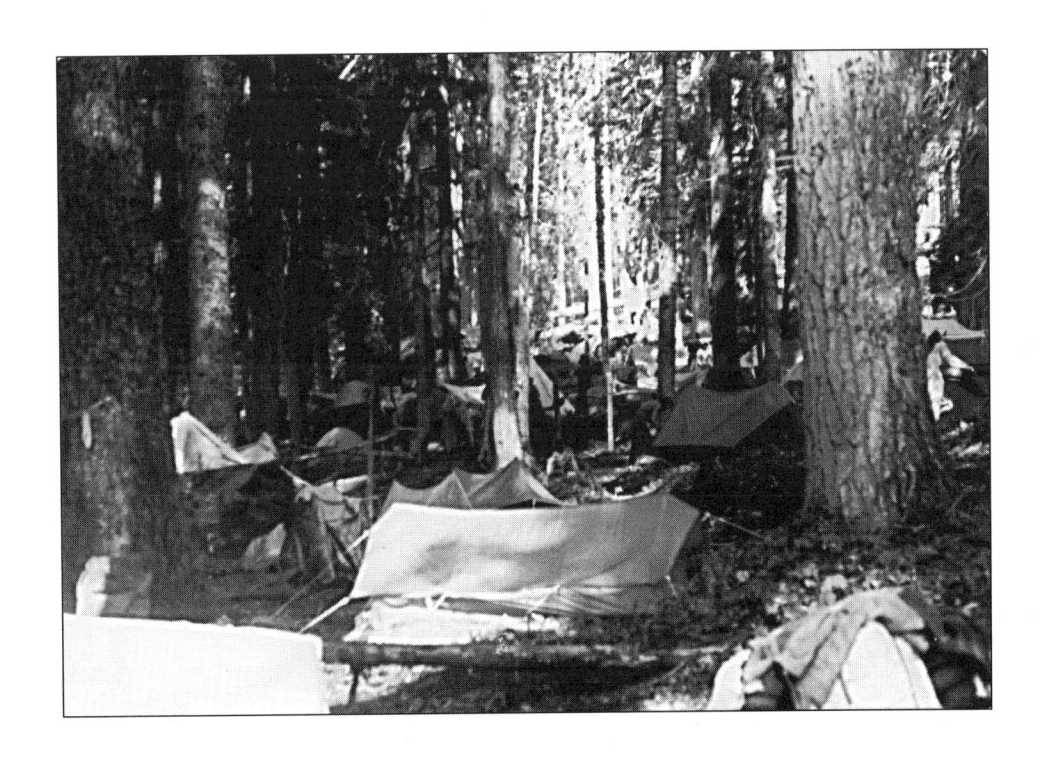

two gnome spirits had vanished. I cried, "Did you see them?" Their heads nodded yes. A rush of relief melted through me. I didn't tell anyone this story for years. I knew it would be mentally hard to believe. It was a gift that renewed a childhood fascination with the fairy world, the little people kingdom.

As an almost pure-blooded Welsh person, the lore of the little people moved in my bones. One of my favorite books as a young girl was *WATER BABIES*. A book that shared a story around water, the animals, amphibians, plants and fairy kingdom that inter related with each other. So, a trampled belief in the little people and plant and animal spirits, gained a new vitality. My time at the farm had been filled with remembering of good relations with trees, plants, butterflies, and the Earth speaking through me. To witness the little people was phenomenal.

Many of the current new age and environmental authors and speakers were present, including political folks. Ram Dass, my hero author who wrote *BE HERE NOW* and *THE ONLY DANCE THERE IS* showed up one afternoon in a meadow wearing a beanie propeller cap. I stumbled, stunned from my fairy exchange, and proceeded to walk right into Ram Dass and a small circle of people.

Within minutes I hesitatingly asked him to elaborate on relationships, commitment and specifically what did he mean that "life was a living orgasm." It was as if time stood still, the doors of clear communications opened, we listened and exchanged and deepened. The options for real intimacy roared its mighty face within my inner mirror. Relationships and all their woes seemed to be the ongoing broken record in my mind. I knew I wasn't any good at them and I needed help to get well in this area of my life.

Lion Heart showed up with his girlfriend and her husband, a man that was as close to me as a brother. He and I were in an emotional fog over marriage commitment and broken morals. The four of us represented the farm at the international peace festival. My heart was working overtime at the Rainbow Gathering.

Though the week was filled with great gifts, the wild Idahoan within me was ready to leave early. No matter how considerate and conscious a group of people are with the environment, that many people living so close to the Earth quickly begin to pollute the beautiful origins of water in the high mountain valley.

I felt the poisoning, and even though I gained some treasured insights, I vowed to never participate in such a large event again. Upon returning to the Magic Valley, several of us felt driven to broaden our commitment to our community and state whether that was by being political and running for office, teaching at the local school, doing cottage art, providing a healthy truck farm or opening a store front. For myself and two other Farm members, we pooled our resources and applied for a small business loan to open a book store in our community.

In my effort to work with my health, I either had to go to Boise, 110 miles away to find endocrine system information or I would order my own books. In the valley that I lived, the largest town, twenty miles away had no bookstores with the exception of a small religious storefront.

In May of 1978 we opened Book Magic in downtown Twin Falls. It was a wholistic book store that offered education in many areas.

By this time my extended family was quite healthy. Still alienated from my blood family, the new family created with children was very important. I did not want my son to go to a public child care center, so four families with five children started a cooperative to attend to our children's well being. One day a week we would each have the children.

We were able to maintain consistent discipline, lots of play and exploration. Plus our dear woman friend, who had suffered brain damage, son received some special mothering.

Each of us were independent store owners—jewelers, an artist, leather and clothing dealer and myself, a book store owner. We were there to help each other be free enough to express ourselves, yet responsible for the physical and mental well being of our children.

"SUZI" AS A CHILD

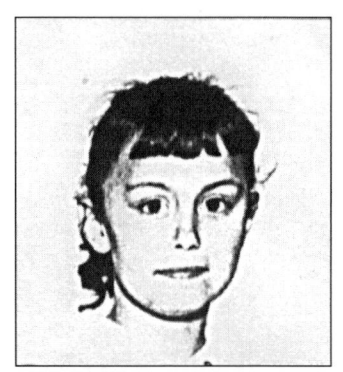

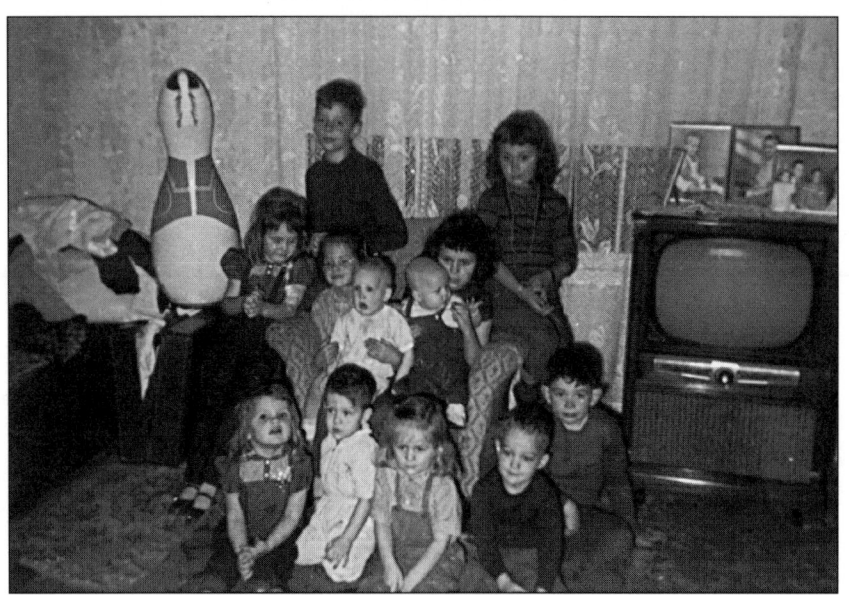

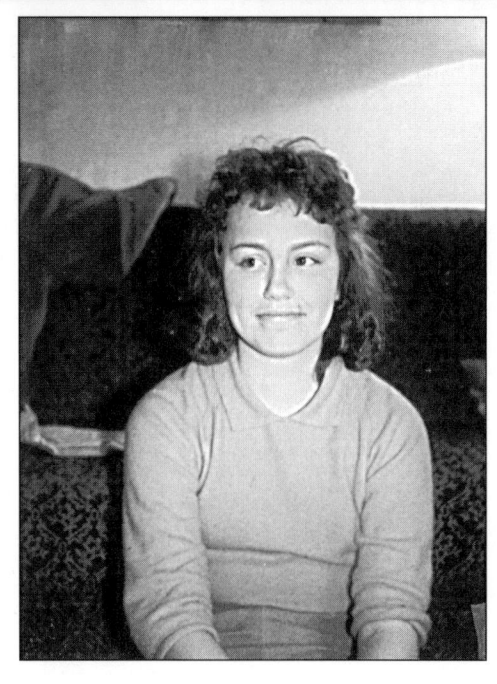

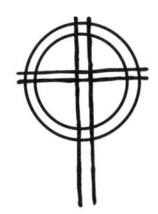

"YOU ARE A CHILD OF THE UNIVERSE, NO LESS THAN THE TREES AND STARS; YOU HAVE A RIGHT TO BE HERE. AND WHETHER OR NOT IT IS CLEAR TO YOU, NO DOUBT THE UNIVERSE IS UNFOLDING AS IT SHOULD"

FAMILY PATTERNS - 1978

I now could recognize that to this point I had not been willing to see or speak to the destructive family patterns I learned from early childhood. My view of successful relationships between a man and a woman were greatly tainted by my blood family, a husband that barely tolerated his less than perfect wife, berating her constantly, and a father pushing to make the perfect child, the best in both the body and the mind. Outside our family home, my dad spoke only of his "perfect family with perfect girls."

Of course the fifties and early sixties were characterized by *Leave it to Beaver*, with June Cleaver as the perfect mother in the model home. The television showed us for the first time how families looked. My family did not get a television until I was in the fifth grade, but I saw that we did not fit that model perfect image of the typical, lower middle class home.

The firm words of wisdom my mother espoused included "Never trust a man to touch you above the knees and below your neck." "Never trust a man." My father was famous for the heralding of his "perfect family" to his friends and students, yet the reality at home had us unworthy and not good enough. If I brought home a report card with all but one `A'; he saw only the lower grade and impressed upon me to do better.

My father was a man responsible for three beautiful daughters and who strutted the lie that everything was just great in his life. While his family desperately tried to act the role in public, we lived behind the closed family doors, a life involved with alcoholic despair and violent spousal fights. We were taught from a young age to live a continual 'white lie' outside the home. This distortion deeply instilled the need to stay separate, not trusting any one inside the family or out. Stressed with roller coaster emotions, strained to breaking, we lived on the precarious edge of self-destruction.

Each day I heard my mother's broken recital of how tough her life was when she was my age. My mother's mother committed suicide when she was five and she quickly gained the 'evil step-mother.' She also was raised among continual strain, pain and emotional hurt. We frequently watched and felt her break emotionally. My father seemed to enjoy other women and my mother was continually devastated. She told us about it, constantly. Often we would be so mad at our father that we would call him Mr. Lewis. We joined in the marital fight and, I am sure, hurt my father back. Our family was always warring and yelling and back-biting.

I became accustomed to being told how I could be better, smarter, faster, thinner, prettier...better than who I was just then. When I turned fifteen, my first wooer, Lion Heart, wanted me and I was such a good ugly duckling, it was my second nature.

Now, I had my father telling my how I could look and achieve better and a boyfriend who continuously criticized me.

Lion Heart basically didn't like who he was. Repeatedly I heard him say "I am a bum, I am no good." In our capitol city, he was known as one of the toughest fighters in the area. He was mad at a social system that had not allowed his own family life to be easy. My parents did not like my first boyfriend.

Trying to save him and prove my parents wrong about his character became my teen-age drive. The alcohol abuse at home surged. My dad would beat my Mom, my mom would beat my eldest sister, and then she would pound on me and our little sister, who would become enraged and hurt herself. I was the one who cried for all of them. I could see my sisters becoming the victims of our mother's own hurt.

Little did I know about the hormonal changes that occurs when one is a teen. My father was the head coach and science teacher at the junior high I attended. I can still see myself in junior high, cloaked in large, bulky sweaters, slumped shoulders, afraid, lonely, disbelieving in love and kindness, searching for a true friend.

Entering the school system undid my mental/emotional systems. I did not attend kindergarten and was a very young first grader in the public school system. The kids teased me for my shyness, calling me 'scared-y-cat' and I would cry and cry. My big sister often came and rescued me from the bullies. She was tough. She could easily deliver a few good punches.

In the third grade, I was one of the few strange girls who was not invited to the popular girl's birthday party. I cried a lot. This same year I remember many headaches and frequent bellyaches that would force me to go home from school. These were usually the same days I would be asked to take a test or perform.

When the young teenage boys started noticing me my father would quickly squelch their attention. I remember telling my dad about a young man who was walking me home and teasing me because my slip showed. I later learned that my dad at school 'leaned hard' on the boy. Never again did that teenager walk me home. Since my father taught and was the primary coach at the same junior high I attended, he easily had access to any person at the school.

I did not know Lion Heart in junior high, but my father did. They had feisty run ins. Both my dad and my ex have retold stories of forms of abuse like my dad slamming the rebellious youth into the wall and the teen fighting back.

The sixties in the public school system were tough. They did not 'spare the rod.' If one got in trouble, the vice principal or coach would administer swats to teach a lesson that would not be easily forgotten.

The summer I was sixteen, I was fitted for contacts and removed my thick glasses. I worked as a lifeguard at a local swimming pool where Lion Heart began the hunt to capture me. I was afraid of him; he had such a bad reputation and he strutted and puffed how mean he was. His history told of almost killing a man while in a drunken rage.

At our high school he was a top athlete and a negligent scholar. Rivalry between the city's two schools was intense. There was an extraordinary push towards academic achievement in the sixties. After all, we were in an international race against Russia and communism to get to the moon. Scientific and mathematical expansion and growth was needed nationally.

My parents' fervor to break us apart, propelled our intimate union. My oldest sister, was more outspoken and rebellious. She broke many of the family's rules, marrying young, a fellow coach on my father's staff. Much of my parents' fierce anger went towards this sister. I was not being hit as often. During my last year at home, my younger sister became more and more the focus of both of my parents' physical rage. More than once upon arriving home from a date I'd find my sister battered, a crying wreck. My mother would say she deserved it and my drunk and boisterous father would be in an arrogant stupor.

Anger oozed in every direction my last months at home. I remember the night Lion Heart's older sister wanted to crash her fiance's bachelors party at a local bar. I was under age, yet she insisted I accompany her. Among the bachelor's guests were my father and some his old teacher drinking buddies. I can still see my father's face when his best friend ordered and bought my first glass of champagne. This was the same man who had intellectually challenged me as an eighth grader, taken me skiing, sold us his 'baby' of a car when I was a twelfth grader and who ultimately created a teaching position for me right out of college. A very awkward situation erupted, as I belligerently stayed at the bar and drank the drink. My dad abruptly left.

Upon arriving home I faced one of the ugliest scenes of my teens. A verbal abuse and condemnation of my character occurred. I remember being called a whore. I can still hear my words declaring that personal worth was based on one's own inner knowing of morality and that they could not tell me of my inner character worth.

My mother in a fit of rage pleaded for me to go somewhere else for school and to get away from my awful boyfriend. I didn't agree and she pulled out a gun and waved it in front of me vowing that she would kill him. That same night, in the early morning hours I heard someone coming into my room. I turned on my night light and there was my father. It was as if he was in a trance. His eyes had this strange faraway glazed intensity. I asked what he was doing as he proceed to get into my bed. I demanded that he leave. Fear pounded in my chest and my mind reeled. He finally left, no words just intense eye exchanges. Tears and terror racked my young woman's heart, soul and body.

A couple of nights later, he returned and this time refused to leave the bed. I ran to my parent's bedroom and demanded that my mother come get her husband. She refused.

The next morning, feeling crazed, I knew I had to leave the household and I did so, never again to be a child to those parents.

My boyfriend's eldest sister provided me with a basement room and her husband helped me get to school.

I applied for and received a college scholarship which I maintained throughout my years of higher education. Within six months, we married. My parents attended the wedding, but barely participated. The wedding was grim. Part of me was committing to a marriage for the rest of my life and another deep part of me screamed in outrage. A voice inside wailed "It won't work."

It's very important to share the significance the Viet Nam war had on my getting married at nineteen. For some odd reason from grade school on I was very politically conscious. I identified with Eisenhower and his grandchildren; they were like a grandfather and siblings. In junior high, John and Jackie Kennedy exuded the romantic, fairy tale life that I feverishly wished I could live. I was keenly aware that my home life did not include love or respect or integrity.

The warring against the spread of Communism, the Cuban Missile Crisis and the religious involvement with Viet Nam continued to keep our nation disturbed. My blood

"SUE" AS A TROUBLED TEENAGER

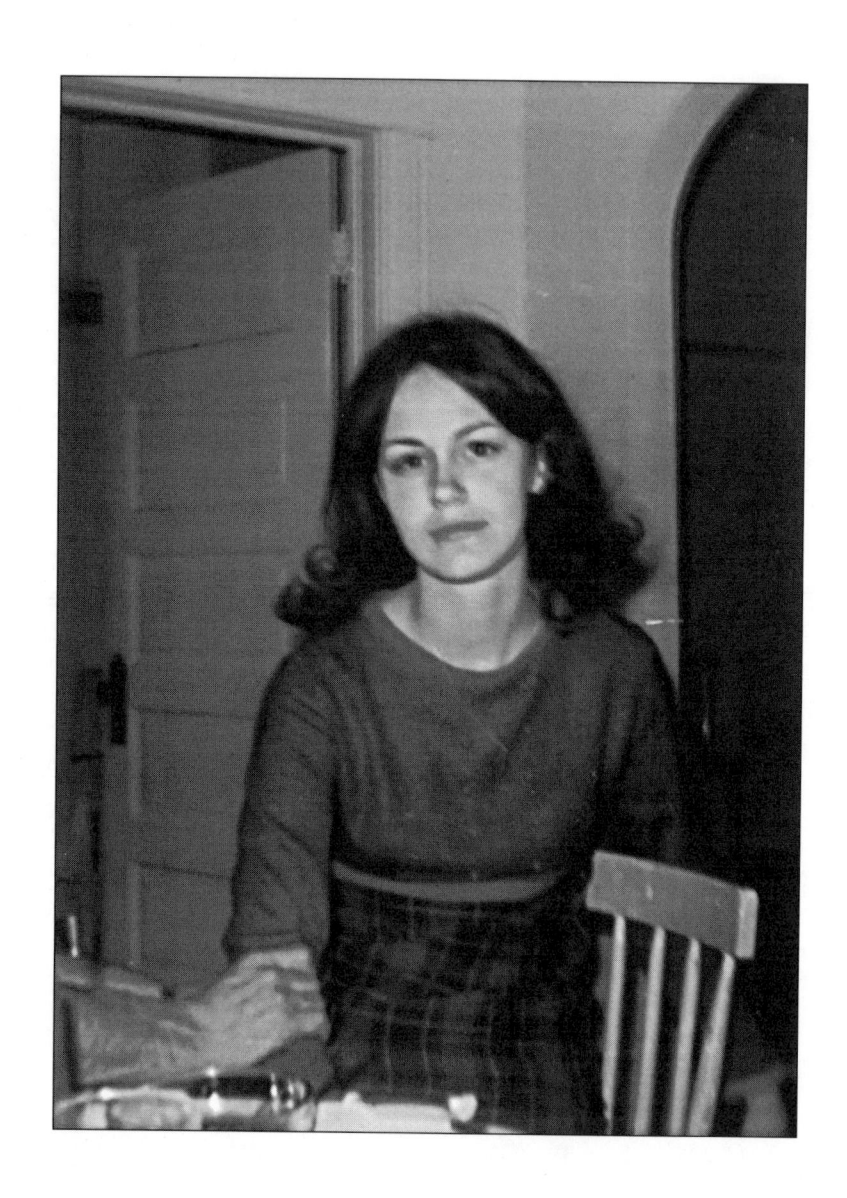

family were conservative, die-hard Republicans. It was unsafe to express my adoration of this youthful Democratic president.

The death of President Kennedy occurred simultaneously with a series of tragedies for me in junior high. My closest friend developed cancer and lost her leg. A dancing, rocking teen in love with the Beatles instantly crippled. My younger sister had a serious accident and almost blinded herself. After the family tragedy and long recuperation, my father's drinking accelerated, as did the family violence.

By the time I arrived in high school, Viet Nam was showing it's ugly teeth. Money, the Catholic Church and male aggressive acts of force polluted everything. As I graduated, older students were starting to come home dead from Viet Nam. I was adamantly against the power trip the U.S. was doing. Political and religious discussion in my father's family were horrendous for me. I was in the minority of a very conservative native Idahoan family. My family had no tolerance for blacks or democrats. My family joked about the stupidity of the above.

Lion Heart was also against the non-declared war. After graduating from high school, those who went to college were exempt from being drafted. So he went to College. Then those who were in college and married were not drafted. As a political maneuver to protect my beloved male friend, I agreed to marry. Just when those who were in college, married and with children were exempt, the lottery number system was enacted. Luckily my mate drew a big number, for he was not willing to have a child, though I wanted one the entire time we were married.

My father had coached me to get aegree in mathematics because it would pretty much guarantee a woman a good job. Of course, I did as my father advised. I did not have the courage to even discuss with my dad the love I had for books, literature, reading and writing. I loved the ability to journey somewhere else with good descriptive writing.

How would one get a job as a writer or even worse yet in area of communication? This was a flaky area where one could not possibly earn a decent living.

It wasn't until my last semester of my senior year that I discovered the world of art. A play course in pottery became a real joy for me. By then I was devastated that I hadn't focused earlier in my college years in that direction. During my senior year of college, in an Abstract Algebra class, it felt like my mind was taken beyond its limits and blown apart by the intensity of this upper division, multi-dimensional math class. My rational, logical intellect was devastated. Man was going to the moon, but my brain felt blasted out to outer space and lost in a strange orbit.

I was so serious, in 3 1/2 years I graduated from college with a Bachelor of Science in Mathematics with a Secondary Education option. I had to get out quick. I needed to prove myself. I had to earn money. So, by the age of twenty, I was back teaching in the same junior high I had attended.

The entire ten years that I was married to my first husband, he practiced women's liberation. Based on the premise on 'an eye for an eye,' he translated the concept to money. We were each responsible for equal contribution to our material life. Also my mate had a great desire to earn monies quickly and retire by the age of thirty. So, with the help of a kind brother-in-law, we began the workaholic mode of gaining money, money, money.

All the while Lion Heart cultivated his peer group that I called the BIFC Boys Club. Meeting often they would pursue meditation, Zen philosophy, and multidimensional living. I would spend hours creating gourmet delights to earn their praise. Seldom would I be invited to participate with their philosophical growth.

Meanwhile my husband continued his extra-curricular female relationships. He could not help it that his persona attracted women. He was quite honest as he shared explicitly his growing intimacies. So, daily I heard about the strength and beauty of the various other women in his life.

Part of me listened closely to hear what it was in the other that so attracted this man, my husband, to them. More often than not he responded to fun-loving, non serious types. Ones who adored him and placed him high on the pedestal. Women who needed guidance and deserved his quality love.

My blood family was blessed with a love of loud humor. My grandfather kept a little book of jokes cut out of *Reader's Digest.* Some of those I actually understood. But my uncles were infamous for prejudice, slurring jokes aimed at blacks, women, and Democrats. I found it difficult to laugh at hurtful stories, so I became the brunt of many jokes at various family reunions. Constantly I was labeled slow, naive, quaint, and serious. I still find it difficult to laugh at someone, race, religion or political party that is being wounded by words and intentions

I tried to remember jokes; I prayed to maintain the punch line long enough to make an impression with my mate. I was an intellectual with that degree in math and science. Humor was connected to hurting others and I knew personal pain too well to perpetuate it. Most of the time I failed and again found my self being ridiculed and laughed at for the wrong reason.

We did not talk about divorce, because we were married in the old school of thought. Married for life. I spent long hours alone down by river trying to put my inner emotional, mental house together. I began to question the worth of even living.

From junior high on we had another couple who mimicked our life patterns. The woman was one of Lion Heart's conquests. She was fun loving and sensual. Quickly the focus changed; I was being asked to change my moral structure and also shift away from monogamy. My mate wanted me to benefit from other sexual love exchanges and not focus so much attention his way.

Under the influence of too much alcohol, smoke and badgering, I allowed myself to swap partners with this other couple. Within minutes of coming together with my only other good man friend, a thick, deep sticky grief rolled through me. I was bad. I saw that my husband and the other wife could not get enough of each other. They did not see or understand my grief—her husband and I shattered together. It was a bad, bad situation.

The next few days were a living death. My moral code was destroyed; I wanted to die. An easy way to end my life became clear to me. I put myself in front of a car and fell off my bicycle. I remember the squealing brakes, the swearing voice, the eyes looking down at me, the pain and I was still alive and still being told I was a stupid woman.

Within weeks my husband recognized how intensely I was broken and arranged for us to take an extended walk into the high country of Idaho. It was on this trek in nature I learned how to meditate. After days of walking and seeing and hearing only the inner dialogue that chattered constantly about how wrong and bad I was, I finally learned how to stop that internal noise. I saw nature and the immense beauty of the green and rich brown earth and rocks around me and the all embracing depth of powdery blue skies. I was discovering peace inside through watching nature.

"SUE" IN HER TWENTIES RETURNING TO THE HIGH COUNTRY

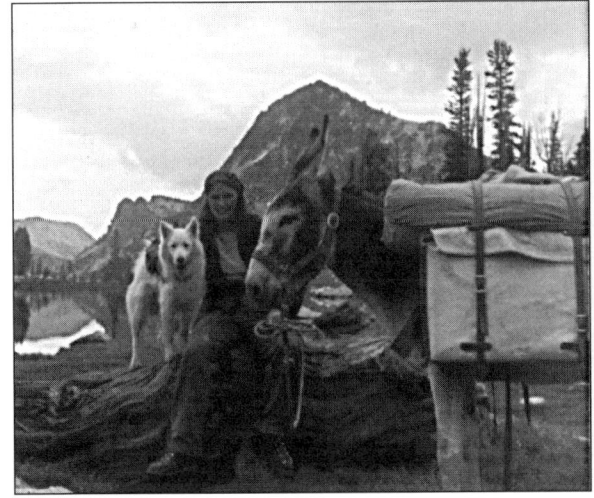

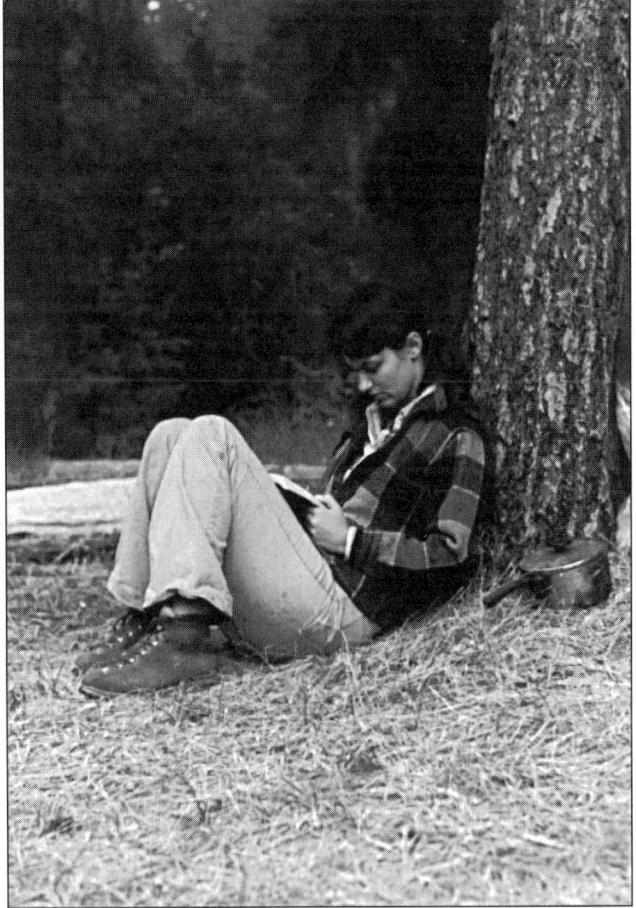

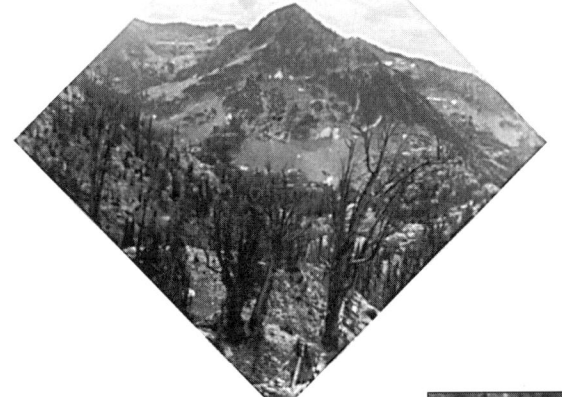

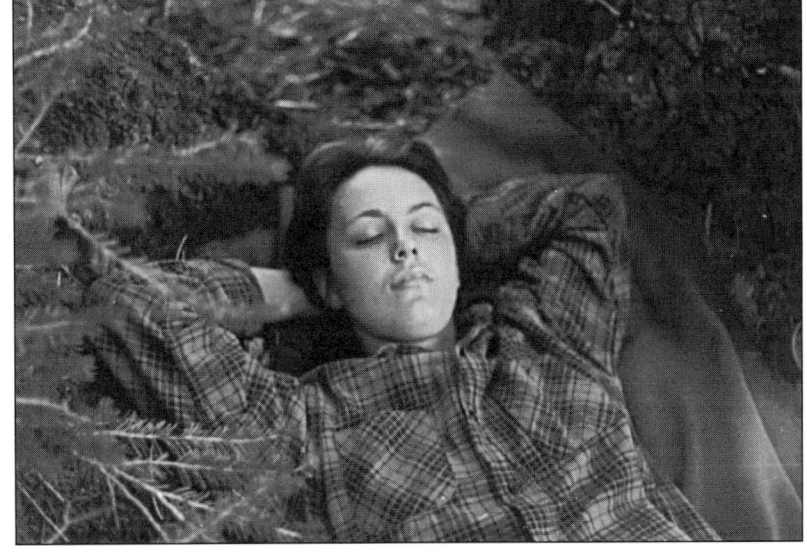

Many years later in the late seventies, I sat reflecting on the patterns of relationships I had lived with others and felt empty and broken. I did not know how to be myself in outside relationships. Until I learned how to love me, it was clear I wouldn't be able to love others.

Through my son, I knew a quality of love I had never experienced with anyone else and that was good. yet, I still held a deep grief and shame for being a single parent unable to meet and walk beside another adult who was male. The last thing I would have ever chosen was to raise a child alone. That was a sin in my moral code. Slowly, I was learning it was better to be a healthy single parent than a broken married parent. This was a very bitter medicine for me to take. I was learning how to witness my own needs that deserved to be met.

I was living in a small, very rustic home with two other men and a very young boy child who was born ancient. I was haunted by how I was undermining the form and values I wanted in a relationship. The veil of confusion over being a monogamous person lifted. I knew practicing 'poly-monogamy ie. love the one you're with' philosophy, did not fit my moral fiber.

The image I had of myself was being stocked on a grocery shelf. Man came along and would chose to sample the product, the nectar of woman; before choosing to commit. Both men said our 'relationship' wasn't the 'soul' mate they were looking for. They knew if our relationship was 'right' they would know it, and they didn't. Therefore, were actively participating in the 'meat market' approach to intimate coupling.

I discovered that engaging in more than one intimate relationship at a time brought in anxiety, judgement, and comparisons that what I shared with one I didn't share with the other. Together the two relationships 'fed' me better than the monogamous union I had held for ten years with my ex. I wanted someone that could walk beside me, proudly, willing to mirror the other. Being in a sexual exchange with more than one man was just a barrier to a true commitment that I felt called to be in. Immediately after my divorce I had vowed to never marry again, but that too did not fit my true yearnings.

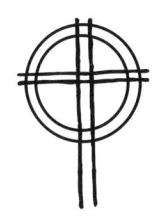

"BE YOURSELF. ESPECIALLY DO NOT FEIGN AFFECTION. NEITHER BE CYNICAL ABOUT LOVE; FOR IN THE FACE OF ALL ARIDITY AND DISENCHANTMENT IT IS AS PERENNIAL AS THE GRASS."

EARTH CELEBRATION - TWO RAVENS AT TALL PINE - 1979

My friends who sponsored the Two Rainbow Community were planning an earth festival for mid-summer high in the mountains of Idaho. Our farm group was asked to help in the process. Since we were on the land and close to crops and having recently formed a food co-op, providing the food for the first festival became our way of helping with the festival. The objective of the festival was to get the finest of artisans who appreciated a healthy relationship with the Earth, out of the city and into a natural sacred cathedral in the heartland of Idaho's mountains. Dance, music, family communions, tai chi, healing arts and Native American natural spirituality were to be shared.

As the time for the festival approached, my friends who owned Miracle Hot Springs asked me to present Idaho to a couple of massage therapist that had moved to the Magic Valley from a successful massage practice in Colorado. I felt one of my prayers for a 'touch' teacher had been answered. They were going to start a class in the fall and I was ready to study other than from books and doing. I immediately invited them to come and participate in our first Earth Celebration.

Some of the finest musicians attended the Two Ravens at Tall Pine Festival. A pianist called Spencer Brewer not only performed on our hand hewed meadow stage, he also taught what he called Sound Therapy. He asserted that the human body was an instrument that could be tuned like body electronics. My studies of chakras and yoga had introduced me to this language. I knew that the seven chakras each had a tone and frequency and color that they resonated with.

He mentioned an association with a fellow musician, Stephen Halpern, and the research that was showing the medicinal value of reducing body stress and tension by letting go and being free through music. He had us go into what we called the cathedral of a tall circle of ancient evergreens and choose a tree and go to it and melt into an embrace with it. Next we were asked to hum or sing to it. Our ears, which were melting into the trunk's bark, were to hear the tree respond back. We were to spend about ten minutes communing with the tree. My eyes grew big with the instructions. No one had ever asked me to do this; yet, early childhood flashes streaked in my memory of listening to trees.

Much to my surprise, as I willingly allowed myself to hear, I did. It was so wonderful. I was hearing a vibration, a frequency through my whole body. I closed my eyes and got lost in the toning. Then Spencer asked us to leave the trees, continue our humming and join back into the circle, singing our sound.

SUZANNE ON THE FARM — 1978

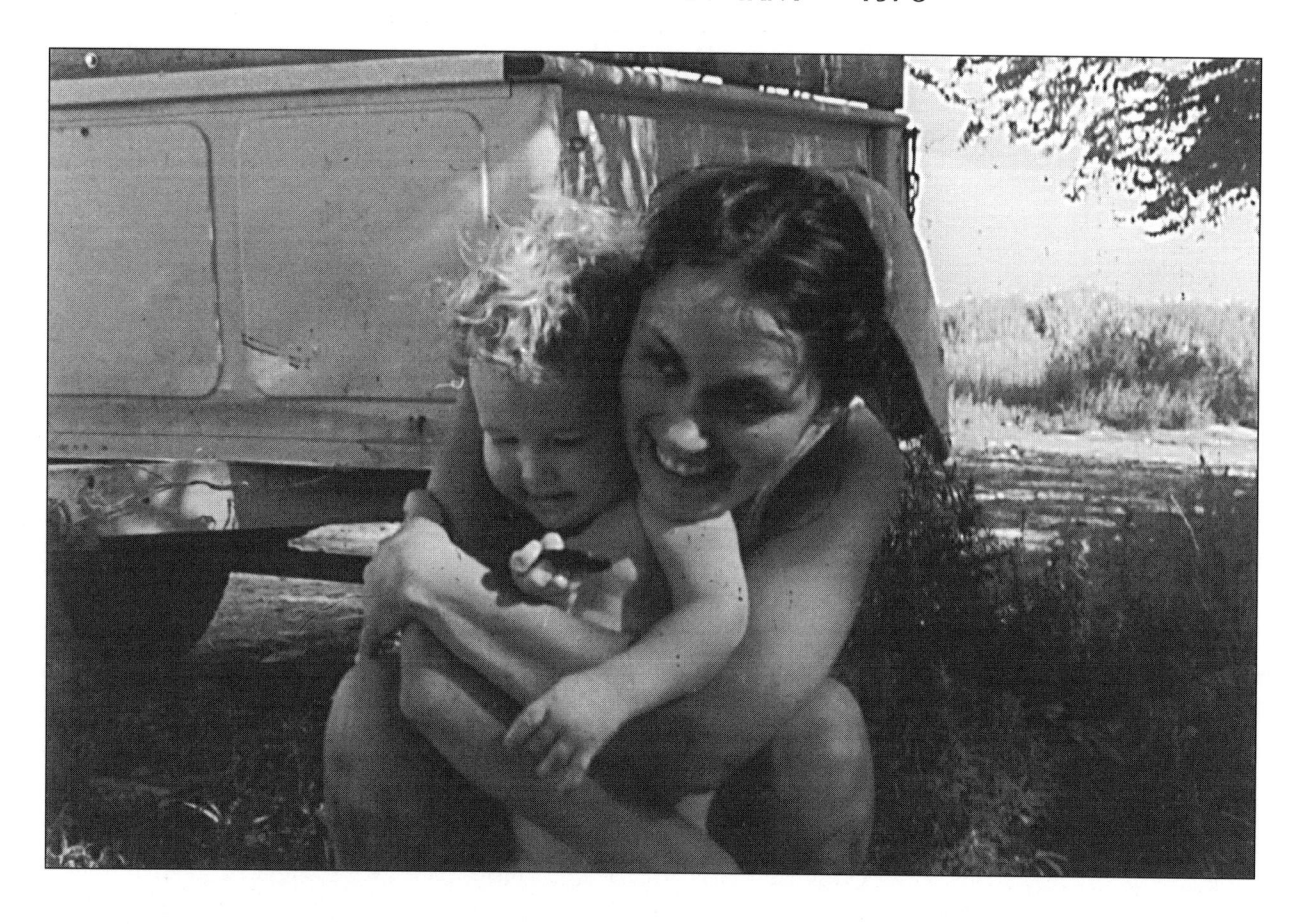

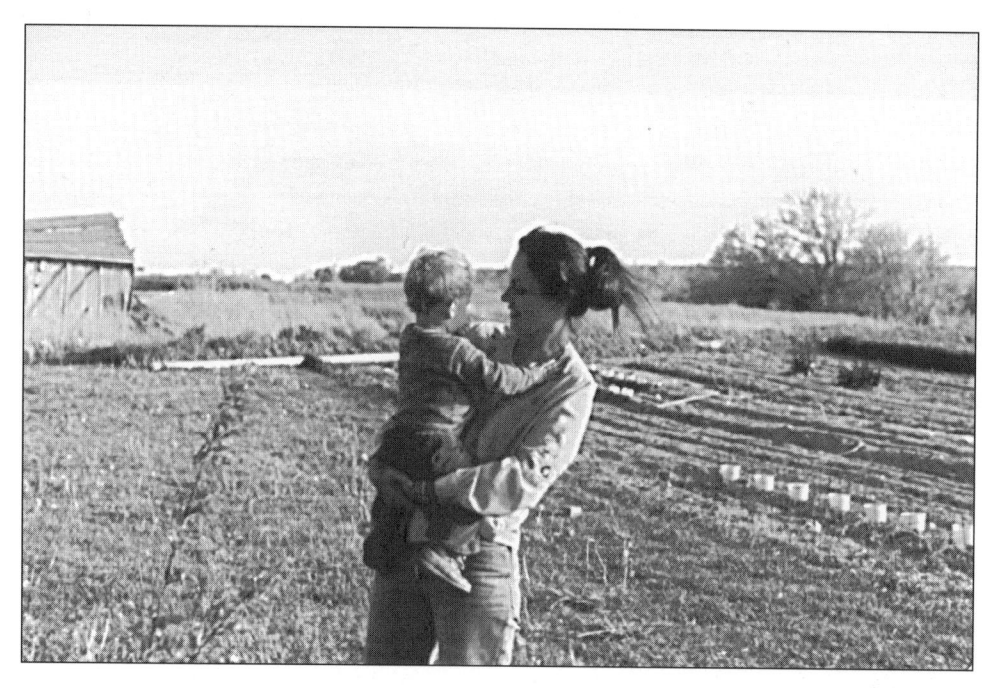

Hesitantly we rejoined, and soon heard the harmonizing our sounding made. It was beautiful and moving. He explained that the earth was truly harmonic. In musician terms he said it was C minor chord. He stepped us through other revealing ways to respond to our senses and integrate nature inside and out. Nature would assist to heal and soundly vibrate.

The setting for the music and dance was on a hand hewn log stage, overlaid with tarp flooring. The artisans from Salt Lake City brought an entire bus filled with sound equipment which required us to have a generator to provide the power. The performance time was as the sun set over tall pines, where hours later a full luminous moon would cast her beams. It was nothing less than magical. The dancers came from all over the world sharing from classical ballet to interpretive dance theater.

My two year old son preferred to hang out with the 'belly dancers'. There was something that fascinated him in watching that circular bare belly rotation. He was not alone. I too was amazed at how they had such a flexible pelvic region. I did not. That was the area of my body I was especially embarrassed of. All the way back to grade school my bulging belly had been criticized. As I look at pictures, I was not fat: I had a collapsed posture that tilted my belly forward. To dance in public was terrorizing for me. I knew that everyone just stared at how bad I looked and moved. I was envious of these relaxed, belly exposed Eastern dancers who seemed to love their dance art form.

We would continue helping with summer festivals for five years, often inviting Native Elders to come and share there values and visions. We were hungry to hear their stories. It had just become legal for them to share some of their earth medicine and natural spirituality.

Some of us were trained survival experts. We trained people to be more conscious in the wilderness. Our intent was to honor all of the Earth's family.
At this festival True Creed shared the seven concepts that he had been given. First he spoke of *honesty* so complete and open within oneself and those others we interexchange with. Next he stated *create your own reality.* Meaning that each person is completely responsible for his or her individual life, thoughts, attitudes and actions. Then he said *recognize a supreme being* by whatever name one chose. He believed it was the recognition of and interaction with this supreme being, the *God* of one's heart, that bonded all existence in harmony. Fourth, he prescribed *prayer* as a medium for one's personal communication with the supreme being. The resulting power from prayer would be a tangible force in one's life. *Meditation* was next, a time of quiet listening, equally as important as prayer. By listening to the prompting within, one could receive insight and clarity of purpose. The next concept he spoke of was *be here now.* The only reality which will ever exist is occurring right now. He asked us to become consciously aware of how we were living every moment. Lastly, he prescribed *positivism*. He asked us to live our life in a positive directed and loving manner, for our world would correspondingly respond.

This was a man that often quoted St. Germain speaking of a violet ray. Holding these festivals was not just for pleasure for True Creed. He was a visionary doing his part to help educate people to love the Earth. He said he was a dog soldier, a medicine society of natives who would lead the way for others to safely travel. Dog soldiers were scouts who often were sacrificed in times gone by. He often would find other dog soldiers; it seemed that the times were calling us to unite. I felt honored on one hand to be recognized and pained on another because the concept wasn't widely understood or acknowledged.

A chosen few participated in a sweat ceremony that True Creed facilitated. I was becoming more accustomed to the language of the *Medicine Wheel*. He elaborated at first through the unique traits for each of the four direction, north, south, east and west. He described the South as the home of innocence and trust; the heat of the Summer's sun that causes good green growth on this sweet Earth. The South's talismans or power animals were the mouse and snake. Both creatures could not see far, but were so close they felt and sensed their life with the Earth. This south direction reflected physical healing and love and communication with all the family of Earth.

The West is the place on the wheel of death and rebirth, a time of introspection and intuition and the fall of the year. The West is a time of harvest in nature and the release of what no longer serves to go back to compost on the Earth. Often the language of waters relate whether it's the rivers of emotions, the ocean and all it's cyclic waves especially as it relates to an individual's journey deep into emotions or the 'caves of darkness' or the 'night space' with it's worlds of dreams. The bear, owl or mountain lion often represent the West, as they either literally go into their caves or come out at dark.

The death and rebirth connected with this direction doesn't mean physical death. It usually reflects a chapter of transition in one's life. An aspect of our dysfunctional/negative life patterns is intended to be released so one can return to the place of original grace and belief that this truly is a good, healthy world to exist with.

Next on the Medicine Wheel as a clock turns, is the North. The North is the time in one's healing cycle when we are most likely to walk alone. Knowledge and wisdom, the key strengths, are illustrated by the symbolism of the buffalo trudging through deep crusty snow, leaving bloodied footprints as it heads for the destination that he instinctually knows he to go to. In human terms, it is the time of prayer, persistence and meditation.

A deep cry for atonement and oneness with the Maker of all things, God, is demanded. External feedback won't be enough a security and individuals must feel and know it within themselves. Often we hear the North as the place of the crone or elder. It is said that a person either learns to 'walk his/her talk or one could literally die. The North is the winter season and statistically a time when many do chose to leave the Earth plane and go over to the other side camp. Sometimes the North is the place of Death, the location of facing one's greatest fears, whether they be physical death of choice or truly being in aliveness.

So when one comes full circle and now faces towards the East, the place of the rising sun and the spring time of the year, we perceive a freshness, a new beginning. illumination and enlightenment speak to the East a time of visioning, valuing and goal setting. Often the Medicine wheel is translated through analogous Earth reflections. The Springtime is when one plants one's seeds of intentions. Native Americans believe in the Greeting of the Sun each day to invoke inspiration and direction as do the East Indians who also exercise and pray daily to the sun. Affirming to begin again in the highest good, the brightest light.

The Eagle and The Red Tail Hawk are often characterized as East medicine talismans for they represent those who can see great distances and with fine clarity. Often people vision quest by journeying to an Eastern facing bluff just as the sun is to rise and sit in quiet praying and sacrificing for divine guidance. Miracles occur with patience and when blinders are removed. Having the eyes that can see and the ears that can hear allows the miraculous to give strength to balance the negativity and distrust that permeates those on the Earth who have forgotten why they have chosen to return to this Earth plane.

The circle is a common symbol to most cultures and religious traditions. It stands for balance, harmony and all-encompassing wholeness. The Medicine Wheel is complex and many layered. The above account is greatly modified by True Creed who impressed that different tribes and cultures depending on their own location on this sweet Earth would associate various concept, symbols and colors, and animals with the different parts of circle. He challenged us to personalize the wheel within our own being before espousing it outward.

The center of the wheel has often been called the spirit channel, or the tree of life, or hub of the wheel. In life we visit many of the directions, or sometimes we hang out in one direction most of our life. The challenge is to have compassion with detachment for all the directions. That is the place of being in the center of the wheel: to look out and know the life experience another is traveling without getting sucked into their script of life. This is about being whole, holy unto one's self, in good relation with the maker of all things.

Saturday night, the long awaited piano concert was to occur. We sat close to the stage excited by what was going to happen when my son, overtired and needing attention turned into the whiny, demanding two-year old I knew too well. I ended up leaving just as the piano performance was to begin, anger fuming through me that this child was keeping me away from the only fun or desired thing I had allowed myself to anticipate this festival weekend

By the time I walked up the hill carrying my crying child I knew he needed some prime time with his mother. Sitting up at our camp, I began massaging his head and neck. I found myself holding the top of his spine and rotating his head clockwise and then counterclockwise. It felt like I was unwinding him. He couldn't stay uptight. I was learning the beginnings of what I now call craniology.

From the long strenuous birthing process with my son, I gained a sense of what his brain and it's cranial bones went through in order to be born. It had to have hurt badly. It took me three months after the birth to be willing to even think about this event.

It was a horribly painful process. The placenta previa was like a rubbery plug that prevented my son's head from sliding down and out. His poor head had been stuck for that way for too many unnecessary hours. Instinctually, I gently worked the suture connections between the bones this sunset evening high in Idaho's mountains.
Because of my own illness within my brain, I was keenly aware of the two hemispheres, the left relating to the masculine, orderly father influences aspects and the right relating to the feminine, sensing, instinctual creative, artistic parts of a person's mental process. If, through injury, birth process or mental stress patterns, circulation is limited to parts of the brain the body can not correct and maintain a healthy system.

I knew that the anger I experienced during my pregnancy reflected the energetic level of my son. I knew high strain and so did he, even before he was born. My son's intensity ran people off. Did mine?

He was a live wire demanding much continual attention. When I touched his neck and skull my own brain, especially behind my left eye, just at the base of my skull throbbed with his. Often inside my brain it felt as if something would swell and the resultant externally felt pressure would almost blind me. Meditation was a constant tool in mending my irregular sized pituitary gland.

1979 TWO RAVENS AT TALL PINE FESTIVAL

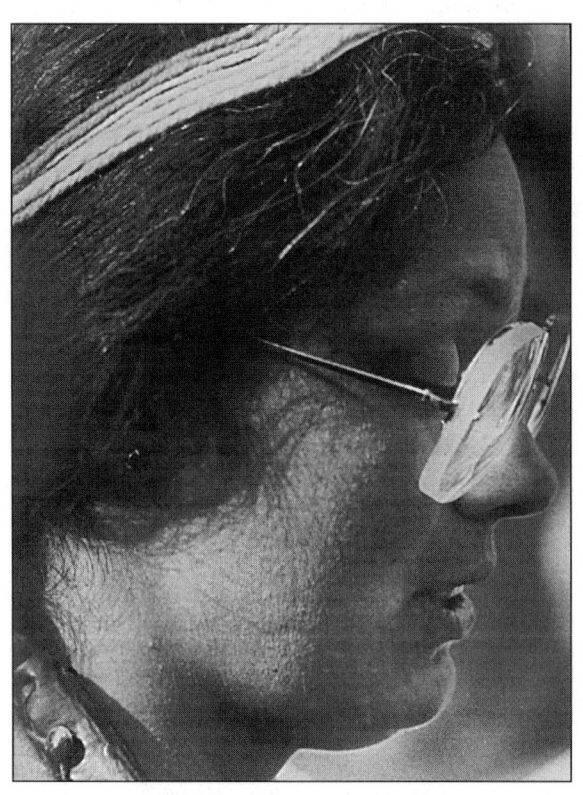

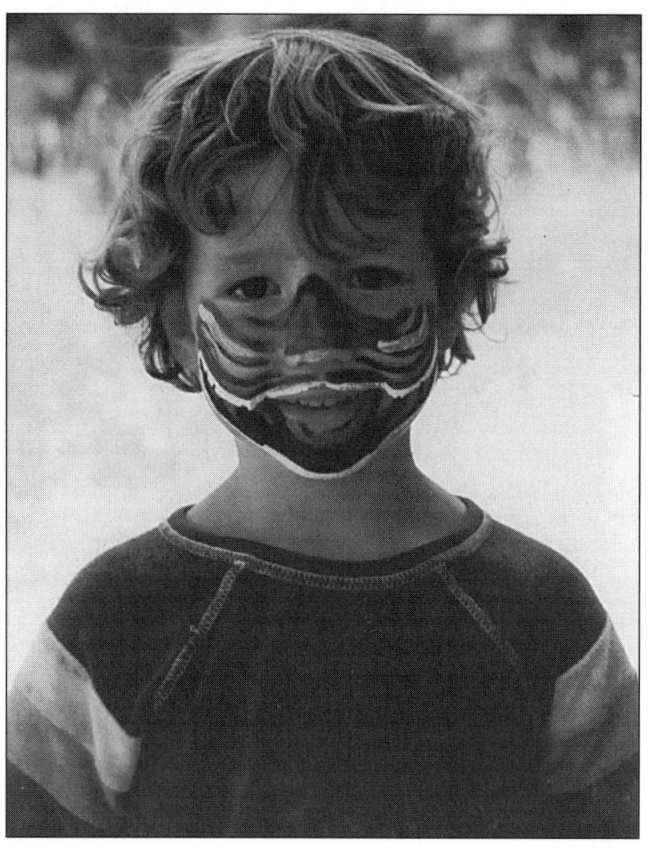

1979 TWO RAVENS AT TALL PINE FESTIVAL

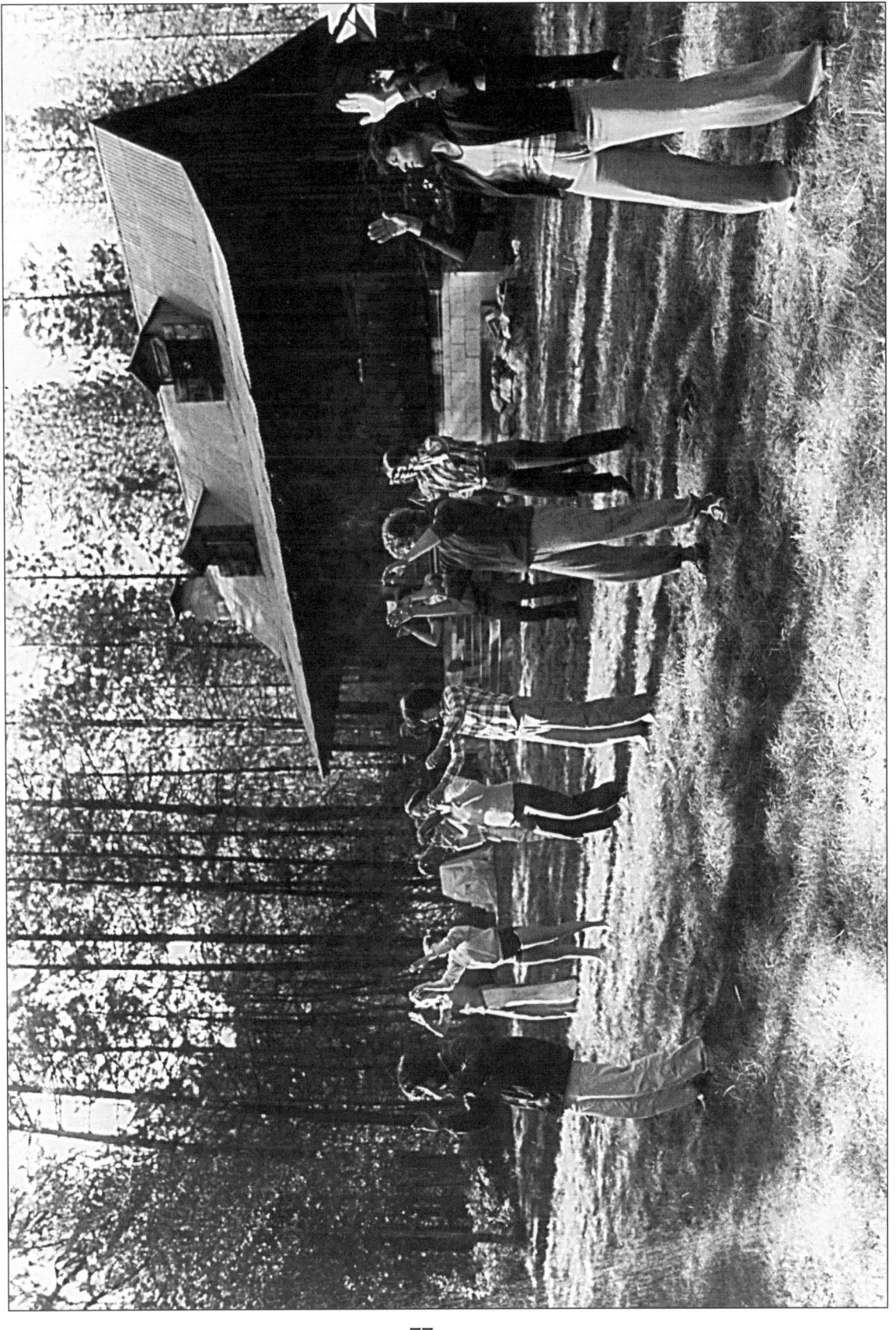

Daily I would push and press on my own skull with great passion to help relieve the pressures. Some days it was so intense that by mid-day I would be flat on my bed no longer able to hold my head up. I consumed aspirin daily. I'd go through bottles when my head pain was relentless. My skull would bulge and I knew my pituitary was still growing.

No one had formally instructed me on the brain finger techniques; I knew it instinctively. Now, I know about the Oriental Shiatsu approach to all the body's bones, nerves, organs, muscles, posture and emotional balance that are connected to points on the head. Later, the course in *TOUCH FOR HEALTH* would further explain the neuro-lymphatic release points. But for this time in 1979 I trusted instinct.

By the time the last Sunday morning meal was prepared and shared I was wiped out. I lay on the hillside aching. True Creed beside me, questioned what fun had I really had this weekend. I had worked way too hard and my son was a suffering ragamuffin.

I came home from this earth festival exhausted, I had overdone it, again. My head, heart and body ached. I was disillusioned because I was doing something good for the Earth and her Peoples and I still did not feel well.

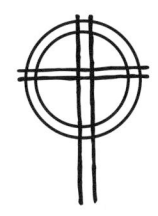

*"YOU ARE A CHILD OF THE UNIVERSE,
NO LESS THAN THE TREES & THE STARS;
YOU HAVE A RIGHT TO BE HERE."*

BOOK MAGIC—1979

As others on the farm were dedicating themselves to be either a politician or jewelry makers, three of us set forth to bring a wholistic family bookstore to our valley. Our farm group spent over a year applying and going through the multitudes of steps to qualify for an Small Business Administration loan to open a bookstore in our rambling country neighborhood. First timers at owning a business taught us how to do the research to validate the potential of a book store in this farming community.

We had lofty goals to bring books to this community to assist in expanding one's self education, no matter what the field of interest be. Within the first year of operation, two other bookstores opened in our town. One was run by several rich doctor's wives and the other was a B. Dalton chain store. We discovered that the timing was truly right to open, but not with so much immediate competition.

We bought enough books the first year to supply the community; however, we shared the season's earnings with the other two stores. Our finances were challenged immediately. It wasn't like we jumped into the business unprepared. One owner had experience in managing a bookstore, but we felt confident and competent. Going through the S.B.A. system required many steps and surveys to assure the soundness of our business adventure.

Another partner became the store manager as I was teaching at a junior high the book store's first year. Going to the store and working only part time was truly delightful. I called the bookstore my office. It was a place I could practice the growth of my spirit and the mandates to maintain peace and health in my self. My number one objective was to greet each person who walked through the door and assist them to find that gem of a book that would meet their unique special inquiry. I was practicing unconditional love with everyone I met. I did not judge their requests or appearance, but was abe to be neutral and helpful. We were proud that our store was a family store. There were no books on our shelves that were of poor content or racist.

One of the first books at our new store that 'jumped off the shelf' for me was Dr. Brugh Joy's book, *JOY'S WAY: A Map for the Transformational Journey. An Introduction to the Potentials for Healing with Body Energies.* It is a biographical story of one cancer ridden physician's path to rediscovering health. He wrote an outline for human transformation. This special book told of his journey from skepticism to receiving special universal knowledge. At this time in my health cycle I was again in chronic pain. The point where this neurosurgeon/author turned away from death and back into life

1979 BOOK MAGIC OPENING

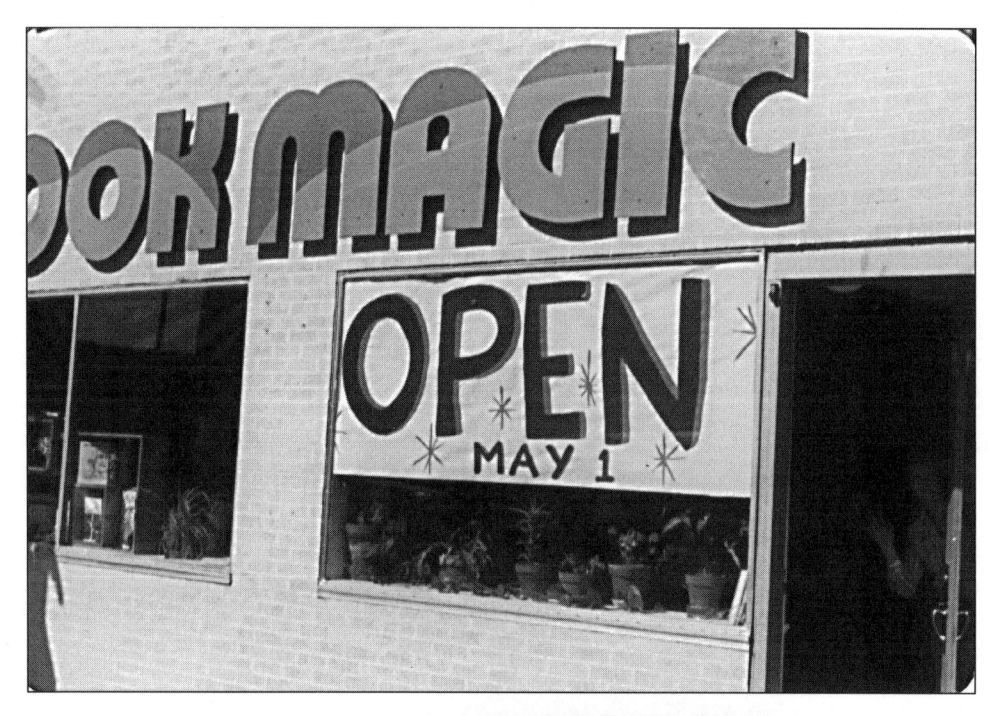

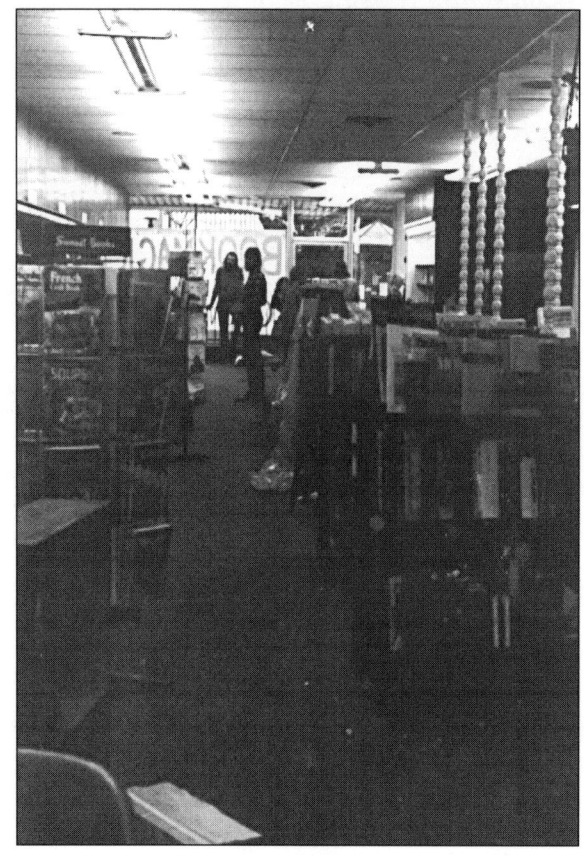

was when he embraced various alternative health practices including concepts that spoke of energy fields.

Dr. Joy in the book stated "If a disease is on a terminating or downhill course, a Transformation Process is manifesting. The obvious transformation toward which that person is heading is physical death, but these may also be a transformation on this side, in the living. If that transformation is chosen and if it is to be effective, the change in the patient's attitudes and life patterning must be as complete as would transpire through death. Halfway won't do it; there is no room for compromise. Marshalling the courage and clarity to make the necessary changes is the real challenge."

"The vast area of our Beingness does not know what death or disease is. When change is called for, often by a disease process or some other serious disruption in one's life, we have a choice. We can take direct action to harmonize our Beingness, or we can block ourselves from that direct action and let our outer minds pretend that we don't understand. Our disease or our psychological knot is doing for us what we couldn't or wouldn't do directly and with awareness."

"When our outer mind cannot or will not manifest the essence of our desire, the unconscious mechanism does it for us. Without our understanding it or willing it, the unconscious mechanism finds a pathway out of the mode from which the psyche desires release. The path it finds may not be to the liking of the outer mind, such as death to the cancer or pancreatitis patient; but it is nevertheless, like death, an effective way out. If the action of the mind obstructs the soul from fulfilling its fundamental life commitments, then mental diseases, emotional disorders and diseases of the body ensue. On the other hand, transformation brings about resolution. One way or the other, through cure or through death, transformation resolves the symptoms and the disease."

"The principles involved in unblocking the soul's flow can be applied universally. In this widespread sense they are the basis of a psycho-physical-spiritual therapeutic interaction called Transformational Psychology. The word psychology, literally interpreted, is the study of the soul, even though current usage restricts it almost entirely to the outer mind. Transformation Psychology is nothing less than the study of the transformation of the soul, the freeing of the soul into its' natural expression. The fundamental focus in the treatment of the human being is the mind that has somehow walked into a closet, closed the door, turned out the light and instantly forgotten all these events."

"Most conventional therapeutic approaches to the mind now recognize the mind-body relationship, but hardly any of them accept experientially the body-mindsoul integrity. A mind cut off from the very source of its essence, the soul, is like a body cut off from its brain. Clearly, the soul that animates the mind is analogous to the mind that animates the body. When all three are in conjunction, the Transformational Process of the human being is greatly accelerated."

"From the metaphysical perspective, a person's body is essentially "perfect" for that individual in any particular lifetime. There may be "built-in" restrictions that act to limit a particular person's physical or mental actions, but no matter how the outer mind conceives of them, these restrictions are always for the betterment of the individual. Once the individual accepts the limitation, and turns to the development of other resources, and the limitation has served its purpose and is no longer necessary in this or later lifetimes. The individual is enriched through the limitation. In any individual the soul is always the most advanced aspect, at a developmental stage, far beyond the awareness of the outer mind or body."

"It is the mind, not the body, that blocks spiritual awareness. The body and the spirit need no education. It is the outer mind, in relationship to the soul, that is undergoing the training and the experience in this dimension. The mind, which is out to be the liaison between the physical and the spiritual, is the only aspect of the human being that has to be integrated. Of the three, the mind is the only portion that can be confused."

"The soul is an individualization out of spirit."

"Transformational Psychology is a tool to integrate the three parts of the triad. One recognizes the client's mind, with its memory bank of experiences both in this lifetime and in many prior lifetimes, is what makes all the mistakes. Transformation Psychology places direct responsibility for physical and psychological disease directly on the patient, specifically upon the patient's mind. The true reality of the soul-andbody relationship, from which the mind is only a bi-product, is literally mind-boggling: it is simply incomprehensible and intolerable to the intellect. Until the mind can accept this status and reposition itself to become the soul's witness on the physical plane, pain and suffering remain."

"Once the mind accepts that the soul's consciousness and awareness transcend the consciousness and awareness of the mind itself, there is freedom. One no longer needs to remain within the confines of the outer mind."

"Transformational Psychology observes three stages in any Transformation Process. First is the awakening to the realization that most of the experiences of life perceived as external to oneself are actually projections of the self. The second stage emphasizes the "owning" of these projections—pulling them back into the individual's mind and integrating them with the concept of self. This stage is the critical one. In it one must learn that the dynamics of any problem are clearly under one's own power and control and therefore changeable or, in terms of Transformation Psychology, transmutable. This second stage is completed when what is really "out there" can be perceived without distortion. Knowing the separation between what is experienced as external and what is experienced as internal are one. There is no external or internal reality to distinguish."

"The Tibetan Buddhist approach to the resolution of problems delineates three pathways. The highest and most difficult is to transmute the problem—that is, to generate an intensity of energy from a higher, more expanded awareness and to use this energy to force a change in the configuration of the problem's less expanded, less intense energy and thus to free the energy that influences the problem. Transmutation implies a change in the form or nature of anything into another form of nature. In this plane, all energy flows from more energetic sources to less energetic manifestations, never in the opposite direction. Therefore, high aspects of consciousness always transmute lower aspects of consciousness."

"The second Tibetan Buddhist pathway is to ennoble the problem, to treat it as a necessary and important steppingstone of experience in one's unfolding. In the West, this process is called rationalization, and it has a negative connotation rather than the positive insight that it has from the Buddhist viewpoint."

"The third Tibetan Buddhist pathway is to go directly into the problem and allow it to manifest completely. There is but one injunction; one must make a portion of one's awareness into a witness that observes the problem. In this way, understanding may come. This last method is considered to be the path of subtle wisdom, and for many people it is a more appropriate pathway than that of direct transmutation..."

"Vitvan, a Western mystic, taught that there were two ways of dealing with problems. One was to transmute the problem, and the second was to wear it out Sometimes it seems that most of us are stuck with the latter method..."

"The Transformational therapist is in a process of working through the filters of his or her own mind. The therapist clearly sees the outer mind of the client, and also enters telepathically into a rapport with the client's soul, thus gaining insight into the particular dynamics that soul is expressing. The Transformational therapist is in contact with the flow not only of his her own soul, but of the patient's soul as well. This particular development of the therapist comes through the meditative process, through working with a teacher or through both."

"The Transformational therapist has developed the ability to heighten his or her own consciousness at will. The heart-chakra center, and usually the throat center, the forehead center and the crown center are functioning in a more refined state than in ordinary states of awareness. The therapist's level of consciousness, as reflected through his or her body fields, induces a similar level of consciousness in the client's energy field, and the client's consciousness shifts concomitantly to form an appropriate fit to the new energy field. Induction is the process by which a body having electric or magnetic properties produces magnetism, an electric charge or an electromotive force in a neighboring body, without contact... Energy-field induction through the heart chakra, manifesting a state of Unconditional Love, lifts the client up, out of the level the outer mind is configuring as the problem, into a state of clarity. (Dr. Brugh Joy. *JOY'S WAY,* pgs.210-217)

Dr. Joy wrote of methods in the book called the spiral meditation or energy field scan of ones own inside. "Meditation is a tool of the consciousness, not an end in itself. Do the kind of meditation that intuitively feels right to do, whether it is a formal posturing or a quiet nature walk. As has been documented time and time again, cosmic awareness happens whether you meditate or not. You don't make it happen; it happens to you. All you really have to do is get out of the way and stop blocking your own unfolding... Meditating while lying in bed in the morning is generally (but not always) ineffective. For most people, the horizontal position is too strongly associated with sleep and the hypnagogic borderline of sleep, which are not meditative states. Some research studies seem to indicate that the sitting position—whether crosslegged, in the East Indian lotus position or even in a chair—increases the alertness of consciousness for meditation." (*JOY'S WAY,* pg. 285)

If the mind persists in chattering away, interfering with meditation, he recommended creating for the chatterer inside a huge auditorium filled with people. Then just tell the chatterer to talk to all those people and to keep them entertained while you go ahead with your meditation. All the chatterer wants is an option to not have to listen; thus, the problem can often be overcome.

"Ghandhi is supposed to have said that five minutes in meditation, contemplating Unconditional Love, would do more for the world than filling starving people's rice bowls."

"Love sent to another soul surrounds that soul awaiting the time when the outer mind of that individual opens the door. No one can open the door for another. ...In general, there are two broad, mutually exclusive approaches to meditation. In the first, one excludes or blocks out from the awareness any outer sound or activity. One simply tunes out everything. This technique requires a quiet space. The second approach is inclusive, and utilizes all sound and action to heighten the meditative state. It is used in the practice of Zen meditation..."

"You are going to perform a series of ten controlled breaths. Seated in a chair or on the floor in any of the ways described, with your shoes off and your eyes closed, begin to inhale slowly through your nose. When your lungs are fully expanded, hold your breath without tension while you slowly count to seven, and then slowly exhale through your mouth, with your tongue touching the front of the roof of the mouth so that you make a slight hissing noise. Exhale slowly and completely, and then start the cycle over again. Repeat it for a total of ten time. This technique is a wonderful way to attune and prepare the awareness for any meditation."

"Breath control can be a meditation in itself if it is carried out for a period of time... After the cycle of ten breaths, one might, for example, begin the contemplation of Unconditional Love, or one might practice a visualization techniques or one could just 'let go and let God'—not focusing or doing anything but sitting quietly, sensing after well-beingness—or one could shift into the spiral meditation." (*JOY'S WAY*, pgs. 186-189)

"Part of the meditative experience is the development of the 'witness state', and Unconditional Love is one pathway to it. In the witness state, an impersonal observer can be found within one's awareness. It simply observes, without reaction to whatever passes before the awareness. It usually cannot be achieved, or further developed, without Unconditional Love... which is totally unemotional and impersonal..."

The spiral meditation came to Dr. Joy " one morning in Findhorn as he was conversing with his Inner Teacher on the subject of chakras. During the meditation, he received an image of a naked man standing with his arms extended out from his sides. From the area of his heart chakra, a pattern of energy began to form. It flowed to the man's left and down in a spiral pattern to his solar-plexus chakra, continued to the right and up to the mid-chest chakra, then left and down to the splenic chakra, right and down to the lower-abdomen chakra, right and up to the throat chakra, and so on in the spiral to the root chakra, the forehead on up to the crown chakra and around on to the left hand, left knee, then right knee, right elbow, on up to the crown chakra and around on to the left hand, left foot, then right foot, right hand, and finally flowed to an area about eighteen inches above the head, the transpersonal point."

The vision was beautiful; all the major and important chakras were connected in a single spiral pattern. The Inner Teacher told me that I was to work with my own chakra system in this same sequence at the beginning of my meditations, and at the end, to reverse the flow and pattern of the spiral, working from the transpersonal point back to the heart.

Joy's spiral meditation directly contradicts classical literature of metaphysics the Egyptians, Japanese, Tibetans and Sufi's all teach that the center of the body is in the abdomen, near or just below the umbilicus. Dr. Brugh Joy contended that "we are preparing for a transformation of consciousness that supersedes the past, moving from the more power-controlled areas, the areas of mastery of the material plane, into a blend with the higher awareness that is associated with the upper chakras. The root chakra, the sexual chakra and the solar-plexus—splenic chakras comprise the lower triangle; it is associated primarily with the physical and emotional planes."

"The heart, throat, forehead and crown chakras are associated with the developing spiritual awareness in humanity. The heart chakra, the fourth level, sits midway between then lower triangle and the main upper chakras. This shift of the center upward will imbue humanity with a sense of relationship, the deeper aspects of which rest on spiritual values rather than on power and control over others... the shift to the heart is a beginning reflection of this actuality, a shift to a relationship between the body and the spirit."

"In a natural pattern, the chakras are awakening in ascending pairs. The second (sexual) chakra is transformed to the fifth (throat), reflecting the transformation from physical procreative activity to such aesthetic creativity as art, literature and music. The second transformation is from the third chakra (solar plexus) to the fourth (heart), reflecting the change from emphasis on power and the emotional aspects of awareness to the more collective and unconditioned states of awareness, imbued with Love. Finally, the first chakra (root) is activated, its energies ascending to the seventh (crown). There are effects on the head centers with the first two transformations, but the third, the root to the crown, represents the unbelievable energy variously called the Fire, the Serpent Fire, the Kundalini energy, the Fire of Transformation. When it is fully activated and begins to ascend through the energy pathways, connecting each of the successive chakras, the process is called the rising of the Kundalini. It sweeps the individual into cosmic states of awareness."

"The Kundalini energy can also be awakened through a willed action. This uncontrolled awakening, in someone who has not prepared the higher chakras for such an intensity of energy, can be devastating, causing not only great physical pain but psychological pain as well." (*JOY'S WAY,* pgs. 195-6)

With my illness centering in my brain, and all this input from the Eastern perspective of a neutral mind, the meditative state, I was aware of not being in it enough. My mind had many voices that chattered and scolded and judged me.

Dr. Joy shared the perceiving of auras and what the color fields meant. Being raised in the sixties with Western, scientific-rational tradition, the view of "What science cannot tell us mankind cannot know." dominated most of our `objective' view of life. Yet all the religious teaching showed Jesus Christ and other spiritual teachers with a halo of golden light. With great intrigue I observed babies and young children gazing at people's outer periphery with delight. Auras to me were like the halos artist always drew and children knew. The energetic field of color a person, mountain, tree, actually anything radiates, exists as auras.

Dr. Joy addressed delving into one's dream space. He shared C. G. Jung's view that "dreams are objective facts. They do not answer our expectations and we have not invented them...We dream our questions, our difficulties. When we reach an impasse where there seems no way out, we should seek the facts provided by dreams....Our dreams are most peculiarly independent of our consciousness and exceedingly valuable because they cannot cheat." He went so far to insinuate that dreams are the "divine at work in the human soul bringing revelations of the underlying meaning of life and, therefore, of God." Initially one's dreams may seem like an illogical jumble of people, places and things. But they are really a hidden intelligence that you can use to resolve emotionally-charged problems. Simply put, we dream that which we cannot work out in day time world.

I had a recurring dream that terrorized me since I was a young girl. Never had I spoken a word of its contents to anyone. It was sexually oriented and my mind knew it to be bad. So now I had this significant doctor say watch you dreams. They are a teacher for that which one cannot work out in the conscious world. I had a horrifying night dream and in the daytime during deep meditations I would see inwardly this

'Garden of Eden'. A beautiful sharply colored, bushy green place where the people were not only physically beautiful but golden and glowing with peace and happiness. I preferred my daydream over my night dream.

Most importantly he shared in his book a theme . . .

"Delete the need to understand,
 Delete the need to compare, and
 Delete the need to judge."

To this day when my intellect gets challenged, I will repeat the above as if it is a mantra. It was turning the responsibility for well being over to a higher power other than my own mental mind. The key term above is 'need'. I began to sense that there is a part of me that did know and whatever part of me that dominated with disbelief, pain and anger deserved to back off.

So deeply did I feel his message, that I vowed to go study with this fore-runner of alternative self health. Joy clearly stated that the higher—or expanded or natural- states of consciousness were merely the attuning of our central nervous system to perceptive states that have always existed in us but have been blocked by our outer mental conditioning and by our dwelling on our physical emotional and sexual aspects." (*JOY'S WAY,* pg. 49) At the same time my dietary sensitivity remained acute and my mental/emotional self was burdened with confusing thoughts. There was some correlation between the pain behind my left eye and the peacefulness of my belly.

Somehow my pursuit for healthy foods attracted a bank official to me who had reserved funds from a defunct non-profit food co-op. Before I knew it I was actively negotiating for a peoples' natural food cooperative to open upstairs in our bookstore. It was a good outlet for our own organic farm crops and an excellent way to assure fresh, organic (non-poisoned) food.

I was acutely aware that our physical location downstream from Idaho Nuclear Energy Laboratory was also attributing to not only my health but the whole community's. My grandparents had raised us with horror stories of the nuclear testing in Nevada. The plumes or mushroom shaped clouds would appear and numbers of sheep and other animals would die and become diseased. It was plain ignorance not to know that we the two legged weren't also absorbing some of the fallout.

With the food cooperative upstairs, we began a series of discussion on various social and health concerns. One of our farm members, also a native Idahoan, chose to run for political office to assist getting relevant health and Earth issues discussed.

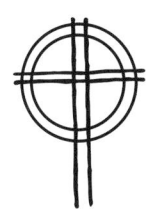

*"BE YOURSELF. ESPECIALLY DO NOT FEIGN AFFECTION.
NEITHER BE CYNICAL ABOUT LOVE; FOR IN THE FACE OF ALL ARIDITY &
DISENCHANTMENT IT IS PERENNIAL AS THE GRASS"*

SELF AND SELF WITH OTHERS - 1980

Our little town was a steppingstone for travelers to get to Sun Valley, an internationally known ski resort. Often lecturers and teachers would present workshops to off set their travel to this high mountain playground.

Michael Murphy, from Esalen Institute, Big Sur, California, came and offered a three day workshop called Self And Self With Others. It sounded like something I knew nothing about but instinctively I felt drawn to participate.

A dozen of us met with him. His form for teaching was through questioning and didactic answering (finding a partner, repeating the suggested question and listening without giving feedback.)

He spoke of how our attitudes bring forth actions that end up creating results. Specifically, if one was hoping for something, they were allowing actions to occur and the result would be disappointment. If one set their intentions, then the person chose what was going to occur and therefore would end up satisfied.

This action diagram helped us to see where we were responsible for our own life and we could not blame our actions on others. Immediately we were asked to list "How we were not doing our life 100%. Then we were asked how one goes about expressing lack of self commitment?" Then he asked, "How do I not forgive myself and what did I make myself wrong for having done?" Getting in touch with these last two question, he reinforced, was essential in order to be able to shift into forgiving oneself for the actions that create karma.

Karma is an East Indian concept that parallels for me the thought in the Bible, "an eye for eye" except that the time line for balancing actions could refer to lifetimes. For an example if one goes out of their way to lie to gain financial increase, the karma or balance would be some period of being lied to and financial loss. The objective is to live a kind, thoughtful, integrity filled existence where one does not deliberate harm to another, including the earth. "If you forgive yourself, it can't come back and get you. You will become immune." he reiterated.

At first the questions all seemed to be the same. Over and over I shared how guilty I felt for being a poor, single parent, a divorced mother. The failure of not being in a healthy male relationship became glaringly obvious with my communing. Michael Murphy contended " that one's heart cannot be hurt if you have experienced that place of living one's life 100% full."

Since we were there to work on our own personal relations and the one's we had with others, Michael shared the three ways most people relate. The first is being "stuck and resisting;" the second, "at the effect of and running away;" (basically, reacting) and the third, centered. We went about listing situations, relationships that fell into the three above categories. We were learning about experiential states of being, or, "modalities of being." He went on to ask, "why be in a relationship with a being who is not willing to work to the degree that you want to be."

The last morning he asked us to list five things that we saw were wrong in our life. Boy that was easy for me; not accepting that I was a sexual, passionate female, not forgiving my father, being a single parent, being distant from all my blood relatives and lastly not being able to commit myself to a deep relationship.

Quickly after we listed our wrongs he pounced on what he called "the wrong cycle." Wrong—guilt—past sentence—continuation of wrong act. Immediately he had us "forgive ourselves for the judgement that we placed on ourselves." He felt that one became a sitting duck for someone else to come up and say you are wrong if we did not accept ourself. He pleaded with us to release the level of personal torture we put ourselves through. He elaborated. "Events don't need forgiving, the judgement does. Karma is an action he felt that was neither good nor bad."

For homework we were to meditate, "I am fully forgiven." He stated "If you forgive yourself for judgement there will be no energy left in your aura to be condemned with." Since so often in relationships we end up mirroring our partner, we started there with a questioning process. "How does this relationship express my commitment to self," and "How does this relationship express one's lack of self commitment."

We went on with questioning what needs to change in a specific relationship in order for it to work, and then, specifically, what each one personally could change to help the relationship. A lack of commitment to self and negative thought patterns created the greatest detriment to self development.

The last few didactic exercises were the hardest. Oh dear me, I thought as he asked us to share "Tell me how I can love you and then tell me how you can love me." Tough questions. The inability to tell people how you want to be loved leaves you deficient. We must communicate a clear picture of what we want and deserve. When we have a commitment to self and the way we want to be loved, it can become common, a happening.

The inner picture I knew was yearning to know 'heaven on Earth'. This was a place I knew only in fairy tales or inner dreaming. Another part yelled at me that God made man and women in order to learn how to walk side-by-side with each other. I knew I was not living this. In fact, most of my focus was on children. I felt they were safe and a joy to be around. My inside record on how to be 'high' or 'evolved' stated 'Least ye become as children, ye will not enter the kingdom of heaven.' I knew that Children loved easier and were more forgiving. I did not know how to live that way with other adults. After the workshop I looked at all my relationships with more scrutiny than before the Self And Self With Others workshop.

I was haunted by how I was continually undermining the form and values I wanted in a relationship. By this time I knew I was definitely monogamous. Being in an intimate relationship with more than one man was just a barrier to the true commitment I wanted. Joseph Campbell espoused that "we all need for life to signify, to touch the eternal, to understand the mysterious, to find out who we are." To know that experience, he would say read myths. Myths teach us that we can turn inward, and we begin to get the message of the symbols. The myth around marriage can tell us what it is. It's the reunion of the separated dyad. Originally you were one. You are now two in the world, but the recognition of the spiritual identity is what marriage is. It's different from a love affair. It has nothing to with that. It's another mythological plane of experience. When people get married because they think it's a long time love affair, they'll be divorced very soon, because most love affairs end in disappointment.

"Marriage is recognition of a spiritual identity. If we live a proper life, if our minds are on the right qualities in regarding the person of the opposite sex, we will find our proper male or female counterpart. If we are distracted by certain sensuous interests, we'll marry the wrong person. By marrying the right person, we reconstruct the image of the incarnate God, and that's what marriage is."

"Your heart tells you who the right person is," he said. "Marriage is the reunion of the self with the self, with the male or female grounding of ourselves. The marriage means the two that are one, the two become one flesh. If the marriage lasts long enough and if your are acquiescing constantly to it instead of to individual personal whims, you come to realize that is true—the two really are one. One not only biologically, but spiritually. The biological is the distraction which may lead to the wrong identification. Marriage is a relationship. When you make the sacrifice in marriage, you're sacrificing not to each other but to unity in a relationship."

The Chinese image of the Tao, with the dark and light interacting—that's the relationship of yang and yin, male and female, which is what a marriage is. You're no longer this one alone; your identify is in a relationship. Marriage is not a simple love affair, it's an ordeal, and the ordeal is the sacrifice of ego to a relationship in which two have become one. There are two completely different stages of marriage. First is the youthful marriage following the wonderful impulse that nature has given us in the interplay of the sexes biologically in order to produce children.

There comes a time when the child graduates from the family and the couple is left. It's not simply a time of doing one's own thing. It is, in a sense, doing one's own thing, but the one isn't just you, it's the two together as one. And that's a purely mythological image signifying the sacrifice of the visible entity for a transcendent good.

This is something that becomes beautifully realized in the second stage of marriage, what I call the alchemical stage, of the two experiencing that they are one. If they are still living as they were in the primary stage of marriage, they will go apart when their children leave. It takes a commitment to transform in the relationship that which is a remnant of a ritual. And the ritual has lost its force. Marriage is not just a social arrangement, it's a spiritual exercise that the society is supposed to help us realize. Man should not be in the service of society, society should be in the service of man. When man is in the service of society, you have a monster state, and that's what is threatening the world at this minute." (*NEW AGE,* July/August 1988, Marriage and Myth)

Complicating the state of relationship and marriage, there was a horrible blight of sexually transmitted health disorders like herpes simplex I and II rampant in my community and abroad; along with the threat of gonorrhea and skin and tissue aberrations. It seemed that every other woman who came into our bookstore desired a better approach to self care, especially around their oral openings. The medical world at this time seemed to judge these disorders harshly. The women I spoke with did not feel the doctors were really listening and then that the male doctors could hardly be expected to know the trials of a woman's vaginal opening and child bearing cycles. People were seeking ways to assist their own healing. I felt alarmed by unresolved women health issues.

Since the mid seventies I had been forced to study the endocrine system and it's affects on the physical, mental, emotional, and even spiritual planes. I was so glad I had knowledge and could share it confidentially.

In my own backyard, a man I was intimate with, (at this time I could count on one hand the number of lovers I had in my own life) came to me scornfully announcing one of his past lovers had told him that she was introduced to a venereal disease. Therefore, as the famous line up of connections went, others were being informed to have themselves tested for this highly infectious disorder. I was outraged.

After being married for ten years and being monogamous, this was the most heinous announcement I was to receive. The first year after my divorce, I vowed to never marry again. I did not know how to make a relationship work long term. I allowed myself to be involved with two men at the same time. Open marriage, with its sexual revolution, was in full swing. After Viet Nam, and the massive disheartenment with the American legal and government system, I saw my generation open to exploring new territories of values and moral exchanges.

After realizing the vulnerable self-scrutiny the sexual announcement put me through, and the mutual unwillingness of my two men friends to commit to a long term monogamous relationship, I decided to end my sexual intimacy with both of them. Since the farm house was owned by all of the farm corporation, it was obvious that I was in too vulnerable a home setting to adequately care take my personal needs. I made my first decision to leave the farm in the fall of 1979.

Leaving the two now past intimate male friends, my ex-husband, and his girlfriend at the remote eighty acre farm, I moved into a small local town close by in hopes of better caretaking myself and my son.

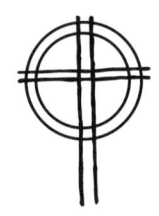

"BEYOND A WHOLESOME DISCIPLINE, BE GENTLE WITH YOURSELF"

TRANSFORMATIONAL ENERGY WORKSHOP

Living off the farm in the old home of my injured woman friend with the young son, I was teaching mathematics at the local junior high and working Saturdays at the bookstore. Journaling was the main avenue I had to communicate and I dared not to show it to anyone else. The bookstore allowed me to share with others what I was most interested in self health. Self health involved how to take care of not only one's physical aspects of well being but emotional, mental and spiritual. All our parts were important to review.

I was delighted to receive an announcement that Brugh Joy was coming to share a very special healing workshop. It was expensive but I decided to definitely attend. I was amazed how I had put a conscious wish to train with this alternatives energy, brain-relating teacher.

We traveled to a downtown hotel banquet room. Dr. Joy began each session with forming a sitting circle, holding hands and experiencing a common current or flow of energy between us that he called 'intunement'. He instructed us to have our right palm up and our left palm down. Dr. Joy spoke of a current much like an electrical charge flow, with positive and negative impulses that our right negative hand would connect with person's left, positive charged hand thus creating a balanced charge between and through the circle of people. When the connection was continuously flowing, a noticeable sensation spread through our palms. Sometimes it created a greater heat in the hand such that much moisture released.

He jumped right into the language of auras. He had us sense this invisible force field through an exchange process where we scanned the person's energy field with our hands. We were to pay attention to the rushes of feelings, or the colors seen with eyes closed or heats as we let our hands travel from around six inches above the head and continuing down to the feet, tuning into the various depths of energy field that emanated from our bodies.

The energy exercises continued to build and inter-relate through the workshop. We would pair up and he would talk us through didactic exercises. He would pair us with a person who would remain neutral and just witness the process, while the other partner would let his/her active imagination play out the script Dr. Joy would describe. For example, he would describe, with emotionally charged language, a situation such as being in the back seat of a car on a winding snowy road and the driver is drunk. The breaks are not working, the car is speeding, and it's not making the corner.

The neutral partner felt through his palms, both upward what the active participant imagined with all the senses. That snapshot of life was registered and then

Dr. Joy would have each person shake it off so to speak and the active participant would then be lead into a differently emotionally charged snapshot.

After living and experiencing several life scenes, the partners would switch roles. The neutral, witnessing participant, reversing the palm direction would now experience through three various emotionally charged snapshots of life. After both people experienced both directions, we were asked to share with the other what we had felt. I was surprised by the heat, the cold breezes, the moisture and tenseness that I could read through my hands.

To this day I share that exercise with people in relationships who are having trouble communicating. This exercise jolts one to authentically know we can read another without words. We feel people. Someone can walk into the room and have had a tough, or sad, or mad or happy experience and upon entering our own energy field we can comprehend where they are at emotionally. This is contradictory to the run of the mill way we communicate and acknowledge our understanding of each other. We need to prove or win or show another what we mean, rather than intuiting through our senses.

The exercises demanded us to know much about the other without words outwardly being expressed. We were being challenged to expand our fields of awareness. I could sense the strength of the energy fields and sometimes even different ranges of temperature with the various participants. Most of the fifty people in this workshop were people I called 'heavy weights' in the alternative healing fields. I felt intimidated and subconsciously did not feel I belonged with such a recognized field of alternative technicians.

With each session, Dr. Brugh Joy would have us lie on the floor and proceed to blast a high volume of music. He contended the vibrations from the wide range of carefully chosen music would activate our chakras. The soul is the bridge that connects the material world of the body, the tonal, with world of the spirit, the nagual. The world of the soul consists of seven (some say ten) special swirls of energy, or sublime forces called chakras. The power of eternal light shines through our "lightbodies", chakra, and we can participate in the cosmic energy through it.

The lightbody is eternal and immortal. One can imagine these energy centers as empty vessels that radiate a different quality of light or energy. (*SHAMANIC HEALING*, pg. 137) and nullify our brain's (ego's) desire to be in control of our reception and thoughts. He also contended that when the chatter in the mind was stopped, in the stillness the brain would secrete endorphins and the total body would heal.

The Eastern tradition of Yoga had first taught me of these energy systems. The first chakra is the root chakra and often relates to issues in stability and security, one's home base. This center is influenced by our family of origin (See Chakra charts, p 14).

The second center, just below the belly button is the home of one's kundalini, one's, life force, vital force, universal force or unseen life energy. The flow from this source is sometimes referred to as "chi" "Qi" or "ki" energy. In traditional Chinese Medicine, pronounced "chee", it means energy that circulates through energetic pathways called meridians, or channels. In a healthy individual this vital energy flows in a balanced and harmonious manner throughout the body. When this energy becomes blocked, impeded, disharmonious, invaded, imbalanced or stuck, one sees the onset of various physical, emotional, and/or mental symptoms.

There is a famous Chinese medical proverb, "Tong zhe bu tong. Tong zhe bu tong." Translated, the proverb means "Where there is flow there is no pain; where there is pain there is no flow." This relates to pain of all kinds, not just physical; however, pain, or more specifically distension, is one of the most common physical symptoms associated with stagnant Qi. Symptoms can include headaches, a feeling of tightness or a lump in the throat, difficulty swallowing, hiccups, stuffiness often with frequent sighing, abdominal distension, especially in the stomach or under the sides of the rib cage and flanks and in the pelvic area and breasts especially in pre-menstrual women.

The word qi, which is spelled chi, does not have a clear English equivalent. Good health occurs when this energy is properly flowing through the body. Ted J. Kaptchuk, O.M.D., author of THE WEB THAT HAS NO WEAVER: UNDERSTANDING CHINESE MEDICINE, suggests that qi can be thought of as "matter on the verge of becoming," or "energy at the point of materializing." "Qi is perceived functionally—by what it does." Such a definition, however, does little to satisfy the Western mind.

The third chakra, located at the base of one's rib cage, strongly deals with EGO and mental processes. The pancreas and spleen greatly influence this center of right use of will. Others refer to this center as the place of the inner marriage, where our masculine and feminine aspects of our being must come into harmony and balance. People coming from unhealthy family traits often feel their stress in this third center, the place where blame, shame and judgement become like blows to the stomach.

The center, or the fourth chakra, reflects compassion and discernment. It is ruled by the thymus, a very misunderstood gland in Western Medicine. Often it is expressed as the home of our spirit and the place of unconditional love. This center responds to time in nature, especially with plants and the sun.

The fifth center, located in the throat region, addresses our trust to be creative and safe in expression. The thyroid represents the endocrine system here and regulates body metabolism.

Just above the eyes, in-between the eyebrows, is the third eye chakra. It address clear vision, often reflecting one's inherited grace. The pituitary gland rules not only the entire endocrine system, but this center as well. The gland regulates the hormonal secretions throughout all seven chakras. Endorphins secreted from the pituitary are often called joy juice and are neurochemical responses that influence our emotions, sexual drive, growth patterns, our ability to assimilate sugars and fats and the ability of the blood to stay healthily balanced.

Dr. Joy said to keep the endorphins releasing and one's total personal health follows. On the contrary, disbelief and negative personal concepts would create the opposite, carcinogens, alias self consumption. The secretion of endorphins brings peace, joy, humor and happiness which equate well being.

The seventh center is our spiritual omniscience, or the bridge with which one is connected with the high self, God in the physical world. A sense of embrace and kindness radiates from this center. I would remember the words from Desiderata:

"GO PLACIDLY AMID THE NOISE & HASTE,
& REMEMBER WHAT PEACE THERE MAY BE IN SILENCE"

The very first night, lying on the uncomfortable floor, I watched my mind scream at me for what I thought to be an outrageous situation. I could hear people banging outside the locked doors and on the ceiling above us, demanding that the music be turned down. Meanwhile Dr. Joy continued to share this intense music with it's tones that activated our various chakras and connected endocrine gland.

I was so scared. I knew we would all be arrested and thrown in jail for disturbing the peace. How could he possibly get away with such an absurd exchange with us! This was not what I expected, to be so challenged by my vulnerabilities regarding the *law and social rules.* How could my mind quit chattering with all this outside interference?

After our music session, Dr. Joy sat peacefully, gently explaining that there were no accidents and those rules just needed to be challenged. He checked in with us and inquired did we stay in the moment or did we shift perceptions? More social fear issues splattered in my face. Later he asked us to watch our night space. The next day he elaborated that we often work out through dreams that which we cannot make sense of in our waking day. The unconscious avails itself through a symbolic language during our night space. I liked this. Everywhere I turned to study I was validated to work with dreams.

Brugh proceeded to relate his dream which he labeled as a group dream. It dealt with a well in a the local community square that was polluted. He, in the dream, had volunteered to go down into the well casing and check out to see what was poisoning the waters. He saw some scientific officials and policemen trying to block the investigation. There was an underlying feeling that the water might be polluted by nuclear fallout.

Dr. Joy then asked our interpretation of the dream. I listened and heard people's perspectives. I felt driven to take the dream literally since I was a political activist against our state's major nuclear plant that is located over the origins of a huge underground river. Our state is the dumping grounds for our nations military nuclear warfare waste. I was ready to elaborate on my theme of taking responsibility for our relationship with this good earth when I was told I was wrong. He insisted that the dream represented parts of our own internal water system, our feelings, that are polluted, afraid of authorities, and needed to be checked into. I did not know if I could agree or not.

He took us through more deep intuitive exercises. To enhance one's own self health, Dr. Joy described what he calls the "Spiral Meditation". He had us image a spiral of light originating at one's heart and then slowly spiraling clockwise out, around and through various organs, chakras and systems until the light energy circled beyond the physical body and became part of the protective glow in the aura field, the energetic field that surrounds one's physical body.

We experienced the loud, specially selected pieces of music, now interweaving the 'Spiral Meditation' in our imaging, releasing and at-one-ment. Each time it became easier to release watching for external physical or mental interruptions and to allow a simple neutral mental and emotional state to be present. My body/mind became responsive to the music vibrations. When there was a block in a center I would feel it and then affirm to let go that part of my life story or responses that no longer served my well being. I desired to heal. Enough with the destructive personal health crisis that dominated my days!

Dr. Joy asked us to do a night exercise. The next day he was bringing in a critically ill person. In our night space we were to talk to ourselves just before going to sleep and ask to journey to this person and then scan the individual, identifying where we saw the illness, particularly noticing colors and feelings. The ill person was willing to have us check into his condition this particular evening.

I cooperated and much to my surprise I did see someone in my night's dream space. I located 'blocks' in his brain and heart and pelvis. In the morning I remembered the intensity of red and black tones as I asked myself first thing upon waking what had occurred in my dream world. I was stunned that I remembered what I had 'seen'. Upon arriving back to the workshop, sharing the circle, tuning in, then meditating to loud sounds, we were ready to participate in a group healing with this unidentified ill person.

Dr. Brugh Joy invited us to come to the cot where the man would lie and with our hands several inches from the person we were invited to share unconditional love. He stressed that if we got emotional over the situation, we were to stay seated. If we had seen something in our night space, we were to direct our hands over the locations.

The healing session lasted several hours. After the man left, Brugh Joy specifically shared the type of illness and where it manifested in the person's body. I was stunned when the locations I had seen the night before and what we were told were the same. The skeptic in me was challenged.

The key concept Brugh Joy impressed was to be neutral and transparent when we share touch or healing, keeping our focus on love, freeing ourselves from being invested emotionally.

Towards the end of the conference, I felt great concern that Dr. Joy seemed to be stuck in what I called the 'God Junior' syndrome that so many of the significant men in my life seemed to continually exude. Men are superior. Women were to be endured but not really valued. Throughout the workshop, I would be caught by the various innuendos belittling women. I wondered if he was just another man angry at women.

During the circle times he was willing to answer questions but I did not feel comfortable enough with the large group to ask him about his male/female view of relationships. Typically, during our breaks he would disappear. The last day I literally bumped into Brugh in the hallway and spontaneously blurted out my inquiry of his perception of man and woman, especially about long term commitment and respect.

His response to me felt shallow. I felt judged and belittled. I sensed he did not like women, especially me. I left the event with very mixed feelings. Parts of me were opened and challenged to grow while the human, woman in me still felt stuck in the same ageless male patterns. An angry side prayed for a woman teacher. I was real tired of male chauvinist 'gurus'.

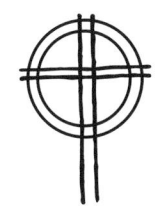

"AND WHETHER OR NOT IT IS CLEAR TO YOU
NO DOUBT THE UNIVERSE IS UNFOLDING AS IT SHOULD
THEREFORE BE AT PEACE WITH GOD, WHATEVER YOU CONCEIVE HIM TO BE,
AND WHATEVER YOUR LABORS AND ASPIRATIONS IN THE NOISY CONFUSION
OF LIFE, KEEP PEACE WITH YOUR SOUL"

BOOK MAGIC —1980

Two years into our bookstore business, we made an additional financial investment and moved our business to the main downtown shopping center. I was racked with continuous inner and outer pain. The manager/partner had broken both her heels while building her home out at the farm and was unable to stand and manage the business. The third partner never intended to be in the store and was of no help.

The store, itself, was truly magical. Those people who walked through the doors had much to share. I called it my office. It was where I could practice unconditional love. The quality and diversity of our books and arts thrilled me. It was a goal of mine to meet each individual and assist them to find just the right reference or book they hungered for.

We had our own version of Saturday Night Live and brought in progressive, leading edge musicians, writers, poets and artists. Plus we were doing a great deal of community networking. Artisans from out-of-state would just happen into our store and then spontaneously share a concert, or a reading, or health tool sharing.

As the Food co-op thrived upstairs in our bookstore, we were helping this community grow healthier and citizens had a public market for their talents to be shared. We attracted as customers the strivers and dreamers. The majority of the old established community people did not support our store.

Growing more concerned for my own health, I was challenged to go back to the University of Utah to study and do research in the health area of endocrinology. It seemed to be a mysterious, poorly understood aspect of people's health system.

The part of me who was trying to become educated on the endocrine system, especially the pituitary gland which is the master gland in charge of the rest of the glands, and the effect of stress on the entire glandular system, searched out books and authorities to educate myself. I became like a volcano, ready to explode as I heard repeated stories of women's health disorders, the chronic bladder and kidney infections, herpes Simplex I and II, cysts, radical hysterectomies. "My God", I screamed inside with each new woman's horror story I was told.

Women's bodies were being destroyed and mutilated by Western medicine. Our female organs seemed to be the battle grounds of white man's medicine. Continual medical stories came to my attention ranging from massive doses of body numbing and consuming medication to advice to ignore the disorder.

There were proclamations that women were hypochondriacs. There were stories of the rapid removal of key organs followed by prescribed drugs for the rest of a woman's life. Women in fear; women who were chronically infected by smelly infections, unsupported pregnancies and confusing medications and complications. An endless script for women of all ages unsure as to what good personal health looked like. The need for an adequate sex health education was a preoccupation within me, yearning to come to some form in the world inside and outside of me.

As a confused, single mother, I was totally uncertain about love, lust and loneliness. Since sexuality had been a tool to harass me by my first husband, I was very ignorant about where sexual intimacies fit into the bigger picture of committed love. I was told 'men give love in order to have sex, and women give sex in order to be loved.'

A younger, gently pure gentleman came into my world. He had a huge grin and loved to dance. He assisted me to move out of the old mold that had me seem to be an elephant in a china closet as far as movement went. Together we entered several western swing dance classes because we moved so well together. In the sexual world, he introduced me to oral sex and thus to the fears which surrounded it, herpes simplex I and II.

As I investigated I was to learn that herpes simplex II was closely tied to herpes simplex I. If a person had an open mouth sore, one through oral sex could transmit and set in motion the potential of a life-time of painful vaginal sores and unsafe physical relations. Furthermore, the possibility of transmitting the virus could occur even though no symptoms were visible for the woman. I knew no monogamous partners in the late seventies. Women were thronging to our bookstore and to me beseeching help to heal their wombs and sacred opening.

We were in an epidemic of unknown, far-reaching influence and interconnections. Yet no one felt safe to speak of it with their doctors, or their ministers. They could only hide in corners of our store and whisper, in intensely fearful tones, trying to gain knowledge of their own sacred body from a woman, myself, who was sharing what I too needed to know.

What activated the mouth sores was stress. If a person was taking on too much in her life and became mentally bogged down or depressed, she was inviting the stomach to get upset and then the whole immune system and blood quality diminished. The mouth sores and the stomach equilibrium went hand in hand.

No matter where I researched my health dis-order, the over-enlarged Pituitary, the mind and it's ability to be peaceful or stressed influenced the master gland of the endocrine system. This system is so intricate, if even one of the seven glandular and metabolic parts moves out of balance, all of them are affected.

The more I learned, the more I was aware of "mind as healer, mind as slayer." I questioned did health begin with one's mental state or did it begin with a peaceful response for why we choose to live on this earth and with its inhabitants? Are people basically good or are we a cut throat, competitive dog eat dog society? Are men and women equal? Are we living to die, or dying to live? And *Desiderata* would speak to me:

"AVOID LOUD AND AGGRESSIVE PERSONS,
THEY ARE VEXATIONS TO THE SPIRIT.
IF YOU COMPARE YOURSELF WITH OTHERS,
YOU MAY BECOME VAIN AND BITTER;
FOR ALWAYS THERE WILL BE GREATER AND LESSER PERSONS
THAN YOURSELF."

Another part of me was responding to teachings I had been learning from Dr. Richard Moss, who was traveling through our country and regularly training in the area of energy fields, healing hands, attitudes, trust and communications with our inner self.

He clearly stated that if anyone was consumed with an incurable disorder, they could do the following:

"From the teachings of the wheel, one could go to the ocean and simply be with the ocean for two weeks. Thoughts were to be on wellness and being one with the ocean. Then the person was to travel to the high country, to the mountains and for two weeks be totally one with the mountains. Not allowing thoughts to be anywhere else. Next, the individual would go to the hot springs, and for two weeks be totally one with the geothermal waters. Lastly the person would go out into the desert and become totally one with the desert."

He declared that if a person did chose that four-part wellness plan, they would be healed. I knew it to be a truth and vowed to take that time to heal.

I announced to my book store partners that in a year I would no longer be physically involved in the store. My health was deteriorating. I named Christmas, 1980 as the time line I would leave the store. The store manager was dedicated and hopeful for this book business and went about hiring extra help to keep our store open. I went about weaning myself from the store.

In the meantime, a familiar new age psychic came to town bringing an instrument called a Nuerophone, called Dr. Flanagon's educational toy. Dr. Flanagon was a brilliant scientist who developed the MX Missile, sadly. When I was hooked up to this little, brown box on an electronic machine that used sound vibrations to tone through a person's brain and bring the hemispheres into balance. Learning suggestions came into the box from a tape player in which one inserted a pretaped subject such as positive affirmations, how to learn Spanish in 40 lessons, being in pink, loving light, and so on.

I chose to experience a past life regression. With Stephen Halpern's *SPECTRUM SUITE* and *ANCIENT ECHOES* integrating with the basic Neurophone pulse, I sensed a deep recollection of 'going home'. Home went back to Egypt. This hair-raising experience moved me deeply. It took only minutes for me to start experiencing a movie showing me inside a pyramid. I was aware of the geometry of the structure. I was aware of the presence of others, draped in loose clothing.

Lights flashed with gem like brilliance. It felt like I was being taught something about crystals and huge transparent , glowing rods of stone. When the tape ended it was time for me to come back. Like a rude jolt, I discovered myself back in the sitting room in our bookstore. Upon sharing my experience, the psychic said it sounds like you went back to Egypt. She suggested that I read the book *INITIATION* by Elizabeth Haich.

After experiencing the ancient remembering, I knew I was to be caretaker of one of these nuerophone tools. I had been meditating for almost a decade, yet my health and mental state was extremely stressed. I knew I needed this new yet old tool. I purchased this costly instrument. This was not the first electronic health tool to

frequent our store and my scrutiny. This little brown box of an instrument was magnetic. Twenty minutes was all a person could be on the frequency tunings daily.

The Neurophone MK XI is an electronic hearing device intended for stimulating the nervous system with an electric field to produce auditory sensations. It consists of electronic circuitry into which audio signals from a microphone, recorder, etc. may be fed, and a pair of metallic output electrodes, each surrounded by insulating materials. Tests of the Neurophone on more than 1000 persons, including some totally deaf subjects, have produced intelligible auditory sensations in all cases through the skin. You actually hear through your skin.

The clue to how the Neurophone actually works, is contained in the skin vibration artifact, which was discovered at Tufts University. The original Neurophone used a high voltage amplitude modulated carrier wave to create a molecular vibration in the skin itself. The skin became the diaphragm of a biological electrostatic vibrator.

The skin is piezo-electric. That is, when the skin is stimulated by an electric field, or by a photon field, it will contract and vibrate with modulation of the field. If it is mechanically stimulated, it will generate its own electric field. In Russia blind people have been trained to 'see' with their fingertips; and in Czechoslavakia, deaf people have been trained to 'hear' with their fingertips.

The skin is the largest most complex organ of the living system. As we develop in the womb, all organs of sense evolve from the skin. The skin involutes and convolutes to form eyes, ears, etc. Dr. Flanagon's research indicates that the skin itself has the latent potential of performing all functions of perception.

The Neurophone stimulates and develops this latent ability. The skin is the organ which receives the signal from the Neurophone, and converts the incoming signal into a modulated molecular vibration which is then interpreted as sound.

As all acupuncture meridians are present on the surface of the skin, Dr. Flanagon found that the Neurophone stimulation balances all the acupuncture meridians by activating the skin.

The result is a new modality for coupling information to the brain, using the skin itself as the receptor. Bone conduction vibrators will not work as a Neurophone, because the vibratory signals are too gross; the skin itself must vibrate in a synchronous mode in accordance with the time encoded information.

Dr. Christopher Hills, in his book *NUCLEAR EVOLUTION,* states that the skin is a second brain, and is the basic organ of spiritual and psychic evolution. He states that the skin can be trained to develop powers of perception such as telepathy, etc.

The Neurophone is an electronic audio information processor designed and sold for experimental and entertainment purposes. It is used primarily in conjunction with an ordinary cassette recorder and then used with music, motivation, nature sounds, and learning tapes. The sound is then fed into the Neurophone and out through the electrodes, giving input directly into the human brain, while bypassing the normal eighth cranial nerve system.

Dr. Flanagan is the Founder of Source of Innergy Inc., of Tucson, Arizona and much of the research being done on the neurophone is being conducted in his laboratories there.

Dr. Flanagan invented the first neurophone when he was 14 years of age and now finally 22 years later (1980) the patent was approved and the Neurophone became available to the public.

At Source of Innergy Inc., they are currently in the process of making special tapes for Neurophone users. They have found that an external stimulus at the correct frequency will stimulate the same response found in meditators who have been meditating for years. The result is a stable left-right brain balance, and an acupuncture meridian balance. If used over an extended period of time, this balance becomes stabilized against environmental stresses that tend to throw us out of balance. The synchronization of brain rhythms is believed to accelerate the natural positive evolution of the nervous system and relieve stress.

Some of the future projections for the use of the Neurophone are tremendous, and research is beginning on some of the following possibilities:

1. Increase in telepathic awareness;
2. A brain-mind link between two or more people. Thomas E. Bearden has developed a mathematical formula that indicates that the combined mind power of group of people will multiply exponentially if these people are linked in a unitary consciousness;
3. Subliminal learning may be accomplished by playing subject material through the Neurophone at a low volume level. No conscious effort is made to learn the material. This could even be accomplished while the student is asleep;
4. Conscious learning may be accomplished by simultaneously listening to tape recorded data by means of Neurophone and headphones. In this way, the learning centers of the brain are being accessed by at least two separate channels;
5. Positive subliminal programs to alter undesirable habits: ie., weight control, smoking control and creation of positive mental attitude.
6. Control the aging process by means of positive cellular programming via the Neurophone;
7. Totally deaf people being able to hear the recorded audio;

(Source of Innergy, Ltd., P.O. Box 18224, Tucson, AZ 85715)

EXTENDED FAMILY'S CHILDREN

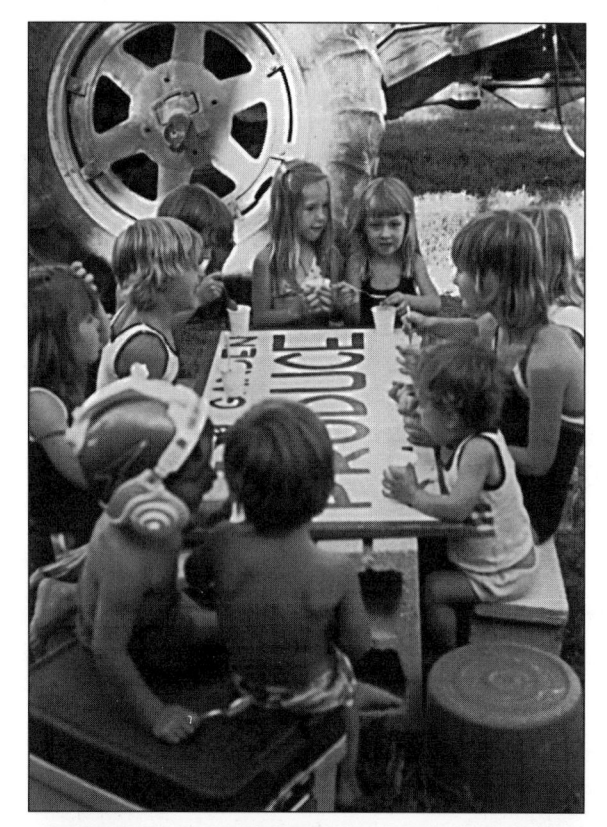

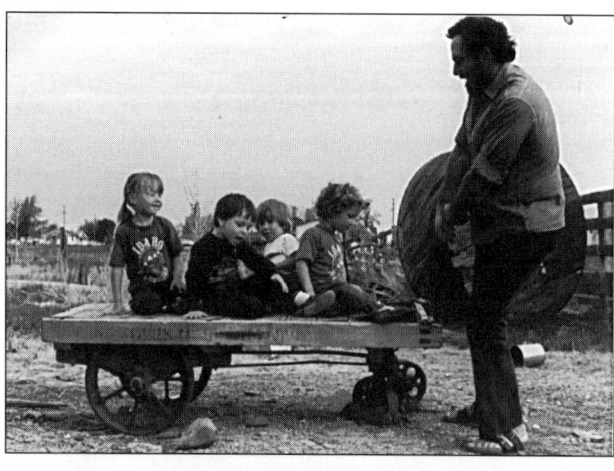

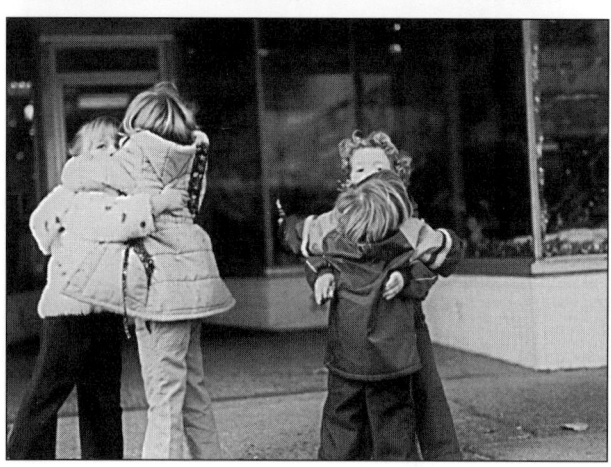

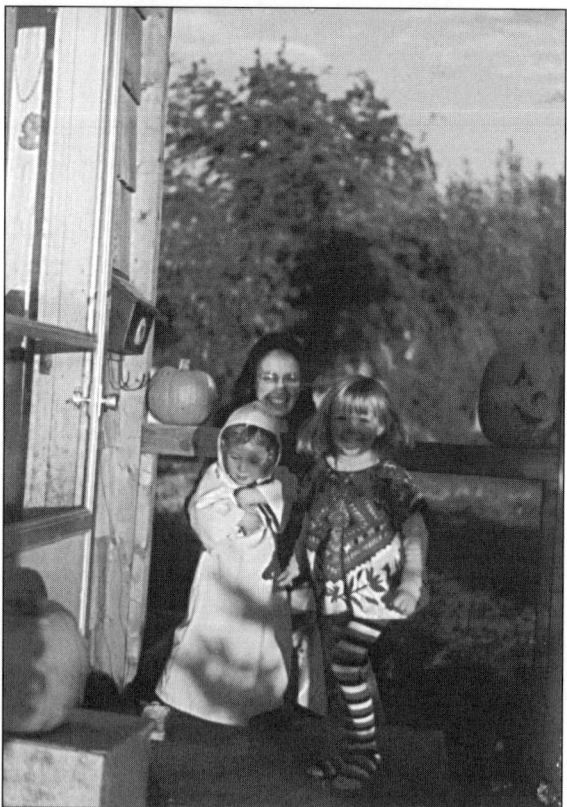

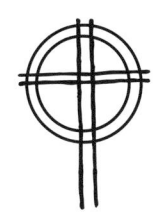

"ENJOY YOUR ACHIEVEMENTS AS WELL AS YOUR PLANS.
KEEP INTERESTED IN YOUR OWN CAREER, HOWEVER HUMBLE
IT IS A REAL POSSESSION IN THE CHANGING FORTUNES OF TIME.
EXERCISE CAUTION IN YOUR BUSINESS AFFAIRS;
FOR THE WORLD IS FULL OF TRICKERY.
BUT LET THIS NOT BLIND YOU TO WHAT VIRTUES THERE IS;
MANY PERSONS STRIVE FOR HIGH IDEALS;
AND EVERYWHERE LIFE IS FULL OF HEROISM."

SPIRITUAL EMERGENCY—1980

Now as I reflect back I understand better that abnormal period in my life. Each time I would meditate with this machine, which claimed to balance the left and right hemisphere of the brain, I would experience another dimension of being. Much like the channels on a radio, it tuned me to another frequency in ways I could only intuit but not quite verbalize. To transform it into the educational tool I needed, I would connect a cassette to the neurophone with the subject matter I wanted to absorb. Whether it was Spanish in three easy lessons, releasing grief, past-life regressions, whatever, the two machine would blend their pitches and I would receive them.

I now know that I was expanding my consciousness at an extremely rapid, abnormal rate. My friends around me were not keeping up. My body developed more symptoms. Lumps at the base of skull, tracking pains from my heart to my hands, shortness of breath and very irregular heart beats. Many walks I had with key friends holding my hand, begging me to go to a doctor, go to the hospital. Whatever it was, was within me, the bigger me. I knew that this machine was balancing my brain but more than that it was helping me in the primordial, natural and spiritual realms my brain yearned to acknowledge. My illness was more than just physical and I did not trust Western Medicine to do more than cause me longer hurt.

For those familiar with the term, I was igniting my kundalini, my internal spiritual fire. I was sure at this time in my life that I was ill and the only thing that would heal me was a spiritual awakening/birthing. I needed to transcend to a place of knowing that all I was love and light.

By this time, in 1980, I was divorced with a two year old boy, living back on the farm with two other men and feeling death haunt me. Through the New Age Journal I had discovered a little news brief about a whole group of people called the Spiritual Emergency Network that worked with people who had developed traits similar to that of having heart attacks, alternating anxiety and bliss attacks, intense headaches, deep feelings of separation and on and on. I fit the list of qualities so I immediately corresponded with this network started by Christina and Stan Grof, and John Price. Upon joining the SEN organization, I started receiving newsletters from this non-profit organization that supplies information and support to people like myself who were troubled by their psychic and spiritual experiences.

According to surveys done in the 1980's by the University of Chicago's National Opinion Research Council and the Gallup Organization, 42% of the American adult population reported contact with the dead, 29% had visions, 67% experienced ESP and 43% had a mystical experience. In comparison, a 1973 survey showed only 27% reported contact with the dead, 8% having visions, 58% experiencing ESP and 35% having a mystical experience.

A huge number of people all over the world were opening up to the paranormal. Unfortunately, many of these people didn't understand what was happening to them. Instead of using their encounters with the unknown to broaden their awareness and enrich their lives, they became fearful and confused, concerned that they may be physically or mentally ill.

The Spiritual Emergency Network provided people with accurate information and guidance so they could integrate these experiences into their lives in a constructive manner, rather than assuming something was wrong with them. SEN knew that support groups were needed both for individuals going through spiritual emergency, and for the professionals treating the people in psycho-spiritual crisis.

In the early eighties the written word that came through the newsletters was my only connection with others in my state of growth. I treasured each correspondence as if I were sitting down at table, exchanging with a trusted, well intended other. I knew of no one else in Idaho, or specifically Southern Idaho in my state of growth or rather disintegration.

In a time of spiritual searching and experimentation, and upheaval of religious beliefs and traditions, SEN served a much needed function by striving to provide creative intervention, safety and nurturing care for people going through psychospiritual crisis. (Mary Milczarek, N.D., Regional Coordinator for SEN in Washington, and naturopathic physician, *THE NEW TIMES* 1993)

Life at the farm took on a Zen like quality as I took care of my personal and health needs. Since I was distant from my blood family, the community associated with the farm and our business was very important to me and my son. The terrible car accident with dear sweet Sonja had tightened our extended family connections. We developed a child cooperative and four days a week one could share child tending. The young son of Sonja's gained four mothers.

At such a young age these children were also around her as she laid on a hospital bed in the living room of her home. It is still very heart rending to write about it. The compassion shared of gentle foot rubs, soft songs and deep prayers.

During this time I became very aware that I could communicate with Sonja in a nonverbal manner. I would stand next to her, hold her hand and look into those piercing hawk-like eyes and send her love and she would begin to cry. Since my experience on the farm during the Feminine Energy Workshop, I felt without doubt a closeness to this very wounded woman.

Now, I would have to pray for understanding as to why, through man's intervention, they brought her back to life more than two times. To what? A life as a living vegetable! Her husband wanted to believe with enough love and attention she would recover; after all she had survived this long. I, too, wanted to believe in the miraculous, but the mother in me railed, "Why should this occur between a mother and her love child and mate?"

In time, the life support was removed and she still stayed alive. She did not die until 1993. Something kept her alive that we did not understand.

Even more significant was sharing positive celebrations with our children and family of choice. My favorite holiday season of the year was Easter. Out on our magical land, the changing season brought lots of good feelings for me, especially spiritually. It was a time of a well planned Easter Egg Hunt in a yard to be envied for great egg hiding places. It was a time we shared together with lots of animation and fun. It was a time to break bread and be thankful.

Most importantly, it was a time to reflect on Jesus, a man who was the son of God and the son of a Virgin Mother. A man I felt who had the same sense as we do but came as a messenger to assist us to be in better relations with one another and also in attune with this dear Earth. Inside I was knowing him as a brother for Jesus asked us to "Pray ye for one another and what I can do you can do and more."

I was constantly deepening my comprehension of Jesus and the various Marys in his life, especially Mary Magdalene, the woman of many names, the one who stood beside him and knelt at his feet at his death. She who was the one to be called to go to the tomb and see him resurrected. She understood through her womb, her instinctual woman center. To me, this is one of the few areas in the written form of his words, where women are at least somewhat acknowledged as wise and spiritual.

This intense inner dimension added to my commitment to celebrate the Easter season, especially to pattern good relations and love for one another and trust that the days to come would be bountiful and good. I knew we were giving our children positive traits and that was validating.

1980 EASTER ON THE FARM

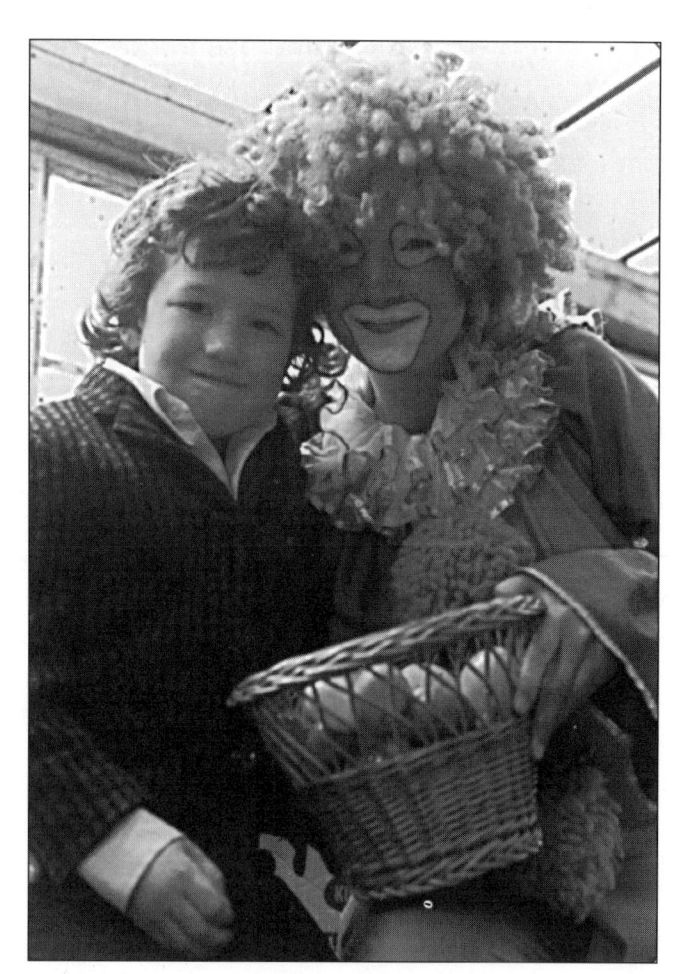

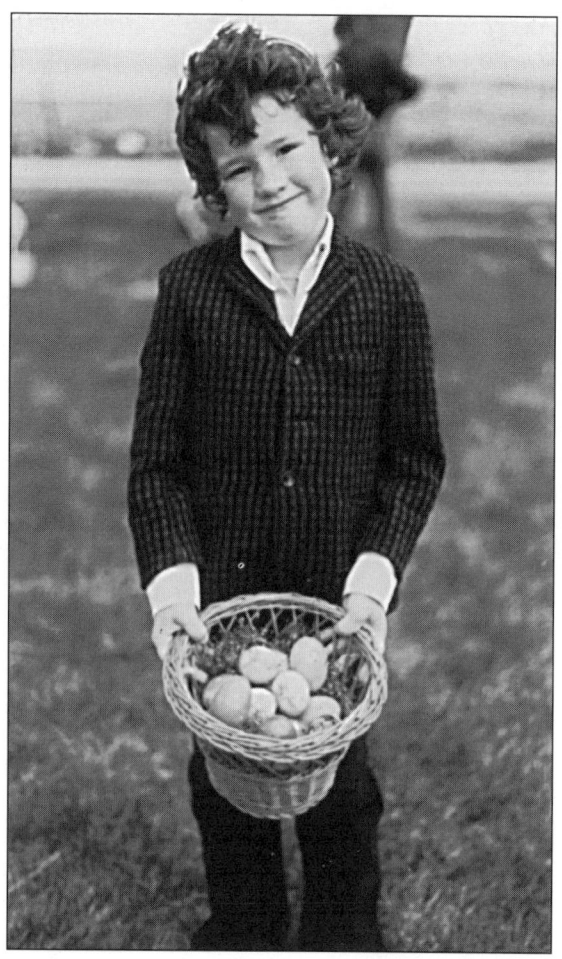

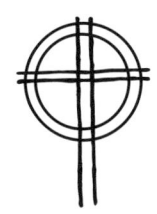

"NURTURE STRENGTH OF SPIRIT TO SHIELD YOU IN SUDDEN MISFORTUNE."

RIVER JOURNEY

Now that I was not working at the bookstore as much and my mental activities were being circuited anew for a greater sense of peace, my hands longed to get back into pottery. I wanted to be creative. A friend invited me to share her clay center, so regularly would I work at centering through the outward process of dancing and molding wet, moist earth while inwardly I would be challenged to turn off all the outside conversations and chattering so the clay, the wheel and me, the artisan, could create a form that had sound structure.

Often in my past, I could register how balanced I felt by baking bread like my Grandmother had done, up to my elbows in flour, relying on my sense of touch and texture to assure a good loaf of bread. Throwing pottery demanded that same sense of balance. Any distraction of thought would collapse my desired project, whether it be a bowl, plate, cup, or whatever. Much to my delight, over the course of time I successfully threw a whole clay table service, a goal I had set almost a decade before in college.

A rare opportunity came my way as my potter friend announced that there was an opening on their boat to float the Middle Fork of the Salmon River. Their names had been drawn and would I like to go in August with their Eastern U.S. family. This was deep, long held dream of mine to float through the high, heartland of Idaho.

Being a Native Idahoan with a father who was a forest service ranger, I grew up watching him challenge and explore every river and mountain top in Idaho. I had longed forever to float this spectacular river in the heart of rugged Idaho. It was a rare honor as well as an expensive trip. So, in addition to being on the edge psychologically and spiritually with the Nuerophone, I chose to challenge my life on this River of No Return.

We rendezvoused in Stanley, a tiny town crowned with ragged Sawtooth Mountains. As we awaited the departure to the landing of the Middle Fork, some of us visited a private hot springs. While soaking in the ancient waters memories flooded me of my youth and I knew that I had learned to swim underwater in this same pool. I remembered being tossed in the water, sinking down, looking up and becoming like a tadpole wiggling through the water. These were some of the positive stimuli that came from my parents.

Deep in contemplation, I observed this three-boat float party. Besides my pottery friend, I knew no one well. Most were strangers. Her grey-haired father sat in the tip of the six person boat, constantly fussing over the safety of the women on our boat. Before we were through the first bend of the journey, he had tumbled backwards and headfirst into the rapids and was sucked under the boat because he was too busy in

1980 MIDDLE FORK OF THE SALMON RIVER

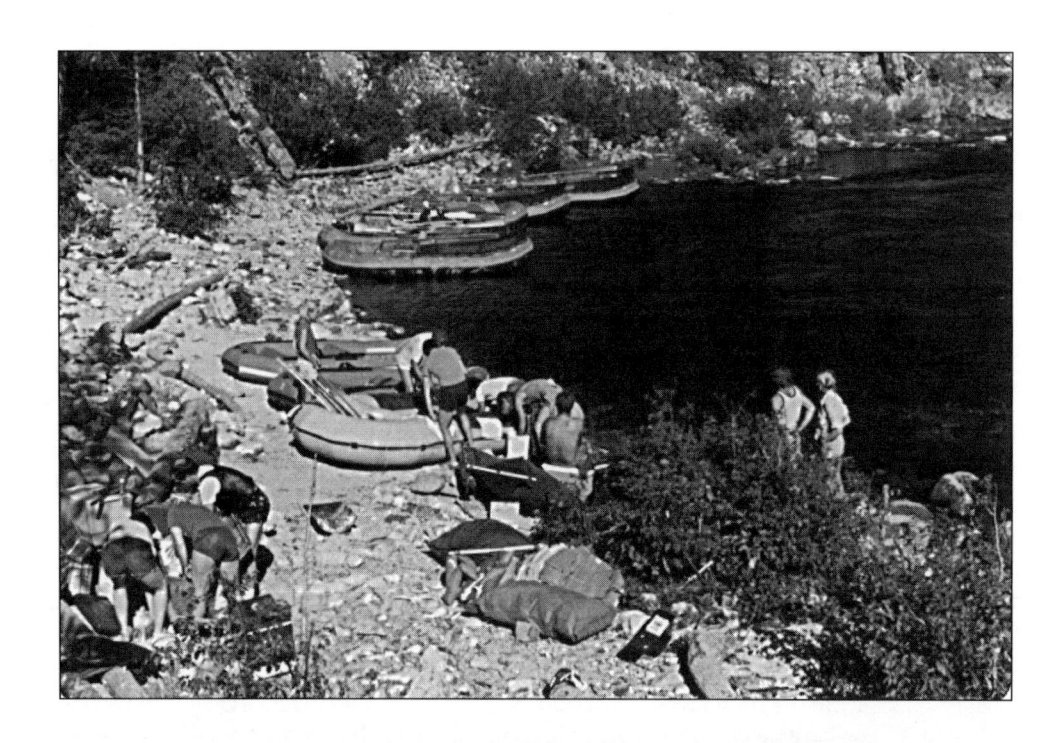

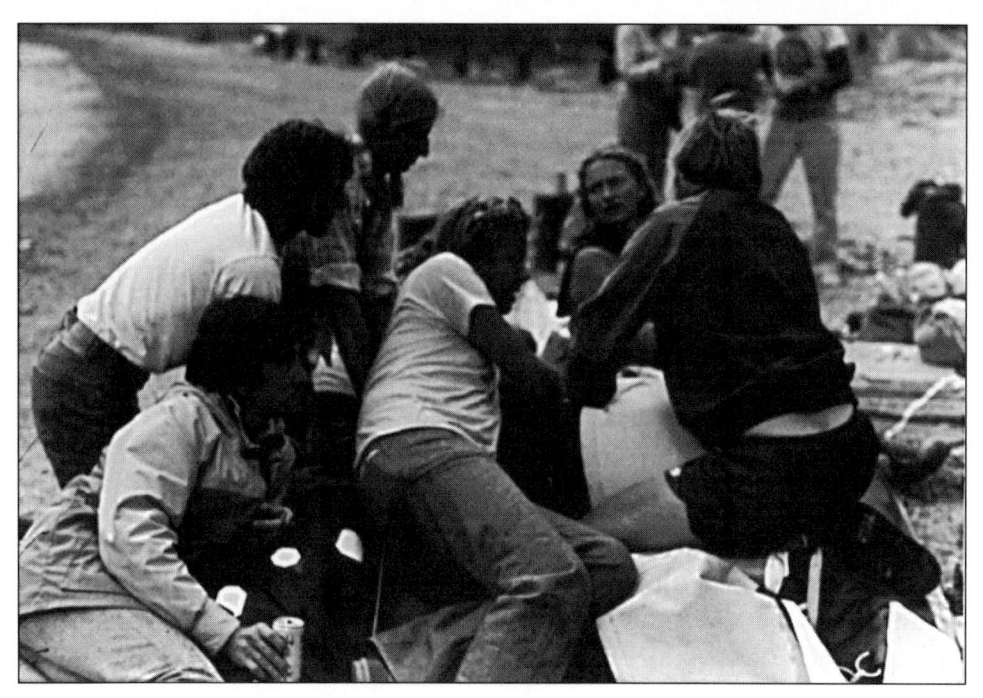

other people's business and not enough in his own position. Not a good omen, I thought.

The second day our boat again had a calamity when in the blasting heat of this August afternoon, our vessel exploded underneath us, as we slowly inched our way through a shallow, rock strewn portion of this amazingly diverse river. Here I was with preconceived notions of this peaceful, grand journey with no hassles. No way. Almost hourly, cast into an amazing script, was some great challenge that again in my life was crazy making. The boat captain and I stitched the blown out side with a very unique patch and continued on our journey. How was it that I was continually so handy, starting the fires, keeping the boat on course, and saving the trip with fancy stitches.

An eccentric veterinarian commandeered the second party. He loved to scare his girlfriend by going backward, sideways, whatever through rapids for the thrill of it. The third four-person boat was captained by a gentle, perfectionist optometrist. He made the journey down this challenging river look like riding a tricycle on a very safe path.

We lost our only map of the river the day before in the exploding boat calamity. Our river float had become quite precarious. We stopped whenever we heard roaring, rushing waters and scouted the next bends of this gorgeous, sometime deceptive river. Our skins were sun baked and our butts were blistered from sitting on the black, rubbery sides, but we were having fun, weren't we?

Frazzled with fear, the veterinarian's girlfriend abandoned her boat, swearing she would walk home rather than ride with the maniac captain any more. Our boat captain surveyed the situation and suggested I change places with the intimidated woman. I was a good team rower and I was strong enough not to let the teasing of this vet get to me.

Within minutes of boarding this four-man raft with the crazy pilot, the lead boat got stuck in a tight channel at Tappen's Fall. Since we were following so close we quickly were forced into an alternate opening in the river channel. Our boat plunged into a mammoth, pointed rock.

My memories hear the tremendous explosion and like slow motion I see me falling backward, catching sight of the towering height of the three story slate granite rock walls. Then the deepest, green swirling hands of the waters sucked me to it's bottom. Churning, my feet in my face, I felt the grips of death as water filled my screaming lungs.

My mind reeled before me options, quick flashes of my life. The cry of my precious child overcame my own scream for a mother's help, the warrior mother in me catapulted through to command a super human strength. Propelled to fight back I asserted my self to break out of the spiraling straight jacket of an undertow and clawed myself upward for what seemed like hours to get back to the surface and gasp in air.

When my head finally bobbed to the surface, my first thoughts were to save the paddles. This being the first rule taught when we began the river Journey, "Never let go of your paddle." Immediately I reached, grabbing more encumbering things, sinking back to the arms of the wild, swirling waters. On one of my bobs up, the potter's father screamed, "For God's sake Suzanne, save yourself." Save myself. What a funny thought. Then a part of me finally shifted and said okay.

I finally gained a handhold on the steep rocky shore, on the opposite side of the river as all my other members of our float trip. Without thinking I scrambled upward through brush finding a place still warmed by the sun and immediately stripped. Quaking like a leaf, I collapsed on the rocks, crying and breathing. It was way too much

NAVIGATING WITH A WILD RIVER

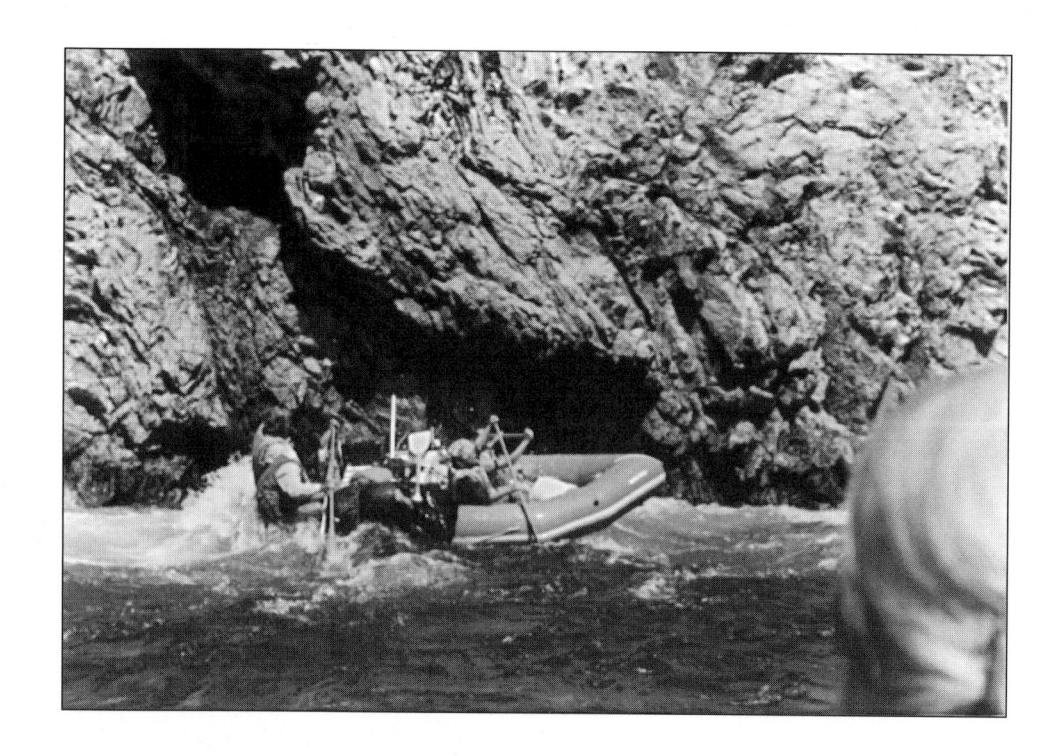

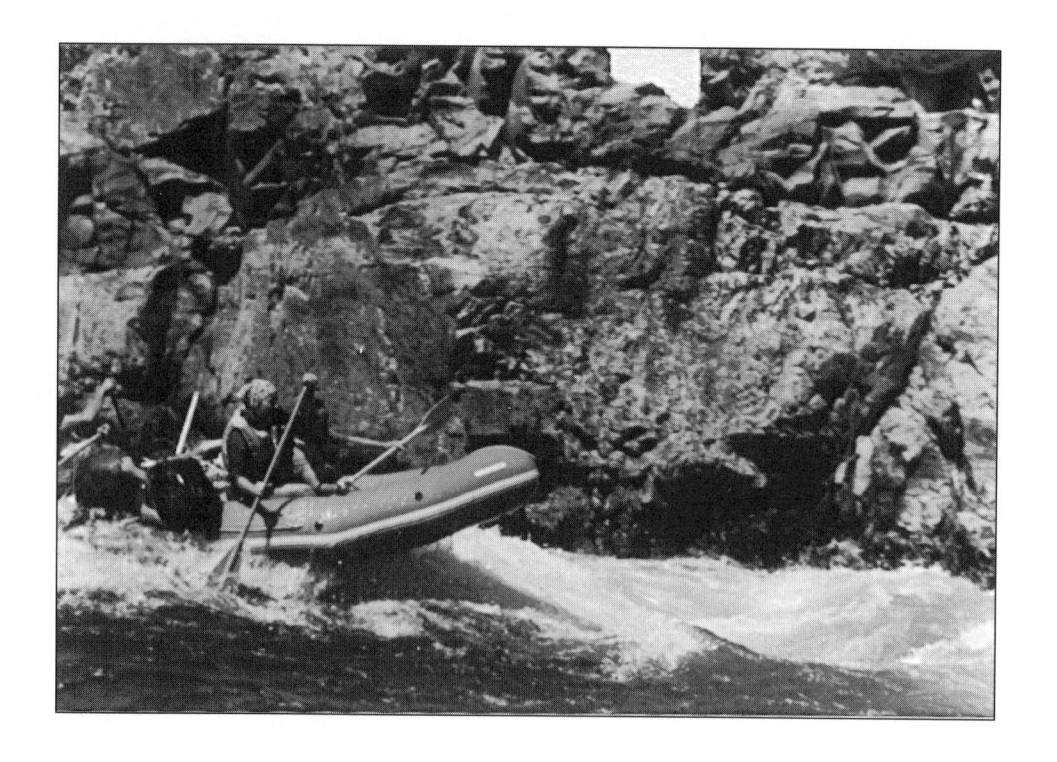

for my brain to compute but I was alive and I wanted to get warm.

Meanwhile the rest of the party collaborated on how to rescue me and the boat stuck in the narrow channel. The captain of the float climbed upriver to the one remaining boat that had not yet traveled through the narrow passage. Heroically this man leaped from the small boat and onto the rock with the downed boat. Every other person filled the largest boat and challenged the strong rapids to cross to my side of the roaring river. As I rested I could hear them in the distance trying to lasso the punctured boat, plastered against the rock. It became apparent that after the boat was tied back to the river's bank, that they needed my strength added before the boat would budge. Every other boat member united could not budge the swamped boat.

I stood trying to regain my balance and then I collapsed again tumbling down through the brush and rocks. Crawling up to my clothes, I dressed and went downriver and took hold of the rope at the end of the line of rafters and pulled. It was a long moment in time that none of us will ever forget. It took every single one of us, giving our total strength before the collapsed boat would budge enough to be retrieved. This was a very big teaching.

Hours later, when we went about setting up camp, all I could do was cry. I could not even start the fire. I looked around and no one else seemed able to emit any emotions. A rage filled me. I had been a crier all my life. I cried when my sisters were beaten, I cried when my mother was hurt, I cried when I was scared in the dark, I cried when I felt someone else being embarrassed or hurt. I was the scapegoat crier. From this moment forth I vowed to not cry for others. I became numb.

The rest of the river journey was anticlimactic.

I did vow to never go on another journey, whether in a boat, car or whatever, without knowing the personalities of the other participants. I'll not go blind into something again just because it fills an unmet need.

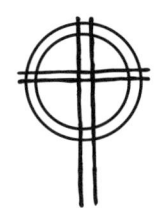

"BE YOURSELF. ESPECIALLY DO NOT FEIGN AFFECTION, NEITHER BE CYNICAL ABOUT LOVE; FOR IN THE FACE OF ALL ARIDITY AND DISENCHANTMENT IT IS PERENNIAL AS THE GRASS."

TRUE LOVE

On my September birthday, a tall distinguished, lawyer softly approached me while at our book store. He was a Southern gentleman working in the Magic Valley for six months arranging right of ways for the oil pipeline coming down from Alaska. He brought me roses and gifted me with wonderful music. He treated me like a gentlewoman and I was swept off my feet, in love like I had never known or felt before. My deepest wishes were being filled. I was ecstatic.

This created some strain with my two co-hearts back at the farm. The repeated pattern of attracting men who were not monogamous haunted me. My father, my husband and my closest men friends all lived poly-monogamously. Love the one you're with. Live and love in the Now. In my view, our generation who went through the Viet Nam war seemed to tear the whole conceived institution of marriage into threads and then we spit on it with distaste. At least the ones who were in my peer group did so.

My lawyer friend asked me to marry him. He announced that he was chosen to be part of the United States Ambassador program and would be called to Washington D.C. at the first of 1981. Intensity surrounded me. I had already announced that I was leaving the bookstore at the first of 1981 and now it looked like I'd literally be departing my home state and friends to go back East and then abroad, if I chose to marry.

At Christmas I went back to Georgia to meet his family and get a feel for where home would be after his sojourn as an ambassador. I left my young son in Idaho. Once in the South, I was overcome with eerie, old and unsettling feelings. There was a part of me that innately knew I could not live there. It felt so old and indoctrinated with unacceptable social systems and patterns about women and minorities, that I could not embrace living out my years there.

When my Southern gentleman's family home's plumbing quit working Christmas day, it became a minor catastrophe for all of them. For myself, I could disappear in the nearby forests to eliminate, but his family became hysterical and drove miles to a gas station's bathroom. I did not dare expose how uncivilized I could be. It was difficult for me to share with my dear man friend my cultural concerns.

His family had strong beliefs that they came from the stars. Both my fiance and his father had intricate ham radio sets. Nightly, I would overhear them communing with the beyond. I thought I had heard of everything, but I was wrong. To my understanding, they felt they were not from this Earth planet, but from the beyond. They were 'walk-ins' this lifetime. I knew I could not speak of this to anyone, but it felt crazy. Why did everything I associate with turn out weird. My belief system was sorely stretched, again.

My gentleman lavishly adorned me with clothing, perfume, roses, all the niceties that honor woman. He pledged his support, for he had plenty for both of us. I was not used to being gifted with things of beauty.

Upon returning to Idaho, my fiance announced that it was important for him that we have a year of just being together. He asked that I have my dear son live with his father for a year and then he would welcome my son into our family unit. His primary desire was to establish our relationship.

A part of me died. There was no way I could imagine giving up being a primary parent for my son. The history of my dear child put me in the main custodial position. Within days I collapsed. My heart was broken for I truly was in love with this gentle, kind man. Words could not form thoughts. All I knew was he wanted just me, not my son and not my family of friends.

I felt like his prize possession as he tried to isolate me from my extended family of friends. Deeply emotional, with racking head pains dominating my days, I left my lawyer wooer.

In my broken state, the words of one of my teachers, Dr. Richard Moss, came to me. If one wanted to heal from any illness there was a sure cure. "Take yourself to the ocean and for two weeks be totally there with the ocean. Then journey to the mountains and exist for two weeks totally in the now. Next, one could go to the desert and be there wholly for two weeks. Finally, one could go to the hot springs and be there fully for two weeks." He declared if you did this, any illness would be cured.

I decided to do this immediately. My problem was that the hurt was so great in my brain that I could not drive. My dear co-heart, the Sunshine of My Life, a person who had stood beside me when I left my husband of ten years, and the man with whom I had a 'yo-yo' relationship with for several years thereafter, had been watching my life from a far and he volunteered to drive me the first leg of my healing sojourn.

Throughout our years of association, he consistently believed that I truly had worth and value. He said that he and I were simply not soul mates. "We would know it if we were, and we weren't." He believed we were part of a tribe that had come together to help the Earth.

As an active 'journaler', my writings became like a therapeutic counselor, yet the few entries I entered the past few years focused on this male/female relationship I had or did not have with the 'sunshine of my life.' The following excerpts are examples of a few of those entries.

"SUNSHINE OF MY LIFE,"

"Seldom have I shared on paper my feelings, cares for you! Tonight as I was `reviewing' my diary, some understanding came my way. A Rimmer quote I've kept is 'the secret to a man's sexual enthusiasm is not because the woman is a stranger but because of the adoration in the eyes of a woman who he knows cares about him.' This may seem a simple statement, but with thought much meaning comes forth! I know that love can build and build. Once one has learned 'it' to a certain point, it can easily be expressed, shared with another open person. In a relationship growth occurs with consistency of the communication planes."

"For you and I, we have developed in my opinion an amazing amount of non verbal communication. In fact, I feel that is probably the main reason we still have our special closeness.

I desire a consistency in our earthly relationship. My inability to be centered with our expression is hard. In the workshop last year on relationships, one of the questions Michael asked was "why be in a relationship with beings who are not willing to work on the relationship to the degree that you want to be?"

"Dear Sunshine man, I see with us that I desire changes in you in order for me to be more at ease. Just being able to state this is a release! I know I do not have the right to work on you for these changes. I apologize for any and all energies I have directed towards you in this way."

"I am praying lots for a way for me to work through this deep, fine love I feel for you. Guidance will come for each day I am more and more at peace with "gypsy, single, Sunshine Man". I am not willing to match those energies. I do not want to mirror you. I want a home. I want a consistent, proud mate. I want to be a family."

"On your journeys, please pray for guidance concerning `us,'. Like I've said before I feel our physical lives will be close this lifetime whether we share it as a brother and sister or as mates. I am ready and anxious to live my desired life. You're such a precious soul—I am willing to give all I can. I just know youare seeing a being who is almost `maxxed' in giving."

Then again in April of 1980 I wrote:

"Whew, three years I look upon my journals. In some ways I've felt great motion, movement. In others, I feel, sense I am still the same.

"My sexual, physical self is subdued. I am just getting beyond an ugly stage of being cranky and not liking myself. I am also not hungry for the male/female market place."

"My stage of life with `the sunshine man of my life' still finds me achy and sad. The questions I was asking two years ago are very similar to those I am asking now. As Sunshine Man left for another short trip, he asked me `whether my love for him stemmed from trying to conquer his sould or self; or whether it comes from true love of who his is. A good question. Often times I find myself empty. I seem to sense a need to feel fuller. But then, I seem to `stay overweight', out of prime condition. Slowly, so slowly, I recondition this tired soul. Sometimes it's very difficult to feel young, romantic, believing in the unbelievable. I know I have taken a mighty big bite to chew. All I see happening is that my jaw is getting stronger. All these things demanding my attention, Sunshine Man, Book Store, Food Coop, School Health Programs, Nathan, Sue; oh yes, where did Suzanne fit in. As a man said `As long as you're happy.'"

"Happy. What does that mean? Jesus with his heart embedded with thorns. Mary, the mother and the loved one. Love. Agony to ecstasy. Responsibility and Commitment."

"Oh, Sunshine Man, why haven't I given up yet. It's been three years. Even though we don't fit and we're not soul mates. I feel the time has been very turbulent."

"Freedom is just another word for nothing left to lose."

From my studies in the late seventies, I had yearned to be Healthy, Happy and Holy. A common motto for those who trained in Eastern Philosophy. I know for myself I had jumped into the beautiful psychological and spiritual premises, fibers and had failed to resolve the 'lower' issues in my self. All that emotional energy had been frozen and was now starting to melt.

The Eastern Buddhist idea of right livelihood is a broad based spiritual philosophy. It seeks to integrate our heart values, inborn talents and the internal quest for self realization with our work and daily life. Right livelihood seeks a mindful, focused approach to all work, especially the jobs we hate, and perseverance, self mastery and the attitudes of service and selflessness to integrate into our very way of being.

The Buddha said we become enlightened by sticking with mundane tasks. We use tiresome, repetitive work as a mirror.

For myself, it was clear my 'work' this lifetime dealt with relationships. As each day is fully the Sabbath, and I am walking on the altar of my belief system, learning to stride peacefully with longevity beside a man was extremely important.

When my farm co-heart, not my 'soul mate', volunteered to drive me to the ocean, this too brought strain with it. He had a camp to do later in the spring in California so he agreed to take me if I would then journey up to his survival school obligation in San Francisco. I agreed.

Within a week we were gone, traveling due south to the closest warm ocean in Mexico. The first night in Mexico our car lights quit working. We were forced to park on private property. My man friend was fried with the strain of driving and then putting up with the demands of a young boy child. So as the dense darkness settled in on our temporary camp sight, he left to walk into the cactus strewn desert.

I was started to see movement; someone was coming towards us bearing a light. Then I saw another light. Fear trembled through me, my worst fear was that of the 'boogie' man coming for me in the dark of night' and it was occurring. Terror filled me, I grabbed my son and ran away from the camp to hide in thick bushes. I waited to see who was tracking us, because we were on private property. The light got brighter but no one appeared.

When my friend finally returned, I felt like I'd experience a chapter from Carlos Castineda's science fiction books. I was ready to put down this fear of the unknown, and put it down now. Fear almost strangled the life and breath from my heart and body.

Camping on a remote peninsula, we lived on a sun filled beautiful ocean front away from all of society. Slowly I began to regain inner worth. On what first appeared to be a deserted beach, we soon learned that we were co-habituating with an American Chinese family. The mother, full Chinese became a wonderful ally for me. Her three tiny children and my precocious son were great companions as we were.

We established a daily regime of running on the beach, tai chi balancing exercises, meditation and truly wonderful story telling and cross cultural philosophical exchanges. She taught me how to glean seaweed for food and how to cook a three course steamed meal in one kettle. She taught me how to make chapatis and I would massage her back and reflex her feet. We loved each other more and more each day. Her faltering English was rich with short proverbs of deep worth.

The cultural experience of hearing first hand of her early life in China is etched in my inner sacred film. I too, told my stories and her Buddhist background began to neutralize the extreme of my inner pain, grief and mistrust. I also was beginning to recognize that I was not the only person in life to suffer grueling, painful chapters of life.

My greatest success while being at the ocean was drawing. I had always wanted to do portraits. My inner mind said I could do anything if I just put the time and

SUZANNE LETTING HER HEART ART OUT

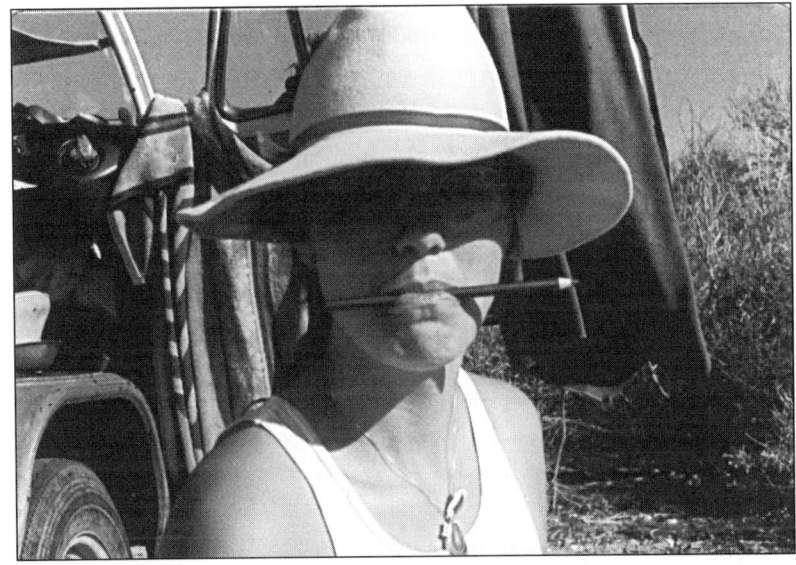

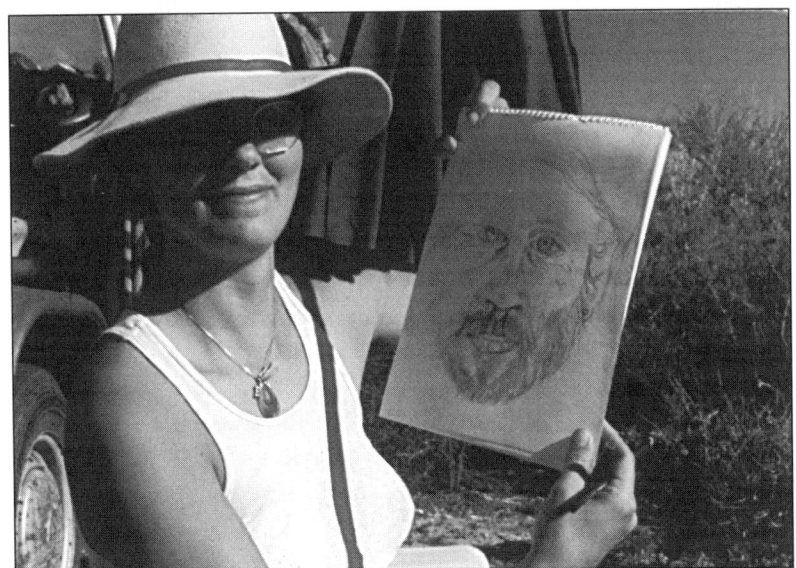

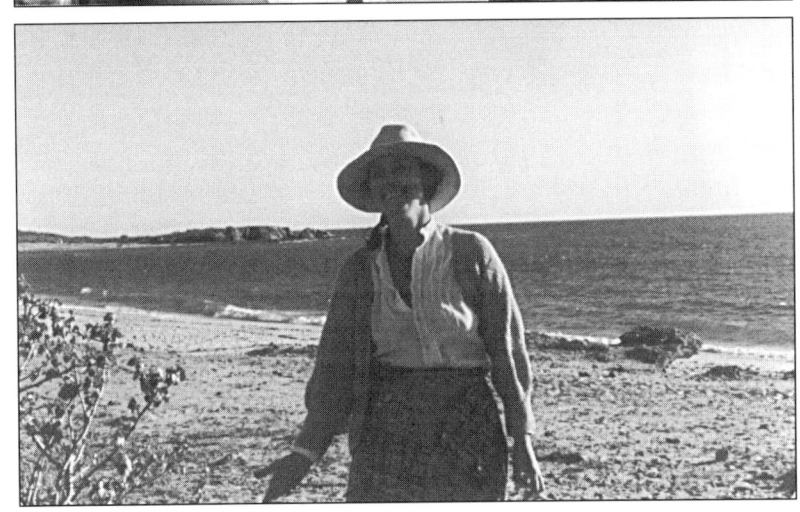

intentions to it. Doing one's heart work allows one to be a true artist. Feeling the artist come through was allowing my heart-mind to heal. My rational mind that was critical was being stilled. Daily I would ask a child or an adult to pose for me. I could do portraits that were recognizable. As the mind perceiveth so shall it be. I could draw, I could do anything if I truly wanted to and if I approached all of life in a prayerful, attentive manner.

    I did not want to leave this peaceful setting but we were obligated to be in San Francisco at a prearranged time. I pleaded with my chauffeur to call the States and see if things were still on schedule. But no, we were on a committed schedule, so sadly, I left my wonderful woman friend and her playful alive family, the sanctuary beach cove and off we went North to San Francisco after a month of bliss and simplicity.

    Those weeks on the warm beach were wonderful.

    The heart artist arrived in me and a deep feminine friendship was honored.

COMPANION ON THE OCEAN
First phase of Dr. Moss's prescription for health

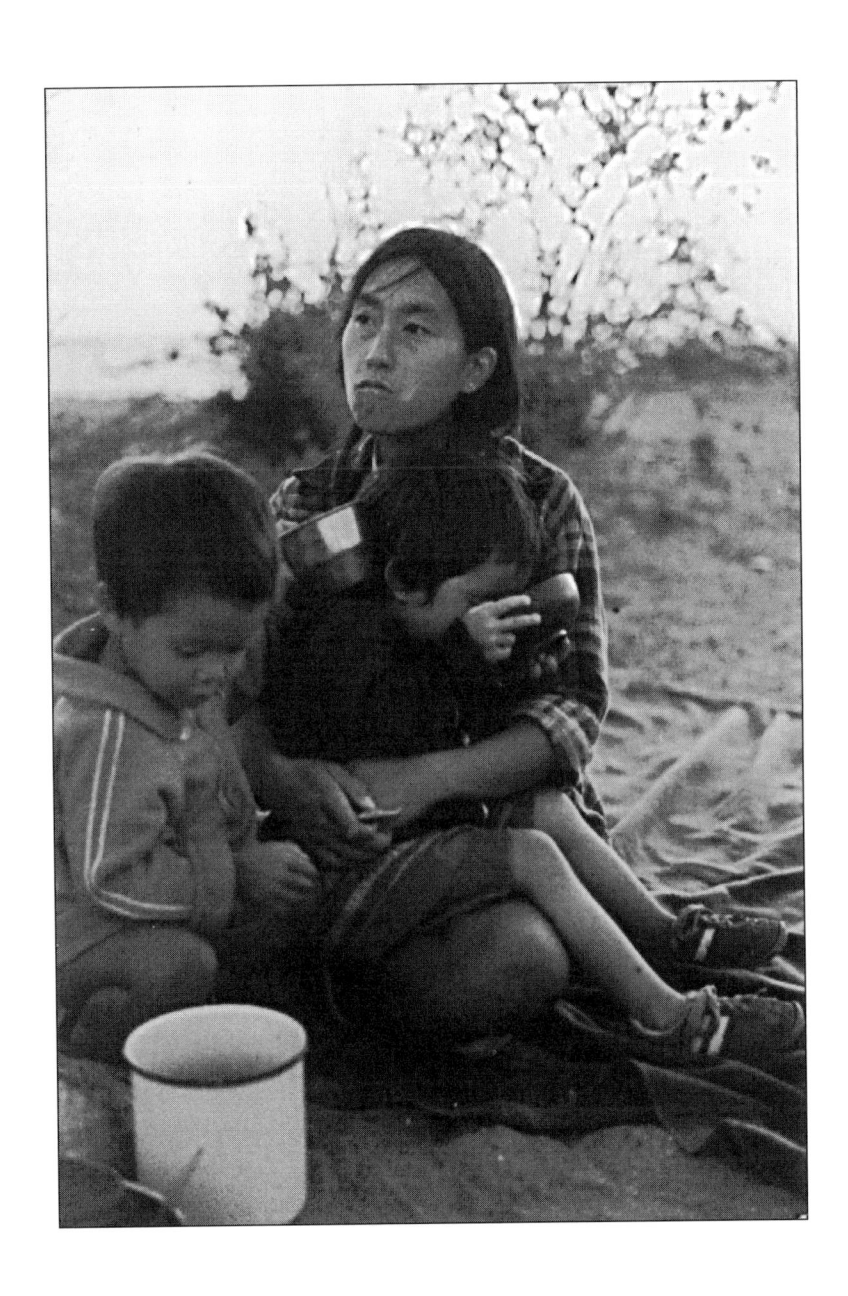

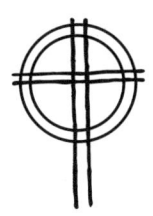

*"GO PLACIDLY AMID THE NOISE AND HASTE,
REMEMBER WHAT PEACE THERE MAY BE IN SILENCE"*

SAN FRANCISCO SURVIVAL SCHOOL — April 1981

Arriving in San Francisco, we drove immediately towards the Golden Gate Park. Just as we were midway over the bridge the car started faltering and we barely coasted off this major eight lane structure. With the car acting very sick, we met the organizers of the survival camp and found out that the prep work hadn't occurred and there was no camp.

Governor Brown had requested this training to help prepare organizations and people for a potential earthquake like the one fifty years ago that had been so devastating. We were encouraged to stay in San Francisco and help organize and make the camp real. We had been unreachable in Mexico to be informed of the delay. I was so frustrated. I felt this possibility while on the beautiful Mexico beach, but my male friend had discredited my 'secondary' senses.

The program was not to occur for another month. A lodging was arranged with an eccentric, wise man. His home in Pacific Heights was a mansion was a like a very classy museum that outclassed any I had ever visited even in Mexico City. Just walking into the four-story mansion initiated another existence this Idaho born girl had never fathomed. A musical, circus clown turned and welcomed us as we approached the curved banisters which were lined with exotic furs. The walls were hung with famous art works Everywhere one looked was a stunning piece of art or a collector's pride and joy.

The owner had a fascination for Oriental artifacts, and a collection of sacred Japanese priest robes, religious tools and much more. There was not one ordinary wall, fixture or stairwell in this home.

We had entered a new reality. My mind was renewed to the roller coaster of altered states. The lump at the base of my skull swelled and I was deeper in pain.

I began writing in the corner of a mammoth library. During the day the owner would hire out certain rooms to do triple X film making. One never knew exactly how many people were his guests. Strange sounds came from under the staircase at night and it seemed like there was ghosts in the walls.

Though my son was in heaven, I felt like life was a dream, much like the movie, *One Flew Over the Cuckoo's Nest.* The top floor had a tremendous view of the bay and the telescopes brought us eye to eye with the boats and waves. I was like a secretary, contacting the Red Cross, the Police, educators, doctors and on and on. I recall a meeting that occurred in the mansion with a half dozen powerful women. As our discussion deepened, we philosophized that until women regained their voice and became politically involved, the masculine aggressive stance would dominate our families and country. We estimated that within ten years women would be much more prominent and respected and assisting the course of our nation. I felt deeply humbled to be in attendance with these fine women. We promised to connect again in 1991. We committed to taking positive steps for women.

I was traveling with the man who at one time was the 'sunshine of my life.' The man I knew was not my 'soul mate', but was one of my dearest friends. Also with us was True Creed, another hero in my life, and a third man, a dark-eyed Indian guide quiet and steaming with passion. And I do not minimize the involvement of my young son who strongly walked beside me. He must have pirate blood, for he loves the ocean and the journey.

I met my first woman healer, a lady trained by a kahuna in Hawaii. The month of retreating did not meet the pressure of the preparation for this workshop and the unsettling living situation. The pain in my head and neck throbbed. Sometimes I could not see straight. The lump in my skull continued to swell. I thought I was dying. The life I was living was so far out of my imagination, that I knew my existence was crazy. With this intensity of witnessing my life, the gentle healer began to work with the pain in my head.

She would introduce me to 'Wave Therapy'. This was a technique of inducing rippling pressure through the cranial bones and internal endocrine glands. Laying on the floor, eyes closed, her palms tightly applying alternating pressure to either side of my skull, I could feel the energetic waves move through the area of pain in my brain. The rippling wave current would cross the hemispheres of my brain, only to have the opposite hand block and then receive the wave and then initiate a return wave back through my cranial region. I was thrilled. This wonderful tool has become a major gift I now teach and share with other.

Just as we were ready to facilitate the Survival camp for Governor Brown, I received a call from my book store manager, partner announcing that there was an out of state investor that wanted to buy the bookstore. This was an answer to our prayers. All the while down in California I had hoped to find an investor for our fine bookstore back in the boondocks of Idaho. I had never drawn a wage for my participation in the book store, plus we were all at the burned out stage of well being and financial reserve. I promised to return as soon as the camp was over to sign the papers to release my involvement with the bookstore.

The workshop was a tremendous success. We held it at the Golden Gate Bridge Park. The setting was majestic, the people responsive and involved. One facilitator was an Olympia trainer, Durveka Spino, who staged various running and movement exercises that enhanced one's knowledge of group dynamics and force. One exercise, Durveka initially had each participant run alone, then we formed groups of three, then five, next seven; each time having us feel while running the geometric formations and total strength of performance. We noticed a dynamic increase in our personal force field and endurance of the total team. The experiences reflected a bigger message surrounding team work.

We went on to set up sample communication systems with the various local agencies.

One of the last evenings at the Park I walked alone up on the ridge above the oceans watching the long processional of boats returning to shore. As the sun melting hues drenched the evening sky, I accidentally missed a foot hold and tumbled downwards through brush and against ragged rocks. Scraping my hands, I finally grabbed a stalk that held my falling force. I barely came away with minimal injury except to my inner critic that saw my life as way too precarious.

Within hours of this three day course, we were back in the van journeying back to Idaho as fast as possible. My body and mind were sick with all the push to create the school. One of the insights gained from the survival school was that this major city would be an island unto itself in the next major earth event. All highways would be barricaded and the people would not be allowed to leave. This observation after the event left me glad to be a country girl with lots of freedom.

Upon arriving home, I wanted to meet the savior to our precious offspring, the book store. I met this wealthy musician, who oozed ego. This slick artisan strutted his knowledge in every field of endeavor, his gift of providing for a better future, and his financial magnitude. I was glad that a solution was found for our bookstore as we had less than a month left before the bank was going to take steps of foreclosure.

Our financial savior was wooing our patrons and many of our local artisans. The musicians thought that a recording studio was going to be created, our writers thought that a small press would be put in downstairs and we thought we would receive an injection to put back life to our stressed and strained dream store. I heard story after story of how every one's dream was going to be fulfilled.

All this talk of his wealth meant nothing. I watched all these people belly up to this man and for myself all I wanted was sound spiritual health. I was sure money was not going to solve my health problems and broken faith in male-female relationships. I was seeking oneness with God. I wanted to believe. Money was not the solution for me, trust in living was.

The 'slick financier' focused on me. He was magnetized towards my spiritual pursuit. I wanted to do a journey back into several sacred spots in Idaho high mountains to the natural geothermal waters. I had not had the opportunity to digest my first leg of Dr. Moss's health prescription. I knew I had to get back to what I felt were the mother waters or original waters. He quickly adjusted his 'song and dance' and with a dear lady friend we traveled to some of Idaho's high mountain sacred centers.

The second stage of Dr. Moss' prescription was two weeks in the High Country. I was scouting the next leg of my healing journey. The past summer I had revisited a natural geothermal site where as a young child my father had taken us often. I remembered a quality of peace and nurturance that was like a recognition of health for me. In what seems to be the top of the world of Idaho, there are densely green mountains with natural hot springs pouring from the moist, velvety river canyon walls. When I would submerge myself in these waters, it felt like I was returning to some ancient, almost mythic mother. One whose waters flowed symbolically through me and deeply eased my mental, physical and spiritual woes. I knew that the high mountain hot springs two week stay was deeply welcomed.

On returning to our rural farm community with my lady friend and book store investor, I was greeted by the police stating that there was something fishy about this man. The money he had promised had not arrived and my business partner was worried. She had begun to sense something wrong about this person and felt we had been kidnapped.

I was stunned that evil had come to me. I very much believed that through my intentions, I was creating my reality. If I was truly doing this spiritual/health recovery process, how could this be? Of course, there was an explanation, the slick financier tried to convince. I challenged this man to be real. We went from a public defenders office to the bank president's office. This man wove a tale of being with the 'underworld'. The money would have come, he said but because the local newspaper had picked up on this exciting survival of our store, he had gained too much publicity. The big boys that he worked through wouldn't send the money to our community. He told us that if he went to Salt Lake City he could safely and discreetly pick up the money and return to us.

We drove back into the mountains, this time with my son. I wanted to know the truth behind this smooth talker. I felt deeply abused. As we were coming down a steep, muddy mountain road, the car's clutch didn't function, and we careened off the wet, slick corner. I was in the passenger seat and as the car teeter-tottered I found myself staring down the incline, my son was pitched from the back seat over my head and into the door. I heard myself wail Oh God, forgive me, please don't let us die. It was like a giant invisible hand held still the swaying vehicle. As we climbed out the driver side, I heard a voice say "get out, you are loved."

My son collapsed on the road, hugging the earth and giving thanks for being alive. I stared at the teetering car, the broken child, the crazy investor and crumbled onto the ground and began rocking myself. I knew this had to be a bad dream. It couldn't be real.

This man with the confused identity cried and asked to be forgiven. I was numb.

We had help pulling the van back to the road and then we proceeded to go directly to my local bank president. I can still see the banker nodding and understanding this man's laundried money tale. The investor carried on this intense dialogue. I was still in a fog. It was too unreal to be understood.

Somewhere in me I knew he was not going to return. I walked with him out the bank door and I watched as he took off to go to the airport and supposedly retrieve the necessary money. He never returned. In time I would label this my chapter or learning about 'the con,' a game player, going for a person's most vulnerable aspect.

The next day, both our store's manager and the other partner lost it. They walked out the back door to never return. It was my 'baby' to complete. Within a week our store was closed by the bank. Many books ended up at our local library. I stepped through the paces to disperse the books but I was an empty shell. I truly discovered who my true friends were. All those others that were going to be saved by the 'monied investor' projected their loss on me. I was a scapegoat, one more time.

My one lady friend, Symphony, had stood beside me during this short reality of total confusion. In the ten days I had been back from the ocean, she had gone with me on the sacred mountain journey. I felt safer with her near and now she and I locked the store for the last time and walked away. Every part of me felt the weight of this tremendous dream and service thrashed and dead. I wanted her to drop me off in the desert to die. She refused to leave my side. This was the fourth time in less than a year that my life had been challenged. The first was on the river, the second on my trip to the ocean when I slid, cascading down an edge towards the ocean below. The third time occurred while driving with the 'con' on a snowy, mountain road, as he shifted wrong and slid too fast over the edge of a high, windy road. And lastly, when I wanted to end my disastrous life. 1980 - 1981 forced me to deal with death.

Reasons for living were obscure, with the exception of my love for my dear son.

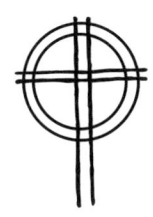

"WITH ALL ITS SHAM, DRUDGERY & BROKEN DREAMS, IT IS STILL A BEAUTIFUL WORLD. BE CAREFUL. STRIVE TO BE HAPPY."

HEALING THE SELF — 1981

My body was running on adrenalin and pure determination. I closed the bookstore with as much dignity as I could muster. Several dear friends watched after me, quietly trying to buoy up the broken shell of a person I had become. Looking back with hindsight, one of the gifts of that tragic time was that I learned who were my true friends.

My massage teacher announced that the next month there was a healing camp towards the border of Canada and Idaho and I should go. Children were welcomed with an interwoven program for the kids to be offered. I felt there was no way I could go back on the road; every penny I owned had been drained by the forced closure of our store. I was still unable to drive. Another part of me quarreled that the third phase of Dr. Moss's healing prescription was two weeks in the mountains and that was exactly where the Health Camp was going to be located.

A friend was getting married in Boise so I journeyed there. This was the sweet and gentle woman who had assisted me during my pregnancy and had attended my 'birthing' process. While in my old hometown I visited with several lady friends. One at a time, they validated me stating that I deserved to take more time out to heal myself.

My dear allies pooled their monies and donated it to me, supporting and affirming me to regain my health and self worth. My massage teacher drove me and our children North to this event that would begin the deep healing of my whole self.

The main facilitator, Paul Pitchford, was trained in the Oriental arts of acupuncture, shiatsu, and five element theory. Paul was introduced to martial arts and Oriental philosophy at the age of ten when he studied with a Chinese teacher from Singapore. He later studied and apprenticed with masters of traditional Oriental healing in Zen Shiatsu Acupressure, acupuncture, nutrition, Tai Chi and meditation.

Paul was committed to practice and teach healing and awareness intensives in which he emphasized guidance by one's spiritual essence. He was a trusted helper with my health. For the past few years he had on a regular basis journeyed to our Southern healing waters and I had received numerous acupuncture treatments and expanded instruction for my organ and nutritional balance.

During the healing retreat, he and other teachers in macrobiotics, tai chi, Reiki, nutrition and herbs, and dance would practice the 'giveaway' of their healing art.

Sleeping in tents, meeting from sunrise to sunset, we fasted cleansed, drank water and herbal teas, shared children responsibilities, danced and participated in the sacred sweat ceremony.

1981 NORTHERN IDAHO HEALING CAMP FOR SUZANNE

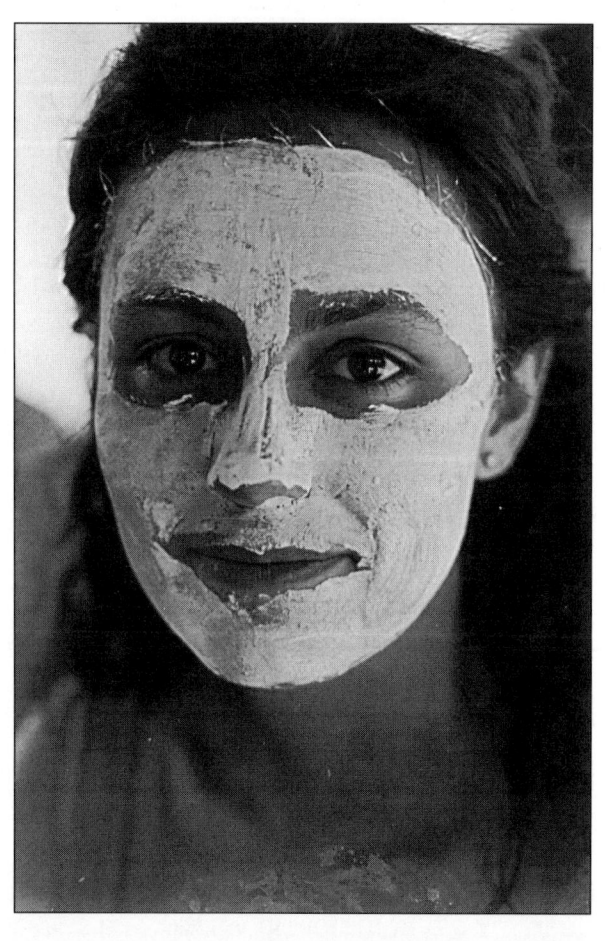

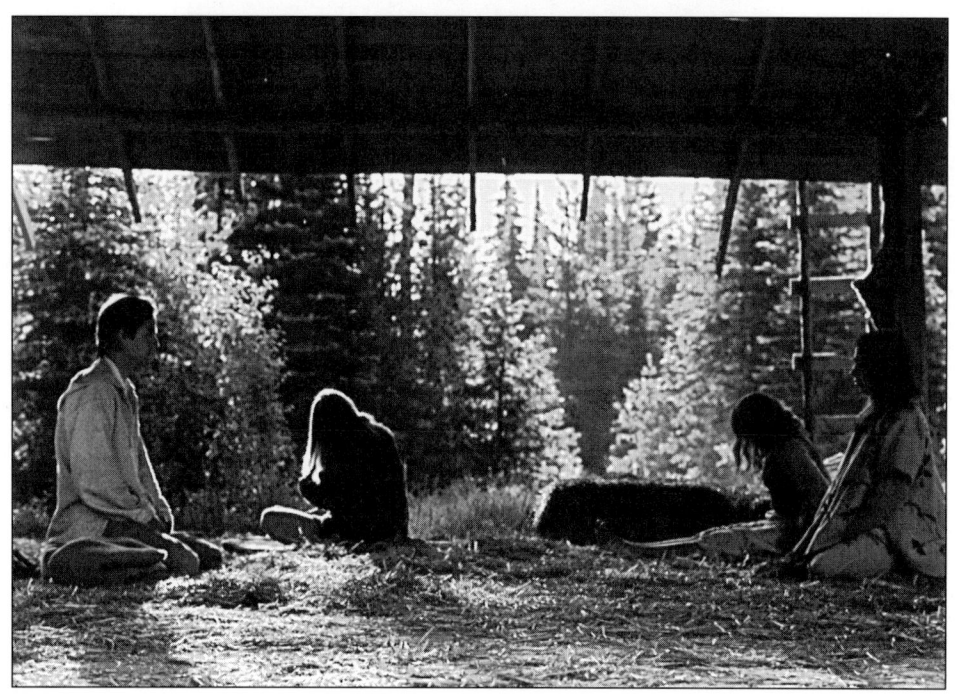

When Phyllis Lei Furumoto, the granddaughter of Takemoto the grand teacher who brought Reiki out of Japan in the late forties, came and presented this natural healing art, I was stunned. As she spoke about this Natural Healing Art that can be translated as "Universal Life Energy", I saw this golden glow all about her shoulders and head. I remember rubbing my eyes, questioning my vision, and finally checking with another in the audience, asking "do you see anything around Phyllis?" I was thankful that another also perceived the glow that `haloed' this dark haired Oriental woman.

This experience marked the beginning of my seeing auras with my eyes open. In the past I had seen 'red' at violent scenes, but only with my eyes closed had I sensed colors around a flame, a plant, or an occasional person.

She went on to explain this Reiki energy flows through a channel providing healing, balancing, relaxation and energizing for both the 'channeler' and the recipient. Since the energy heals on all levels, it treats the source of illness and has a very powerful effect on many varieties of physical, emotional and spiritual problems. Reiki gives the body the energy it needs to ease pain, speed up recovery from physical ailments and aids in the prevention of illness. It's essence is love and peace , helping to bridge the mind and spirit, to transform our lives, overcoming obstacles and accelerating our own personal growth.

Reiki initiates benefit as it calls for one to first administer to one's self, daily. It is both a healing system and a healing discipline. This discipline includes the gift of self discovery of the basic goodness that exists within us all. Reike is not gained through understanding, hard work, or study, but through a gentle daily attention of self treatments that allows us to be replenished and enriched by the energy of Reiki.

Phyllis went on to explain that every one has life force that flows through their palms. Reiki is taught through oral tradition and a rite of initiation. After a Reiki initiation the receiver may notice more aliveness in their hands, as the force field is much greater.

She impressed that words fell short in the explanation of this ancient sacred oriental healing art. She told her grandmother's story of being a student of a Japanese Christian scholar who in the late 1800's rediscovered "the formula" Jesus used when he healed by the "laying on of hands." Phyllis' grandmother brought the art to Hawaii and started her teaching through her granddaughter, Phyllis. Then she wove through words the training from her elder.

Phyllis offered each of us a sample of Reiki in order to experience this healing force directly through our senses. It was good because I had never heard of this healing art. Because of my enchantment with Phyllis, I immediately volunteered to receive a treatment.

We walked up the dirt path to a rustic cedar cabin, high on the mountain top. She and several other Masters had us lie down and with very few words they would systematically lightly touch parts of my body from the head down, front and back. This gentle pattern of hand energy positions created a variety of heat sensation, percolating movement from deep in my body, peace with an intensity that made me feel very dream-like while very awake.

I was fascinated by this mysterious and loving woman. When she touched me it was like 'going home', similar to the sense I had with my neurophone the previous year. This time the sensation was induced through a hand transmitted energy not electronic.

She looked in my eyes and I saw love and peace shower through to me. She impressed that this was a self health tool. One treated one's self first. As often as time allowed, but at least once a day. Giving the Reiki treatment to others was optional. I knew that this form of Oriental art was part of me, but I did not have any money to pay the obligation for learning the healing art. As I left the cabin, I ached to be initiated. Phyllis walked with me for a short distance. I shared how right this felt. She confirmed that she knew me of old and yes this Reike should become my tool.

Since my divorce, money had a nasty feel to me and now was no longer available. What rotten luck. My inner judge lashed through my mind running all the old records of how I was unworthy and wrong, my life was unsupported by reality.

I heard my name being called. It was the golden teacher. She told me that I was natural for this healing art. She could see that I was to gain this special initiation to enhance the flow of 'ki'.

I told her of the closing of our bookstore and my monetary loss. She asked if I had anything to trade. On my neck was a gold necklace that I treasured. I offered it in exchange for the sacred ceremony. She agreed, knowing that sometime in my life money would flow back in and she would willingly trade again. Joy and excitement jumped out of me. Something good was coming my way.

The basic code of Reiki is:

"JUST FOR TODAY DO NOT WORRY.
JUST FOR TODAY DO NOT ANGER.
HONOR YOUR PARENTS, TEACHERS, AND ELDERS.
EARN YOUR LIVING HONESTLY.
SHOW GRATITUDE TO EVERY LIVING THING"

I could honor these vows. These were deep teachings and deep strength to be gained by stepping into these virtues. I spent the next few days training and preparing for my second sacred Oriental ceremony. My 1971 initiation into the Transcendental Meditation movement, an oriental influence, also had an initiation, candles, incense, closed eyes, open palms and lots of trust. It was beyond the mind to interpret, receiving the gift of enhanced life force flow through one's hands. With my mental processes already blown, it was easy for me to trustingly receive.

Paul Pitchford was instructing us in Shiatsu, an Oriental system of acupressure or finger pressure that related to the various body systems, organs, seasons, colors, tastes, and senses. Sometimes it was referred to as the Five Element Theory. He taught us volumes of health knowledge and the hands on location of therapeutic pressure points throughout the body. Each day we learned about the organs of our body and how to give and receive inner-bone finger pressure which related to the parts of the body being studied. Trained meridian technicians were available to help move out stuck or trapped toxins in our systems.

Paul impressed us to improve and balance our nutrition through macrobiotics. He taught "food as medicine - that which makes one well." Our diet during the camp was exemplary. The organs needed certain foods to bring health, whether it was beets for the liver, or aduki beads for the kidneys.

The knowledge he shared was like a graduate course in physiology and nutrition. I took enough notes to write a small book on Shiatsu. Today, I teach and continue to learn from his deep understanding of body chemistry and skeletal muscular/organ inter relations, internally and externally.

Shiatsu establishes information for a plausible prescription to create a body/mind/emotional/spiritual map of one's well being. "The body is considered a sensor, and informational network, a messenger with myriad communication systems- cardiovascular, respiratory, skeletal, autonomic as well as emotional and intuitive." The body uses it's skin and deeper fascia and flesh to record all that goes on around it.

Learning the shiatsu system allows the body to be "a living record of life." The body remembers, the bones remember, the joints remember, even the little finger remembers. Memory is lodged in pictures and feelings in the cells themselves. Like a sponge filled with water, anywhere the flesh is pressed, wrung, even touched lightly, a memory may flow out in a stream." (Dr. Estes. *WOMEN WHO RUN WITH THE WOLVES,* pg. 200)

In the Chinese five element theory every organ has an emotion. Paul taught us what happens when the organ is out of balance. Then the emotions also swing to an unhealthy state. For example when the liver is balanced then one has a strong sense of spiritual grace, but if it's constantly challenged then the emotion of anger erupts. The kidneys, when healthy, know peace and when out of balance register fear and so on. (See insert on following pages.)

Oriental medicine, Paul stated, philosophized that there was no such thing as an accident. He implored us to see the body as a map. Every line, blemish, bruise, or strain reflects an organ or system involvement. A cut at the end of one's little finger is likely to be connected with one's heart or small intestine depending on the location of the injury. He contended the body communicates with us if we can hear it. There is always a forewarning before an injury. This feeling or voice or presence is connected to our spiritual nature. This message was hard for me to receive. Much of me still felt like a victim.

Over and over again I heard him say "Put it down; release whatever is your worst habit. This may be the hardest thing to do, but we must get on with it. Let it go."

My teacher went on to explain that the language of these ancient Chinese system reflects rivers of energy flows which are either YIN (female) or YANG (male). All outside nature reflects our own inner nature. Circulation and balance of the 'chi' energy is one of the great secrets of life. There is a healthy circular flow or elemental flow and a destructive path.

ORIENTAL FIVE ELEMENT THEORY

FIRE	Heart/Small intestines — joy rules tongue
EARTH	Stomach/Spleen — meditation/peace rules mouth
METAL	Lung/Large intestines—grief rules nose
WATER	Kidney/Bladder — fright/fear rules ears
WOOD	Liver/Gallbladder — anger/balance rules eyes

FIVE ELEMENT CHART
The Five categories of things classified according to the Five Elements.

HUMAN BODY

Five Elements	Yang	Yin	Senses	Tissues	Emotions
WOOD	Liver	Gall Bladder	Eye	Tendon	Anger
FIRE	Heart	Small Intestine	Tongue	Vessels	Joy
EARTH	Spleen	Stomach	Mouth	Muscle	Meditation
METAL(AIR)	Lung	Large Intestine	Nose	Skin & hair	Grief & melancholy
WATER	Kidney	Urinary	Ears	Bone	Fright & Fear

NATURE

Five Elements	Season	Environmental factors	Growth development	Colors	Tastes	Sounds
WOOD	Spring	Wind	Germination	Green	Sour	Shouting
FIRE	Summer	Heat	Growth	Red	Bitter	Laughing
EARTH	Late	Dampness	Transformation	Yellow	Sweet	Singing
METAL (Air)	Autumn	Dryness	Reaping	White	Pungent Spicy	Weeping
WATER	Winter	Cold	Storing	Black	Salty	Groaning

FIVE ELEMENTS
CIRCULAR HEALTHY ORGAN FLOW

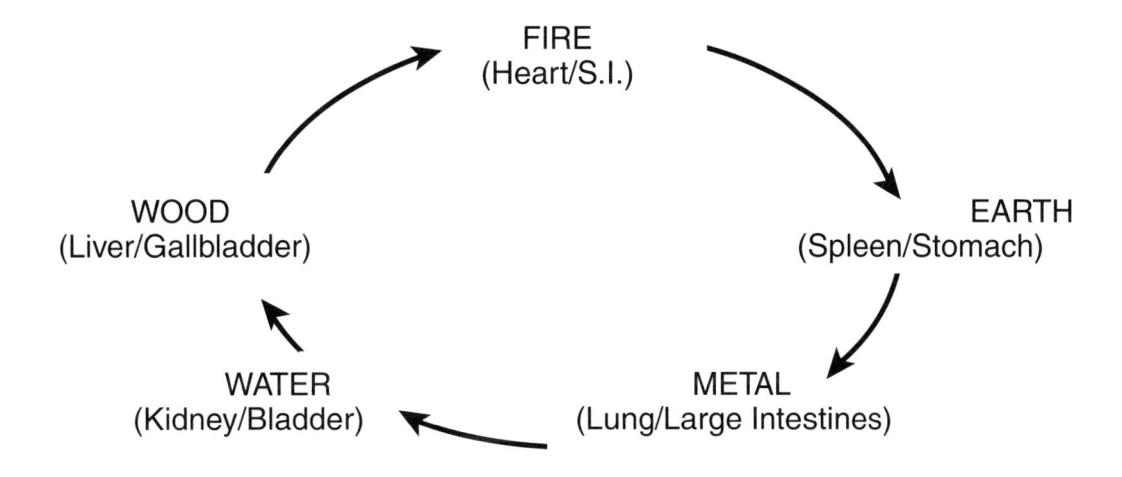

```
        FIRE
      (Heart/S.I.)

WOOD                EARTH
(Liver/Gallbladder)  (Spleen/Stomach)

  WATER           METAL
(Kidney/Bladder)  (Lung/Large Intestines)
```

"The circle represents the "Generation" cycle. It shows how the heart strengthens the spleen, the lungs strengthen the kidneys, the kidneys strengthen the liver, the liver strengthens the heart. It is a circulating process, each organ drawing strength from the one that precedes it and strengthening the one that follows. Improving the state of a weak organ also strengthens the condition of the following organs (its children). Similarly, the weakening of an organ may result in its replenishing its strength by drawing from the organ that precedes it (it's mother).

STAR FIGURE INSIDE CIRCLE IS THE PATH OF DESTRUCTION

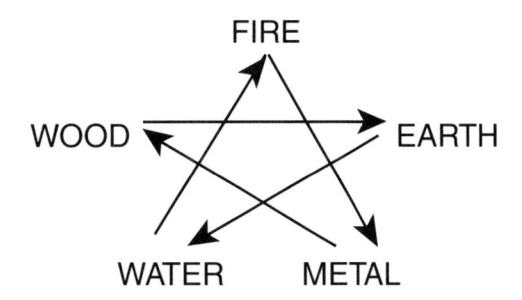

```
           FIRE
WOOD              EARTH
      WATER  METAL
```

The inner star made up by the arrows portrays the Destruction cycle. This shows how overly strong kidneys make a weak heart, an overly strong spleen makes weak kidneys, overly strong lungs make a weak liver. An overly strong liver makes a weak spleen, and an overly strong heart makes weak lungs. There is no circling process in these relationships. For example, if the kidneys are too strong and weaken the heart, the heart alone is weakened. There is no repercussion on any other organ.

Now I know enough to call the inside star pattern that of transformation rather than destruction. "The elements are not themselves energy but energy movements, rivers. They indicate the way energy moves and transforms itself in a natural and cyclical process. For instance:

> Wood burns and produces Fire
> Fire leaves ash, which is Earth.
> Earth contains ore, which produces Metal.
> Metal melts and produces Water.
> Water nourishes plant life and produces Wood.

And thus the cycle is completed. However, in a dispersement cycle:

> Wood destroys Earth by drawing on its strength.
> Fire melts Metal.
> Earth pollutes Water
> Metal chops down Wood.
> Water extinguishes Fire.

When the Five Elements of the Chinese system are positioned on the Medicine Wheel:

> Wood — as the generating force — is in the East
> Fire — as the expanding force — is in the South.
> Earth — as the harmonizing force — is in the Center.
> Metal — as the introverting force — is in the West.
> Water — as the reverting force — is in the North.

Each element is Spirit, but it is not individuated like 'human' Spirit, nor is it a 'group' Spirit, as with animals and trees. Rather, it is a class of Spirit. This is why Native Americans referred to the Elements as Spirit clans.

Each element has identifiable qualities and characteristics:

> Fire is creative, expansive, vigorous, explosive, consuming.
> Water is fluid, adaptable, absorbing, contractive, dispersing.
> Air is boundless, quick, impatient, unpredictable.
> Earth is stable, patient, nurturing, stubborn.

Each Element predominates in one of the four principle bodies of a human being:

> Element of Earth predominates in the physical body.
> Element of Water predominates in the energetic body.
> Element of Air predominates in the mental body.
> Element of Fire predominates in the Soul body."

(Dr. Fred Alan Wolf. *WHERE EAGLES FLY,* pgs. 102-109.)

Woven through our daily camp existence was prayer, thanksgiving and playful exchanges in and with nature. Our children were respected and fed well.
It was everything I needed at this point in my life.

I also watched my massage teacher reunite with an old love, a woman who did sound and touch therapy. I knew he was in relation with another woman back home, but not married. Again I witnessed the philosophy of love the one your with, and, that man is not monogamous. I chose to stay away from male/female exchanges.

I did not know it when I went north to this workshop, but it was an event for the wounded healer. According to the Bible, First Corinthians, Verse 12, we each have a spiritual gift, 'diversities of gifts, but the same spirit.' In our lifetime, each one of us must pursue that gift, and it's not always easy.

> "There are diversities of administration,
>   but the same lord.
> and there are diversities of operation, but is
>   the same GOD which worketh all in all.
> But the manifestations of the SPIRIT is given
>   to every man to profit with.
> For to one is given by the Spirit the word of WISDOM
>   to another the WORD OF KNOWLEDGE by the same spirit;
> To another the working of MIRACLES"
> to another DISCERNING OF SPIRITS
>   to another PROPHECY;
>   to another DIVERSE KINDS OF TONGUES
>   to another INTERPRETATION OF TONGUES;
> But ALL these worketh that ONE and the selfsame SPIRIT,
>   dividing to every man severally as he will."

I was validated in the gift of healing touch. Deeply I knew I was not a masseuse but rather someone with heart felt intentions and willingness to connect at a soul level with people desiring to assist myself and others to 'wellness.' This felt good. I contemplated that there might be a future out there for me in the healing realms.

On the return trip to the farm, I again checked in with my lady friends who had funded my healing retreat. The mother of the boy-child the same age as I mine and the Sioux Medicine person, True Creed, invited me to come back early in the spring and help with the next Two Ravens At Tall Pine Earth Ceremony. I promised to think about it. In the back of my mind I heard the words of a dear elder yoga instructor friend who had called me during the dark days after the bookstore closure, "When one door closes, another will open." She had insisted that I have patience, because she knew opportunity would knock again.

Arriving back at our canyon rim farm, I was met by very unfriendly neighbors. The three other corporate farm partners disliked me. It became clear that I was a non-person. They avoided contact with me. I turned inward, meditating often, doing reiki sessions on myself daily, walking and praying. Children were my focus. Anytime someone's child from my circle of friends would get ill, I would end up touching him or her.

It deeply concerned me that the commandment of the elder brother, Jesus to "Love thy Neighbors as Thyself" was so frayed in my life. I knew it to be an important spiritual code. I was not living in a kind neighborhood anymore.

I would walk the eighty acre farm and feel so alone and cold.

At this time in my life the knowledge of healing with the Earth and her natural herbs and plants was extremely important to me. I was learning how to feed myself as healthy, alive and balanced of foods as possible. A simple chart came to me that helped me in the manner I combined my foods. Often my choice of nourishment had a scrambling affect on my digestion and health. By watching the order in which I consumed made me stronger. The chart is:

FOOD COMBINING CHART

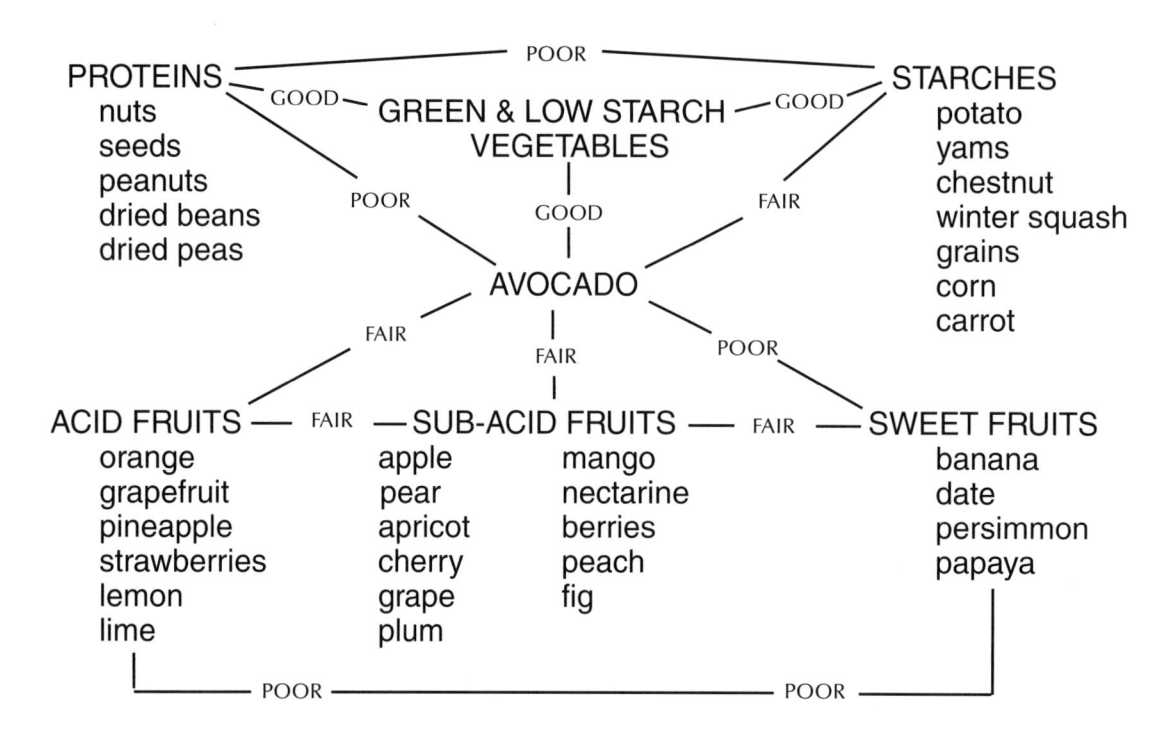

```
                        ——— POOR ———
  PROTEINS ⎯⎯⎯⎯⎯⎯⎯⎯⎯⎯⎯⎯⎯⎯⎯⎯⎯⎯⎯⎯⎯⎯⎯⎯⎯⎯ STARCHES
    nuts       GOOD — GREEN & LOW STARCH — GOOD    potato
    seeds              VEGETABLES                  yams
    peanuts                |                       chestnut
    dried beans   POOR    GOOD      FAIR           winter squash
    dried peas             |                       grains
                        AVOCADO                    corn
                           |                       carrot
              FAIR        FAIR       POOR
                           |
  ACID FRUITS — FAIR — SUB-ACID FRUITS — FAIR — SWEET FRUITS
    orange        apple       mango            banana
    grapefruit    pear        nectarine        date
    pineapple    apricot      berries          persimmon
    strawberries  cherry      peach            papaya
    lemon         grape       fig
    lime          plum
       └─── POOR ──────────────────── POOR ───┘
```

Eat but one concentrated protein food at a meal. Tomatoes may be combined with non-starchy vegetables & nuts or avocadoes. Fruits should be eaten as a fruit meal, unmixed with other foods except lettuce & celery. Melons should be eaten alone.

"Food combining principles are based on the physiological chemistry of the human digestive system. It has been observed that greater digestive efficiency will result when foods are eaten in simple and compatible combinations. This, in turn, helps to secure greater assimilation of food nutrients." (D. Nelson, *The Plan.*)

I had been given a simple herbal manual that became a constant resource in my natural healing process. I am including it for you to have on hand as a nice reference.
HOW GLAD I AM!
I LOOKED FOR YOU BEFORE!

The Female Growth About Champion Fields and Places Well Bordered By Running Water —HERBS. By Janice Areline

CONTENTS:
HEADACHE
STOMACH
COLDS
FEVER
BURNS
TOOTHACHE
EAR ACHE
EYE INFECTION
HAY FEVER - SINUS
INFECTION
SKIN DISORDERS
CONSTIPATION
DIARRHEA
HEMORRHOIDS
RHEUMATISM —ARTHRITIS

Taking an attitude of healing — positive mental and emotional energies that have tremendous effects. Believe in what you do.

Relaxation — the key to achieving good health and promotion of healing—
Learn to release tensions and relax.

ALTERNATIVES

Beverages - serve with honey
    Mints, Sassafras, camomile, pennyroyal, jasmine, rose hip, anise, darjeling, oo lang, mate, yerba buena, mu, red zinger, constant comment

EXPERIMENT WITH

Nutritional aides
    Brewers Yeast . . . B Complex
    Wheat Germ . . . . . E + Protein
    Kelp + Dulse . . . .Minerals + Proteins

Vitamins
    Alfalfa Sprouts . . . . . K - D - A
    Rose Hips + Parsley . . . C
    Milk + Bone Meal . . . . D
    Paprika + Lemon grass . . A

Antiseptic

    Myrrh, Golden Seal, White Oak Bark, Wintergreen

Astringent

    Alum, Myrrh, Tannin, White Oak Bark, Comfrey

Antibody

    Yogurt, Acidophilus foods

Sedative

    Honey, Mints, Camomile, Hops, Anise Seed, Balm

Stimulants

    Cocoa, Coffee, Black Tea, White Sugar, Yerba Buena, Guarana, Kola Nut

SYMPTOMS

HEADACHE
- Tension Headache — spasms + tension
    - Relax, Deep Breathing
    - Massage—upper forehead and lower back neck
        - both sides of temporal forehead
    - Foot Baths + Massage
        - camphor — lavender essences
    - Teas —mint + honey + Pennyroyal
- Systemic headache — Disease + Infections
    - Salicylic Acid = Aspirin
    - Teas — White Willow Bark (salicylic acid), Oak Bark (Tannin)

- Eye Strain Headache
    - Relax — cool packs to the eyes

STOMACH
- Overeating and Nerves
- to calm -honey, mints, balm, clover, camomile (women)
- to vomit - lobelia — finger in throat
- cramps - camomile (women), honey, white oak bark,
    - relax and release tension
- to expel gases - Soda Bicarbonate 1/2 tsp. to 1 cup water
    - Charcoal 1 Tablespoon to 1/2 Cup Water
- to prevent stomach upset - serve with meals
    - Clover, mint, sassafras, ginger, yarrow, cardamon
    - Balance Heart and Mind

COLDS
Rest + sleep + increase liquids
Vitamin C., honey, lemon, rose hips, parsley, mints
coughs - licorice, anise, yerba santa, wild cherry bark, mu, horehound,
sore throat - slippery elm, lemon balm, salt water gargle, apple cider vinegar gargle
mucous breakdown - steam inhalations w/menthols, tiger balm, eucalyptus oil, 'White Flower Essence'
cough syrup
    2 parts mint + 1 part rose hip
    Boil 1/2 hr. add honey and lemon
Mountain Remedy
    1 tsp. cayenne pepper + tsp. garlic powder
    w/tomato juice, salt taste
    one shot sure cure

FEVER
increase liquids — sponge bath
cool packs to head, encourage sweating
A + C — Lots T.L.C.
teas — cayenne pepper, garlic, chickweed,
    white willow bark (salicylic acid)

BURNS
Heat Burns - cold water treatment
    Aloe Vera Gel, Vitamin E
    orally A + C (for skin)
    Avoid infections w/dry dressing
Chemical- water wash — milk baths +honey
Sun Burn - vinegar/water wash
    aloe vera, cool sponge baths, rest

TOOTH ACHE
Oil of cloves, peppermint oil,
  raw garlic clove against tooth,
  marshmallow root poultice

EAR ACHE
Alternating hot and cool packs (stimulates blood flow)
Sweet oils clove, garlic juice, eye bright tea, sulfur

EYE INFECTION
Slippery Elm Poultice — relax
wash 1 tsp golden seal
1 tsp boric acid   steep 15 minutes
1 quart of water
sty - keep area clean —

wash 3 - 5 times daily
hot pack 15 minutes, 3-4 times daily

HAY FEVER & SINUS
local area honey comb (natural antihistamine)
garlic juice with water as nose drop (good drainage)

INFECTIONS
Keep area clean - hot packs
  orally supplement protein, B12 + C + A + E
wounds - poultice w/golden seal, myrrh and castor oil, alum,
  plantain, comfrey
blood purifier - garlic, cayenne pepper, comfrey, fennel + hops flowers,
  borage, red clover, dandelion
cold sores - corn starch (to dry out), golden seal, onion juice,
  garlic clove
boils - hot wet pack w/poultice of golden seal + myrrh -
  drink blood purifier teas, supplement A + C vitamins
  cool baths— When boil come to head, lance, keep clean,
  heal w/poultice

SKIN DISORDERS
Itchy Infection - Poison Ivy
  Keep area cool + dry
  Rosemary flower/sage wash
  plantain poultice - soda bicarbonate pack — keep clean
staff - keep area clean —
  soda solution soaks - gum benzoin — antibody
rashes - cool baths — corn starch — soda packs
soothes skin - witch hazel/rosewater glycerol

CONSTIPATION
Flaxseed, castor oil, bulk foods,
Increase liquids — beverage teas
Fresh raw fruits + vegetables

DIARRHEA
Increase liquids — beverage teas—
Avoid - Dairy Foods + fresh raw fruits +
  bran + coffee + fried foods —
Watch for dehydration

HEMORRHOIDS
Witch Hazel Packs — Warm Baths 1/2 hour —
Relax + avoid constipation

RHEUMATISM & ARTHRITIS
        Exercise — heat oils and Massage—
        Relax - Release tension -
        Vitamin E - Copper Jewelry near joints
        Teas - Chamomile, sage, alfalfa, mints, rosemary,
            comfrey, wintergreen, St. John's Wart

                LIFE IS BEAUTIFUL!

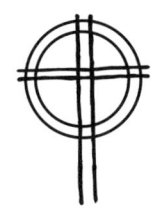

"TAKE KINDLY THE COUNSEL OF THE YEARS. GRACEFULLY SURRENDERING THE THINGS OF YOUTH. NURTURE STRENGTH OF SPIRIT TO SHIELD YOU IN SUDDEN MISFORTUNE. BUT DO NOT DISTRESS YOURSELF WITH IMAGININGS. MANY FEARS ARE BORN OF FATIGUE AND LONELINESS. BEYOND A WHOLESOME DISCIPLINE, BE GENTLE WITH YOURSELF."

NEW AMERICAN MEDICINE SHOW — FALL 1981

My massage teacher convinced me to do another fast and organ cleanser in my course of regaining health. He invited me to attend The New American Medicine Show scheduled in Boise. At the end of my last cleanse I experienced royal belly cramps. Cleaning out toxins involves many layers of release with the body. My illness was like a phantom. First the illness would strike in my head, then my belly, then my ovaries, and back up to my neck.

I chose to do the fourth part of Dr. Moss prescription for becoming well and was spending a concentrated time at Miracle Hot Springs near our farm. I included a fasting cleanse directed at easing some of the stress in my liver/gall bladder and spleen organs. It is often necessary to remove toxins from the lining of different organs and the walls of the large intestines. It is like cleaning up clogged plumbing. Besides a lemon/water/cayenne and maple syrup juice diet for a week, I would take several medicinal enemas.

The prolonged soaks in the natural geothermic water next to the bubbling Salmon Falls River helped draw/percolate unnecessary waste out the pores of my skin. Swimming lap after lap, breathing and gliding in the outdoor pool set in the valley of a narrow canyon close to the Snake River and seeing the beauty of all nature, the birds and kind peoples nourished my body deeply.

I was receiving massage therapy especially focused on my digestive and elimination systems. If the walls of the intestines are contaminated or plugged with that which we can not eliminate, the aged toxins leak into our blood stream.

If a person has unhealthy blood, the kidneys are overtaxed and the adrenal glands get quick continual stress triggers. On a daily basis I tried to consume 'live' foods (those freshly squeezed or juiced) and some form of chlorophyll. I was learning to help strengthen the blood we had to feed it, and consuming chlorophyll was giving both the liver and the spleen help to get back in balance. I had committed to a truly deep cleanse. At the end of my fast I was driven to Boise to attend the conference, light headed and tender from extreme stomach pains and cramps.

Sam Zambito facilitated the The New American Medicine Show with Dr. Irving Oyle, Dr. Paul Erhlich and Jack Schwartz as the headlined teachers who would share with us a new view of health.

SUZANNE LETTING GEOTHERMAL WATER HELP HEAL

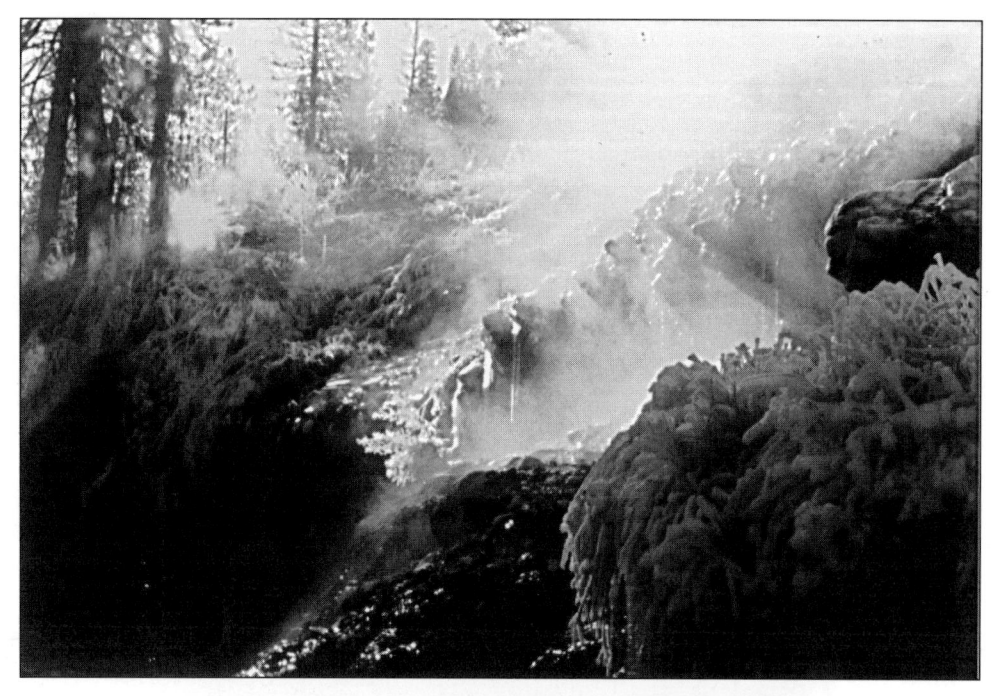

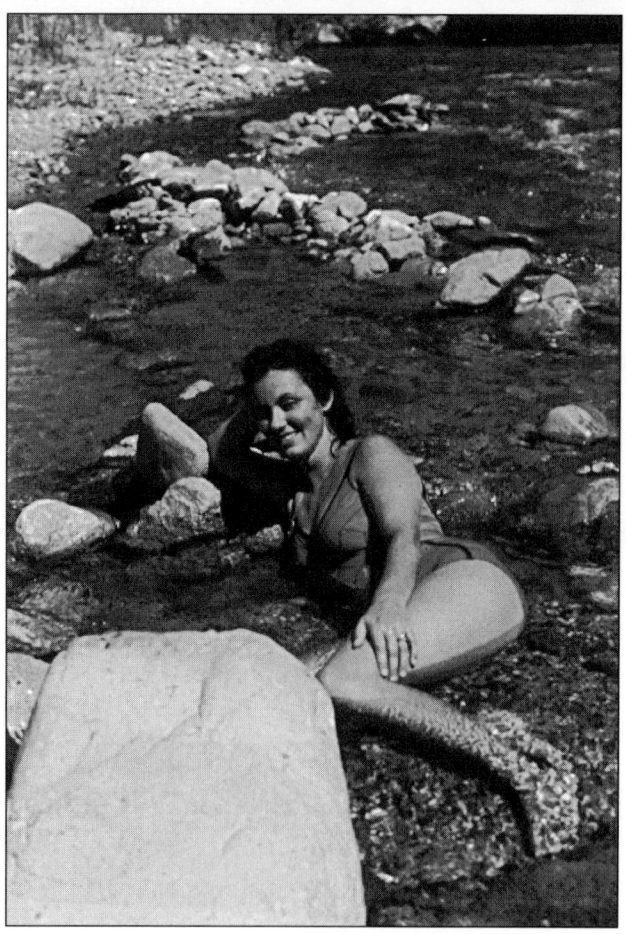

In my newly altered/cleansed state of health, I heard and understood like never before. I especially heard that life was a continual process of death and rebirth. I felt raw from my "death process" of the previous year. I was setting every available intention to be well.

Dr. Irving Oyle, M.D., an author from the University of Hawaii started his sharing with "It's time to end the `magic bullet' theory." He went on to say that his colleagues were killing patients faster than disease was. He impressed that the original physicians were `healer-priests'. The spiritual aspect was known to influence one's well being.

Dr. Oyle went on to explain that germs were mutating so fast that medicines were becoming cost prohibitive. He related that during the Los Angeles doctor strike, the people in the hospital got better by 35-50%. In the New England Journal it was reported that 85% of all disease did not respond to treatments. 85% of disease was related to heart, stroke or mental strain and the remaining 15% was polio, smallpox and disaster.

For quality health a patient's mind over matter was critical. Stress is an energy release in direct association with the adrenal glands which process the here and now, our reaction to life.

ILL meant to him, I Lack Love. The state of total awareness. When sick we're not conscious of what's happening to us. When ill we operate from a different mental component.

For example, sciatic pain aggravated in a man's buttock was often found to be connected with the massive lump of a wallet which pushes inward over the origins of the sciatic nerve. He connected the wallet with the materialism of one's ego.

Next he spoke of how often women have a 'pain in their neck' where the purse burdens their shoulder. Dr. Ehrlick, author of *The New American Medicine Show* insisted that healing comes only from that which takes patients away from entanglement with one's ego.

The heart, a number one source of disease, can be stopped by either the male or female ego.

Type A personalities, in order to survive, must beat everybody else. A measure of success is by the measure of how many things one has. There's very little time for friendship or love just work, work, work.

In contrast, type B personalities believe that the universe loves them and they are optimistic. As Einstein asked "Is the universe friendly?" One's answer greatly determines consequences in all regions of life.

In 1977, the Nobel prize which was based upon the above question contended that one's decision as to what type of universe one believes they live in determines that person's state of health. Do you feel doomed or do you perceive yourself to be still in the garden of beauty? The brain, Dr. Ehrlick contended, is like a gland and it secretes two basic chemicals/juices. The first secretion is induced because of stress stirred by self consumption through judgmental, cynical, negative critical thoughts. This secretion is known as carcinogen.

The second type of brain secretion is know as endorphins, or 'joy juice'. It results with acts of random kindness, joy, love, acceptance and a positive believing attitude.

"What the brain secretes determines one's health." Next he stated that every disease must be recreated, instant to instant. You recreate the body perfectly at every instant. What's important is that everybody in this world has something they're suppose to do. Either get on with it or get sick. Einstein stated "You can do anything you want but chose it!" Therefore, do only what you enjoy doing. Pay attention to everything you do. Watch your body's feedback—closely.

The greatest healer in life rests within each one of us. He went on the impress that a doctor's job isn't to prevent death at all cost. It was extremely important for doctors not to get in between God and the patient. The power greater than the self must be present to be well, even if death is the next chapter of life.

Then Jack Schwartz, an energy healer and tremendous teacher from Oregon, spoke to f.o.c., fear of change. Emotion, he contended was energy in motion. Health is an evolutionary process. Jack implored us to 'Don't believe in God, know God. He felt that there was no language to explain what we know, so therefore allow one's self to heal without thinking.

Dr. Erhlich referred us to a book called *MIND AS HEALER: MIND AS SLAYER.* He contended if we see ourselves as well right now, long enough, we could heal from any disorder. The brain is like a computer. Roger Sperry in 1981 won the Nobel prize for his proof that the left hemisphere of our brain gives us thoughts and the right pictures.

Jack Schwartz was a person whom during World War II was tortured and mutilated. What it took to survive became the medicine he shared with others. He could transcend pain, and wished others to know how. Somehow the emotional charges ignited in our childhood and adult training that were tragic, harmful, or hurting get transferred to the unconscious base of our mind.

Self health, Jack impressed, was how we view ourselves and how we release our potentials. He implored us to open our knowing systems. He elaborated on guided imagery and the importance of reproducing the reception through an inner artistic expression.

In his book *SETTING THE SEEN: Creative Visualization for Healing,* Alan Cohen states "There is a creative power in the mind that offers unlimited possibilities to all of us. This potential has been virtually unused, except by those great ones we laud as geniuses, inventors, and heroes. The irony—and the promise—of this important ability is that it is certainly not restricted to those who have discovered its value; it is available to you and me in equal measure. We can all experience deep relaxation, health, abundance, love, and peace of mind to the extent that we are willing to channel our imaginative abilities in the proper manner."

The essence of the power of creative visualization is this simple formula: "See What You Want To Be."

Cohen also stated it more practically. "If you want to be something in life—such as more relaxed, clear, or loving—you must first get a mental vision of your ideal self, and then nurture this picture with positive thoughts." He also said a series of guided mental images, "mind pictures", can create positive changes in mental, emotional and physical well-being. "These images have been demonstrated to be powerful tools for personal growth..."

Jack Schwartz declared that a rigid mind makes a rigid body and curing is secondary; knowing what is causing the illness is primary. He declared 'Your joy of today is your suffering of yesterday unmasked." One's ability to witness the suffering that has been stored in our subconscious and has acted out as pain and dis-ease and emotional disruption in our lives brings forth better health, emotionally, physically, mentally and spiritually.

Life without stress is death he 'paradoxically' proclaimed. Jack emphasized that lovecould be relearned to mean life only victoriously experienced. His European countenance and brevity of word, made me listen closely.

He too impressed the importance of our chakra system and its interrelation with one's endocrine system. Declaring that self health was how one looks upon one's self, Jack implored us to allow ourselves to heal without thinking. He wanted us to try to recognize all energies in order to have an open system. By all energies he meant emotions, colors, insights and impressions. He declared that a rigid mind makes a rigid body which quickly could become diseased with the likes of arthritis.

Jack Schwartz implored that curing was secondary but knowing what was causing dis-comfort was essential. What was the source of our dis-ease? Discovery or becoming aware of the health issue is 50% of the healing. When you and one's deep self both acknowledge the hurt, injury, soul wound, then we know we are on the path to being wholly well.

He contended that our computer-like brain responds to stress (carcinogens) and joy (endorphins). Currently we only use 1/10th of 1% of our computer's capacity. He encouraged us to get on with our well being alert through the continual questioning process of self health. Joy represents the first stage in healing. Be excited that one is acting upon and becoming ecstatically holy.

The body is the expression of the soul and the soul is the capacity of an individual's energy within the universal self. The mind is the director and guidance to transformational health.

Towards the end of the conference, Dr. Irving Oyle came back on stage to challenge us to get clear on our own personal belief system surrounding living on the earth. Did we believe it was a friendly, supportive place or not? The right side of the brain connects with the outer space and God. He implored us to stop rationally thinking and start breathing. Breathing in divine thoughts and breathing out one's rational, critical negative thoughts.

He then shared the last event of this New American Medicine Show, a guided journey back into our subconscious to regain a sense of our male, female and child allies. He paralleled these to the male—Joseph, the female—Mary and the Child Christ.

As Dr. Oyle set the tone with music and a sense of permission to perceive, he guided us on an inner visualization using a descriptive script with lots of silence. I recall this huge stag that came out of the high mountain peak, somewhat like Bambi's father in the Walt Disney film. I was so surprised. Usually when a guided imagery had been shared with me I only saw darkness. Then we went on to the female symbol, and immediately a golden circle was seen; and then a red rose manifested inside that stood for my child/Christ self. This was the clearest inner sight experience I had ever gone through. To today on my business cards I use the circle and roses to symbolically represent my intentions of spiritual integrity and good relations with the mother Earth.

I heard simple mandates to simplify, unify and purify. I was beginning to relate that the original healers were spiritual healers, the priest of the communities. Dr. Irving Oyle worked to impress within us that the original healer rests internally.

"The greatest discovery of our generation is that humans can change their lives by changing their attitudes of mind," said Will James Harvard. Energy fields and mind over matter did not seem so opposite any longer.

The biggest contribution one can make to life is getting on with it. Live it. Jesus taught "Ye that believeth in me the works that I do shall he do also and greater works than these shall he do."

Intelligence is the ability to discover and accurately interpret truth coupled with the capacity to accept it and consistently apply it to daily living.

The discovery of laws is the beginning of wisdom. (Gibbs. EYES: THE WINDOWS OF BODY AND SOUL.)

Buddha taught "All that we are is made up of our thoughts; if a man speaks or acts always with good thoughts, happiness will follow him like a shadow that never leaves him."

I would write a closure in my journal "I must begin the journey of self awakening. Writing was a way to dedicate myself to my deep healthy self. Love is the only true expression. Take it in — see it — feel it — love it — do it— be it— The mind's journey takes you in takes you out. See it."

Alan Watts' *THE BOOK: On the Taboo Against Knowing Who You Are* explores an "unrecognized but mighty taboo"—our tacit conspiracy to ignore who, or what, we really are. Briefly, the thesis is that the prevalent sensation of oneself as a separate ego enclosed in a bag of skin is a hallucination which accords neither with Western science nor with the experimental philosophy-religions of the East—in particular the central and germinal Vedanta philosophy of Hinduism. This hallucination underlies the misuse of technology for the silent subjugation of man's natural environment and, consequently, its eventual destruction.

"We are therefore in urgent need of a sense of our own existence which is in accord with the physical facts and which overcomes our feeling of alienation from the universe... For this is always something taboo, something repressed, not admitted, or just glimpsed quickly out of the corner of one's eye because a direct look is too unsettling. Taboos lie within taboos, like the skins of an onion. What, then, would *THE BOOK* say, which fathers might slip to their sons and mothers to their daughter, without ever admitting it openly?

"*THE BOOK* I have in mind wouldn't be the Bible, "the Good Book"—a fascinating anthology of ancient wisdom, history, and fable which has for so long been treated as a Sacred Cow that it might well be locked up for a century or two so that men could hear it again with clean ears. There are indeed secrets in the Bible, and some very subversive ones, but they are all so muffled up in complications, in archaic symbols and ways of thinking, that Christianity has become incredibly difficult to explain to a modern person. That is, unless you are content to water it down to being good and trying to imitate Jesus, but no one ever explains just how to do that. To it you must have a particular power from God known as "grace", but all that we really know about grace is that some get it and some don't."

"The standard-brand religions, whether Jewish, Christian, Mohammendan, Hindu, or Buddhist, are — as now practiced — like exhausted mines: very hard to dig."

"*THE BOOK* I am thinking about would not be religious in the usual sense, but it would have to discuss many things with which religions have been concerned — the universe and man's place in it." "The mysterious center of experience which we call "I myself,"
the problems of life and love, pain and death, and the whole question of whether existence has meaning any sense of the word. For there is a growing apprehension that existence is a rat-race in a trap."

"It is a special kind of enlightenment with this feeling that the usual, the way things normally are, is odd — uncanny and highly improbable. . . . This feeling of universal oddity includes a basic and intense wondering about the sense of things. Why, of all possible worlds, this colossal and apparently unnecessary multitude of galaxies in a mysteriously curved space-time continuum, these myriads of differing tube-species playing frantic games of one-upmanship, these numberless ways of "doing it" from the elegant architecture of the snow crystal or the diatom to startling magnificence of the bluebird or the peacock?"

"But the world is in an extremely dangerous situation, and serious diseases often require the risk of a dangerous cure—like the Pasteur serum for rabies. It is not that we may simply blow up the planet with nuclear bombs, strangle ourselves with overpopulation, destroy our natural resources through poor conservation, or in the soil and its products with improperly understood chemicals and pesticides."

"But the problem of man and technology is almost always stated in the wrong way. It is said that humanity has evolved one-sided, growing in technical power without any comparable growth in moral integrity, or, as some would prefer to say, without comparable progress in education and rational thinking. Yet the problem is more basic. The root of the matter is the way in which we feel and conceive ourselves as human beings, our sensation of being alive, of individual existence and identity. We suffer from a hallucination, from a false and distorted sensation of our own existence as living organisms. Most of us have the sensation that "I myself" is a separate center of feeling and action, living inside and bounded by the physical body — a center which "confronts: and "external" world of people and things, making contact through the senses with a universe both alien and strange. Everyday figures of speech reflect the illusion. "I came into this world." "You must face reality." "The conquest of nature."

"This feeling of being lonely and very temporary visitors in the universe is in flat contradiction to everything known about man (and all other living organisms) in the sciences. We do not 'come into' this world; we come out of it, as leaves from a tree. As the ocean 'waves', the universe 'peoples'. Every individual is an expression of the whole realm of nature, a unique action of the total universe. This fact is rarely, if ever, experience by most individuals, Even those who know it to be true in theory do not sense or feel it, but continue to be aware of themselves as isolated 'egos' inside bags of skin."

"The first result of this illusion is that our attitude to the world 'outside' us is largely hostile. We are forever 'conquering' nature, space, mountains, deserts, bacteria, and insects instead of learning to cooperate with them in harmonious
order. In America the great symbols of this conquest are the bulldozer and the rocket..."

"The second result of feeling that we are separate minds in an alien, and mostly stupid, universe is that we have no common sense, not way of making sense of the world upon which we are agreed in common. It's just my opinion against yours and therefore the most aggressive and violent (and thus insensitive) propagandist makes the decisions."

"It might seem, then that our need is for some genius to invent a new religion, a philosophy of life and a view of the world, that is plausible and generally acceptable for the late twentieth century, and through which every individual can feel the world as a whole and his own life in particular have meaning..."

"We do not need a new religion or a new bible. We need a new experience — a new feeling of what it is to be 'I'. The lowdown which is, of course, the secret and profound view on life, is that our normal sensation of self is a hoax or, at best, a temporary role that we are playing, or have been conned into playing — with our own tacit consent, just as every hypnotized person is basically willing to be hypnotized. The most strongly enforced of all known taboos is the taboo against knowing who or what you really are behind the mask of your apparently separate, independent and isolated ego."

"At this level of existence 'I' am immeasurably old; my forms are infinite and their comings and goings are simply the pulses or vibrations of a single and eternal flow of energy."

"The difficulty in realizing this to be so is that conceptual thinking cannot grasp it...At one extreme of its meaning, "myth' is fable, falsehood, or superstition. but at another, "myth" is a useful and fruitful image by which we make sense of life in somewhat the same way that we can explain electrical forces by comparing them with the behavior of water or air."

"Myth, then, is the form in which I try to answer when children ask me those fundamental metaphysical questions which come so readily to their minds: 'Where did the world come from?' and 'Why did God make the world?' 'Where was I before I was born?' ' Where do people go when they die?' Again and again I have found that they seem to be satisfied with a simple and very ancient story, which goes something like this:

'There was never a time when the world began, because it goes round and round like a circle, and there is no place on a circle where it begins. Look at my watch, which tells the time; it goes round, and so the world repeats itself again and again. But just as the hour-hand of the watch goes up to twelve and down to six, so too, there is day and night, waking and sleeping, living and dying, summer and winter. You can't have any one of these without the other, because you wouldn't be able to know what black is unless you had seen it side-by-side with white, or white unless side-by-side with black.'

"In the same way, there are times when the world is and times when it isn't, for if the world went on and on without rest for ever and ever, it would get horribly tired of itself. It comes and it goes; now you see it; now you don't. So because it doesn't get tired of itself, it always comes back again after it disappears. It's like your breath: it goes in and out, in and out, and if you try to hold it in all the time you feel terrible. It's also like the game of hide-and-seek, because it's always fun to find new ways of hiding, and to seek for someone who doesn't always hide in the same place."

"God also likes to play hide-and-seek, but because there is nothing outside God, he has no one but himself to play with. But he gets over this difficulty by pretending that he is not himself. This is his way of hiding from himself. He pretends that he is you and I and all the people in the world, all the animals, all the plants, all the rocks, and all the stars. In this way he has strange and wonderful adventures, some of which are terrible and frightening. But these are just like bad dreams, for when he wakes up they will disappear."

"Now when God plays hide and seek, and pretends that he is you and I, he does it so well that it takes him a long time to remember where and how he hid himself. But that's the whole fun of it—just what he wanted to do. He doesn't want to find himself too quickly, for that would spoil the game. That is why it is difficult for you and me to find out that we are God in disguise, pretending not to be himself. But when the game has gone on long enough, all of us will wake up, stop pretending, and remember that we are all on single Self—the God who is all that there is and who lives for ever and ever."

"Of course, you must remember that God isn't shaped like a person. People have skins and there is always something outside our skins. If there weren't, we wouldn't know the difference between what is inside and outside our bodies. But God has no skin and no shape because there isn't any outside to him. The inside and the outside of God are the same. And thought I have been talking about God as 'he' and not 'she', god isn't a man or a woman. I didn't say 'it' because we usually say 'it' for things that aren't alive."

"God is the Self of the world, but you can't see God for the same reason that, without a mirror, you can't see your own eyes, and you certainly can't bite your own teeth or look inside your head. Your self is that cleverly hidden because it is God hiding."

"You may ask why God sometimes hides in the form of horrible people, or pretends to be people who suffer great disease and pain. Remember, first, that he isn't really doing this to anyone but himself. Remember, too, that in almost all the stories you enjoy there have to be bad people as well as good people, for the thrill of the tale is to find out how the good people will get the better of the bad. It's the same as when we play card. At the beginning of the we shuffle them all into a mess, which is like the bad things in the world, but the point of the game is to put the mess into good order, and the one who does it best is the winner. Then we shuffle the cards once more and play again, and so it goes with the world." (Alan Watts. *THE BOOK: On the Taboo Against Knowing Who You Are,* pgs. 1-16)

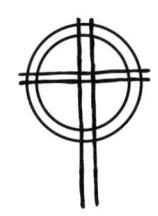

"BE YOURSELF, ESPECIALLY DO NOT FEIGN AFFECTION, NEITHER BE CYNICAL ABOUT LOVE; FOR IN THE FACE OF ALL ARIDITY AND DISENCHANTMENT IT IS PERENNIAL AS THE GRASS."

DECEMBER 1981

Rebirth. I felt raw from my "death process" of the previous year. I was setting every available intention to be well. Winter was settling in at the farm and my ex-lover still lived in the original farm house. The winds were fiercely announcing the cold to come. Huge flocks of ravens and other migrating birds would darken the sky as they journeyed South. I was in deep contemplation of my life after the New American Medicine Show.

During a sweat ceremony held on December's full moon I was embraced by a vision. I felt myself 'journey up a very steep mountain ridge through thick mist, up and over to the other side seeing immediately a scattering of tipis with smoke rising. My attention immediately focused on a circle of elders tightly wrapped in snow covered robes. I swooped so close to the People, I could feel the warmth of the fire on my face. I belonged in that closed circle.'

The sweat lodge became my way of going to church. In the lodge I would pray and pray for a death of the parts of me that were sick and the reunion of my higher, graced self. In this December lodge, I prayed to clarify male-female relationships. I was caught in the drama with my sweet sunshine of my life. He and I had a 'yo-yo' form of intimacy. We voiced a knowing that we were not "soul mates" and we did know how to get along without fighting.

My 'journaling' practice had become my best friend out there in the wind wailing desert edge. Most of my entries were filled with my examination of my relationships with farm members. I was seeking a love outside myself to show up and consistently be present in my life—a special heart companion. "Smile on your sisters and brothers. Love one another right now, right now" was a theme.

I would write "walking through life, being on a graduated time line with an inner knowing of an essence of home and love that doesn't blend with current physical manifestation."

My massage teacher shared with me, "It looks to us, Sue, that when you are weak you look favorably on your Sunshine man and when you're strong and on your own two feet, he becomes unsatisfactory."

I observed the input and watched to see if it rang any bells. The only obvious feedback was sadness. I would write, "When I was masculinely strong I could maintain a relationship with my farm hero. Now, when I feel neither masculine or femininely strong, just healing, I yearned for my home to be a safe harbor where my emotions did not have to be constantly tested. I had proven that I could live with pretty much anyone in this rustic farm setting, but at this time in my life I wanted to live alone.

I had never lived without a male prominently in my home. I had completed the two week retreat with the hot springs. I did not know if I was healed. What was clear was the importance of being true to my personal needs first, rather than every one else's. I was aware of more personal integrity.

My farm friend had stood valiantly beside me numerous times in the past years encouraging my personal growth of self worth, right livelihood, and personal health. We could not commit to be monogamous with each other. Always there was a triangular relationship going on. Either he would have another girl friend or me, another boy friend. Sometimes we'd both be in outside relationships. Never were we able to be a recognized couple, especially in the world outside the farm.

I sensed that in a few months or so after this declaration of wanting to live in separate homes, we'd look back and see this time as when we walked through one door into a clearer, more sensitive rapport with ourselves and others. To me it seemed so much more honest. Now my chalkboard was getting a good cleaning and I would be a clearer energy source. Maybe I could mend this hurt that ached so deep inside me for a healthy male/female relationship.

I had a dream strongly come through me and I wrote "I am passing a house, a three-story stone building whose insides are on fire. At first I try to just walk on by but then I know I must go back and put the fire out. There is already a hose hooked up on the left side so I turn the water on. Meanwhile, an identity to my right also assists in extinguishing the fire. Time passes and again I view the insides of the house and now the house is replenished; no one could tell a previous fire ever had occurred."

Later, in that same dream sequence I meet a man who has two children, a girl and a boy. I would ask myself, are dreams visions of what can become an earthly reality? Maybe that is the quest. First, to acknowledge their existence and then to balance and nurture the dream symbols and archetypes apparent and sometimes paradoxical needs. If they can't be met, death, sometimes sorrow and eventually acceptance occurs.

Life on this plane is real. One cannot put total peace in dreams. Earth has to become peace and joy. I pray to hell with pain and to heaven with joy. Ecstasy for all who will indulge.

Tears of life stream down my heart and vision. Each is directed to live their own statement. Mutual respect and honor extended. Questions are disregarded, trusting the known.

We must be ourself — fulfilling our inner vision, letting our dreams and visions become realities. If the dreams do not become known, faith will fail.

Love and compassion are but a passing notion. The eternal path is guided by a beckoning light and shortcuts are not given, only a step-by step commitment. Earth is an endless unknown; yielding a lack of continuous understanding. The minute one think's they know it, it becomes unknown. The individual self seeks atonement, harmony so that God within equates to God outside."

Music became a way of deep communication for me. The musical themes found in *Take It Easy, Stairway to Heaven, A Horse With No Name, Desperado* or *Knights in White Satin* spoke to my yearnings to attain a peaceful, present, deep, loving relationship with another and with living, period.

My personal life seemed like a wipe out. I didn't feel liked, let alone special to any one. "Humans today hide behind emotions and ego," I wrote. The mind computer is in there awaiting the programming and I was demanding to get into it.

During these early winter days a local paper printed an article about Veteran's Day and how to honor war heroes. It spoke, for what seemed to be the first time ever, about the poor treatment Vietnam veterans received when they returned in the seventies. The article went on to address the Baby Boomer generation born after World War II.

We were a tribe of citizens who saw the space shuttle land on the moon, and saw our heroes, President John F. Kennedy, Martin Luther King, and Senator Robert Kennedy, murdered. Each of these men stood for the values that "this generation believed in...peace and justice, tolerance and equality."

"Those who lived through the sixties aren't likely to forget. The images remain etched in memory, barely faded by time: the motel balcony in Memphis; a dimly lit serving pantry of the Ambassador Hotel in Los Angeles; the televised madness of Chicago's Democratic convention; students smugly occupying the president's office at Columbia University; the clenched fists of Mexico City's Olympics; Marines besieged at Hue during the Tet offensive; the Poor People's march on Washington; Soviet tanks rolling into Prague; clean-cut youth canvassing Eugene McCarthy; President Johnson announcing, "I will not seek, nor will I accept..."; Richard Nixon raising his fingers in the victory sign; George Wallace daring protesters to lie down in front of his car; the bedraggled faces of the captive crew of the Pueblo.

There was Mrs. Robinson, Laugh In, the White Album, Hair, Appollo 8 circling the moon. It was the "Dawning of the Age of Aquarius." It was body counts from Vietnam. There was Watergate and the lies.

The people and events that most influenced the Baby Boomers reflect what has now become named "wounded idealism."

My own search for peace took to me to the farm in 1975. I knew I would either heal or die. Now I knew I had to respond to the editorial in the community paper. I submitted the following letter to the editor, becoming even more vulnerable in our conservative farm community:

ALLOW WAR WOUNDS TO HEAL

"I want to thank you for the thought provoking editorial written on Veterans' Day. I agree that it is time to allow deep festering wounds to heal. For so long, a generation of young people has been faced with burdening decisions as to national respect or moral values, or killing a country's citizenry who were defending their own land. The questions were major. The stand an individual took sometimes forced him/her to be ostracized from the majority's grace.

Today some of our culture's citizens, who are now in their thirties and early forties who have been misunderstood in the past, now wish to be acknowledged as worthy, valuable members of the community. Some have easily slid into social functions by cutting their hair, modifying their spoken language and holding their tongue when jabs have been made to those 'social misfits' who would not condone the Vietnam War and the monies behind the scene.

Others have, with much conviction, kept pace with their own inner voices which have directed them as to how they relate and work within their community. Many who faced the war and the deaths walked away appreciating what has been called the 'quality of life.' This often refers to tight family ties, close earthly reverence and daily health and happiness.

The work process that subscribed to 'working for someone else or system has often been replaced with their own self-defined social occupations.

As an educator, I work with young teenagers who are the children of the young parents of the Vietnam 'error'. I speak with deep concern for this present generation who walk around supporting who's wearing which type of jeans and who's going with whom. I ache when I learn of another ninth grader who is with child. I listen to them seek out love. I know they are hungry for a hero. I pray that in our United States an honest, integrity-filled leader stands true, one who does not bend to the wills of money but stands firm to what the Declaration of Independence represents.

For those of you out there who have not forgiven those 'social misfits' of the sixties, please stop for a moment to consider that a lot of these individuals were upholding the ways of this America's democracy truer than the government of that time was. Let's all try to believe and become better Americans."

Coming into voice with this letter applied a soothing bandage to my mental pain in the late sixties and early seventies.

Easter, April 16, 1996 *The Idaho Statesman* ran the front page story "McNamara Reopening Old Wounds....One Vet says his book should be called "Sorry Bout That."

"Robert S. McNamara's recently expressed regrets about U.S. involvement in the Vietnam War seem to be reopening old wounds and reviving a raw debate that was beginning to slip into history."

"Reaction to the former Defense secretary's revised views, published in his new book, *In Retrospect: The Tragedy and Lessons of Vietnam,* has mostly been relentlessly negative, with little credence or charity accorded his comment that 'we were wrong, terribly wrong.'"
Part of me wondered if the delayed exposure of my book was due to this land-mark exposure by our defense secretary who stood silent to the injustice of the Viet Nam Error until almost twenty years later. Part of me felt vindicated for my outspoken resentment and sadness at the destruction in which we participated.
I truly want to clarify that the men and families who were directly involved in the war are not the issue. I respect them for representing our United States. It was the lying and leadership dishonor that needed to be aired and cleared. Maybe we can now move on to more respect for those who spoke up during those troubled sixties.

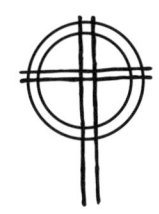

"ENJOY YOUR ACHIEVEMENTS AS WELL AS YOUR PLANS;
KEEP INTERESTED IN YOUR OWN CAREER, HOWEVER HUMBLE;
IT IS A REALITY IN THE CHANGING FORTUNE OF TIME."

EARTH MESSENGERS - 1982

Dark, cold winter was fully embracing our primitive farmhouse that my son and I continued to share with my 'Sunshine'. A home where I felt very alone. So I decided to take my Boise friends up on their offer for me to come and stay with them and help facilitate the fourth fine art festival in the high mountains of Idaho.

Weeks after Christmas I would leave that wood-heated drafty home to go live in a greenhouse room off my friends home near the foothills in Boise. We had big plans to invite to Idaho the Hopi Elder, a spiritual messenger who carried earth prophecies, Thomas Banyaca, and the Planetary Healing 'spokes person' Gordon Feller who would speak to local and global efforts.

Eileen and Peter Caddy from *The Findhorn Community* in Scotland were also asked to participate in our environmental celebration and spiritual union of earth and spirit.

Peter came to visit our project and he emphasized "our radiant energy pervades and gives rise to all life. While it may speak to us through plants, nature spirits or the human beings with whom we share life on this planet, all are reflections of the deeper reality behind and within them. . . essentially, the divas and nature spirits are aspects of our own selves, guiding us towards our true identity, the divine reality within." His involvement helped us to language the importance of an intimate relationship with nature and her aliveness especially through prayer.

We would coordinate with the local university as well as churches and various organizations in Southern Idaho to bring these people in to speak and educate us about the global picture, integrating ancient wisdom and current scenarios in our world.

Simultaneously, True Creed, was also organizing a Sawtooth Survival School with programs in the wilderness. Originally he offered these survival programs for pilots but we mutually desired to expand the school to include challenged teenagers. Since leaving public education, I was outspoken about getting strained youth out in nature, to assist them to regain a confidence and trust within themselves and with the out of doors.

Deeply I felt that by removing youth from the social stimuli of television, cars, telephones and demeaning peers, youth could regain a natural sense of a their birth right of peace, comfort and ease with the earth. Removing the distractions would aid in returning to a place of listening with the inner senses and feeling the rewards of diverse beauty nature gives.

I knew personally how much I had benefitted in being comfortable in the great out-of-doors and I was willing to invest much time to get this program established for the troubled youth in our society. We worked with a national organization that had foster children to set up our youth programs. My work was a gift for the future of the Earth's children and I did not draw a wage.

Until I bore my own child, I could stay distant from my own blood mother. In the generation of Viet Nam and outspoken rebellion to killing people who were protecting their own land, I was determined to help raise healthier, safer children. I knew first hand how painful and fearful it is to be raised around violence, verbal abuse, physical misuse and general critical judgement and demeaning relations both within my blood family and in the cultural as a whole.

I vowed never to raise a child the way I was raised. When I was a public education teacher, I was involved with special programs on campus as a counselor for youth in crisis. I personally vowed to raise a new kind of male person, one who valued woman and would treat them kindly. It was as important as the health of our earth, to me. No wonder, I thought, that the earth was getting savagely chopped, burned, polluted, poisoned and ignored, just as we women were.

I wanted to change that pattern. That's why the Youth Survival Program was part of my internal passion. By helping them regain safety and a trust with Nature, in a way it would also reflect that same kind of response towards woman. In my own simple mind process, I allowed the Mother Earth to be a symbolic 'mother' to me. One that responded when I touched into her. One who was consistent and resourceful. One that sang to me when I was silent, and gave me beautiful gifts like rainbows, flowers springing to full bloom and constancy.

I believed that one is born perfect, radiant and vitally alive, but through life, one can become torn and tarnished, whipped, cold and numb by the severity of life's lessons.

But we were born good.

As background information for the Youth Programs I would write:

"Some of today's youth/young adults have `turned' off their internal `light bulbs'. It's unclear what exactly ignited that move - parents, themselves, schools, television, impending war, killing, sugar, phony foods, baby sitters, discipline, drugs, etc. In order to teach something, first the student must want to learn. True educators extend an invite to share in some knowledge, but the student must also `extend' to receive the information. This `willingness' to learn is what our program directs a bulk of its emphasis to."

"These young adults/youth are children of parents who were young adults in the sixties. The sixties characterized by the Viet Nam error, protests outspoken-over achievers, governmental disapproval and discouragement. These sixties youth were children of parents who experienced the depression and World War II. These present troubled young eighties youth's grandparents programmed `living a better life, improvement, and the American Way, upgrading one's class system. When the youth of the sixties were told to go fight a war based on monetary reasons, much internal struggle resulted. Rights and wrongs, moral and immoral, killing or `right to life', nuclear threats, spirituality or atheism and drugs were issues we all dealt with and are now seeing our eighties youth drowning in."

"Everyone on our staff are either parents or godparents to children that are of the eighties. Also as educators and native Idahoans, we accept the challenge to broaden our perspectives and meet these young people as `fellow human beings' and offer an extended hand to help them sense the worth of living a `good, healthy, happy and peaceful life'. One in which it is worthwhile to make future goals, feeling safe that there will be a tomorrow."

"Drugs, consciousness altering substances presently afford shading, screening of the young people's daily concept of life. By alternating the vision of daily reality, they are postponing integrating with what appears to be the future. Our project offers another option—daily joy of life."

"The young must be reunited with their true basic nature — our babies did smile and glow when they were extended love. They still have that glow; it is just protected, darkened, blocked right now. They are confused. Our school offers peace with the Earth Mother, calm with the Father Spirit and joy with one's self."

"We have a confidence, self-reliance building program. Our efforts are directed to repairing and rebuilding self esteem and balanced use of will. Life is meant to be known peacefully. We commit to meet and work with each of our participants in support and understanding. Once a quiet `meeting or knowing' occurs — meeting the eyes — we then allow the wilderness setting to be our classroom giving the participant the opportunity to identify, befriend and depend on his/her own inner strength. Wilderness is a state of health, a state of total awareness."

"When this stage, the confidence step, is met, then the noncontrived situation (wilderness) presents the participant enough time away from his/her previous life space to re-evaluate him/her self and make positive changes — a transformation rather than a modification."

"Nature, our greatest health (mental/physical/emotional and spiritual) tool has a healing, calming affect which reinforces the participant's newly found/rediscovered will. Taking charge in life, rather than giving his/her power away to peers, drugs, television, money, big people, make believe, sadness, etc becomes the new behavioral pattern."

Living in a glass walled room used as a bedroom at night and an office during the day, allowed me constant access to an electric typewriter. Thus daily thoughts were easily logged.

This was the first time I had returned to the city of my youth after being in the country since 1975. I chose not to call upon old high school friends, or friends from my first marriage.

Magazines like *New Age Journal*, *East West Journal* and the *Mother Earth News* and books like *Aquarian Conspiracy*, *2150*, *Initiation*, *Superbeings* and *The Mustard Seed* became my immediate friends with deep communications.

During the day I would assist with True Creed's Two Rainbows projects.

Descriptive terms like a 'Center of Light and Rejuvenation,' or a 'Spiritual Trust', were given to this effort. Some went so far to call it a "hippie community, a sixties leftover filled with starry-eyed idealists seeking to build a new society."

The Internal Revenue Service considered the Two Rainbow's organization a church, but in some ways it was a spiritual conglomerate. Subsidiaries included a craft guild, a wilderness outfitter, a mountain retreat, an educational foundation and a river running firm.

The founder's philosophy rested on seven concepts: self honesty, personal responsibility, prayer, meditation, living positively, awareness of each moment and recognition of a supreme being.

I was asked to establish *Medicine Camps,* (Medicine — that which makes one strong). Knowing that a state of total health was a state of total awareness, I developed the programs and lined up the wholistic health instructors and guides that would teach in the high country retreat. I was keenly aware that I was establishing a healing program that would weave nutrition, massage and touch therapy, visualization and meditation, movement and exercise, and oriental medicine all in a supremely beautiful location in nature. These were all tools that I too deserved to use in my personal life.

In late February I wrote in my journal:

"I am very aware of watching the ticking of my heart. Nervous-that's what it feels like. Looking, sensing Love, knowing the openness of
it protects thee. Surrendering in to the clarity of the prayer. No room for doubt, just caution — don't leap before you look. Rewritten in my journal was the prayer —

"From the point of light within the mind of God let light stream forth into the minds of men. Let light descend on earth.

From the point of Love within the heart of God, let love stream forth into the hearts of men. May Christ return to earth.

From the center where the will of God is known, let purpose guide
the wills of men. The purpose which the Master knows and serves.

From the center which we call the race of men, let the plan of love and light work out. And may it seal the door where evil dwells.

Let light and love and power restore the plan on Earth."

Oh, dear God, these things I pray.

"As I watch love is there something in this hard headed being that is out of kilter or did you plan for me to be common with love? Am I to declare myself a nun-people lover? Unconditional, non specific love for all? Once the question is asked it disappears?

Oh Dear Lord please send forth immediately that being who is to walk beside me on this path of life."

The next week I wrote:

"It is as I look out at life that we are a continual stage of integrity. We look to one another and perceive what we can conceive. But this is just on one level. It is as though giving up on insecurities also means believing and sensing another. The physical manifestations be an unconscious conscious decision."

Quite the nervous activities!!

There is something... I thought I had fallen in love. In times gone past I felt the martyr syndrome. Any way, the silly rush, the tingling of energy up my spine resonating deeply. I am wooed by the stimulation. I pray to be protected on all planes. Do not hesitate to know love, an inner voice murmurs. Whatever plane it is expressed can be as pure as a crystal mountain stream trickling green water life that tiny creatures nestles in.
I guess that on the most basic of planes, I am thoroughly enjoying the opportunity to melt . . . oh, the never ending anticipation of joy.
JOY. LOVE in TOTAL ECSTASY.

Step off into life aligned, wholly balanced, I prayed.

Writing in mid-March, I titled the entry *Cosmic Relationship*.

"Departure from the norm. Hesitating to try to determine the `make' of the expression. Learning to derive total joy from whatever the love form.
Stopping along the way to determine if enough life is being met. Is there a part that is incomplete? When I wonder about male-female being and internal drives for completion, what would occur if that button no longer ignited? Or what would happen if it got pushed and never returned to normal?"
My farm lover's statement, "It's nicer working for something with somebody than not." A band of energy exists that is far beyond the singular identity. I heard today someone said that "they were whole unto themselves." Why is it that I do not feel whole? I know of my discipleship, but I do not know of my perfection. Something inside continues to long and also yearns to know of a touch."

I felt fragile in the city, away from my farm retreat life where my closest neighbor was a half a mile away. The singular power poles sung during wind storm but did not accentuate like the static from all the electronics in the city and the constant roar of traffic. I wondered how long I could maintain away from wide open spaces.

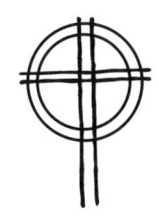

"YOU ARE A CHILD OF THE UNIVERSE,
NO LESS THAN THE TREES AND THE STARS; YOU HAVE A RIGHT BE HERE.
AND WHETHER OR NOT IT IS CLEAR TO YOU,
NO DOUBT THE UNIVERSE IS UNFOLDING AS IT SHOULD."

SPRING 1982

The *East West Journal* in December of 1981 and then again in January of 1982 had a cover story and a focused story about a Native American Medicine Woman called Brooke Medicine Eagle. I felt a prayer being answered. The articles first *"Visions of the Rainbow Woman: Brooke Medicine Eagle's Healing Power,"* and then *"Montana's Medicine Woman"* expanded my knowledge of Natural Spirituality.

Brooke's willingness to share her ancient teachings and her wisdom from Moshe Feldenkrais and others intrigued me. Her desire to stimulate understanding, growth, and healing in her personal life and in turn that of our Mother Earth called for a maturing of the species of two-legged (humans). The messages, the spirits, the energy of our great teacher is calling us to live this out in the world through our own bodies and our own experiences.

I simplistically interpret natural spirituality to mean that all of earth, heaven, all of life is related. The outside of self world reflect the inner personal self. For example, he looks like a bear or she has a heart as big as the ocean. Brooke related that all the two-leggeds are family. People injured, starving or ignored anywhere in the world affect us. Everything on and of this Earth is family. We are all connected by the same spirit. We are one.

It's out of spiritual dignity to be aloof and distant from another's death or harm, whether it be a child, a time honored mountain, a tribe of indigenous peoples, vital waters or sacrificed winged ones. There's no part of nature or life that isn't sacred and special. How to trust in that sacredness is the challenge, especially when harmful patterns persist.

I was educated about white settlers fears and abuse towards indigenous peoples in North America. I learned that until 1978 it was against the law for native peoples to practice their religion. Brooke Medicine Eagle spoke "of `rainbow medicine' which teaches that in order to step across the gap that lies between this age and a new age of harmony and abundance, we must make a bridge, and that bridge must be made of light.

In order for the light to become a rainbow powerful enough to arch across the chasm, it must contain all colors—all people, all nations, all things. If any one color is left out, it will not have the strength to become the arching rainbow bridge upon which all of us will walk into a new time. She would elaborate that these were the same teachings given to her people by White Buffalo Calf Pipe Woman; the teachings of oneness, of unity, cooperation and harmony." (Brooke Medicine Eagle. *BUFFALO WOMAN COMES SINGING.)*

Brooke, a Crow, Sioux, mixed breed medicine woman, was removed from her parents and the reservation and sent to a Christian based boarding school at a very young age. She pursued structured white man's educational system all the way to the last doctoral stage, the dissertation. Her story of intuitively being called back to her own native cultural roots and reclaiming that rich heritage while still endowed with great Western modalities of wisdom was deeply moving to me.

I vowed to study with this great woman. One significant observation I'd seen in the past year was women were courageously coming out of the closet and sharing their deep wisdom and natural strength. I saw some similarities between the Native American's persecution by white male authorities and women's lack of equality and respect in our current male dominated government, religions, business world and political realms.

Women were a scorned minority as were the Native Americans.

It seemed like no sooner had I vowed to train with this Indian medicine woman, than an announcement arrived at the desk of the Two Rainbows. Mercy Medical Hospital's Pain Clinic was offering a two day workshop called *The Body of a Warrior* with Brooke Medicine Eagle. I could not believe me eyes. I knew without a doubt I would find a way to attend this training which was aimed at awakening participants to a fuller sensing through their bodies and thus to create an awakening of one's spirits, ie. embodying spirit.

That a pain clinic was sponsoring this woman thrilled me for I knew pain. Since the third grade I had been besieged by headaches. I could not believe how long I had lived with pain as a companion. Deep inside I feared that I was not healthy enough to maintain a good male/female relationship. Until I got to a place in my life where I was well with no residue pain and filled with deep inner peace, I thought I would probably never find that so yearned for perfect 'soul mate.' When the student's ready, the teacher appears.

Living in the greenhouse office at my friends home was no longer appropriate, so I rented a loft studio across town for my son and myself.

That Spring I worked with the local Red Cross getting our guides and teachers legally prepared for the summer Survival courses and certified in First Aid. At the training a big, red haired, all eyes Irish man watched me closely. He was a photographic guide for a river floating company. Part of me felt his eyes stripping me. I ignored him and his pursuit appeared magnified.

Simultaneously men, attractive, powerful, communicative and passionate men, seemed to be walking daily into my life. Whether at the print shop, at the first aid course, at the coffee house or while riding bicycles, I was noticing these men and strangely they were looking back at me. I did not trust my heart and its responses and as I was truly trying to heal, I allowed them in my life but only as friends.

Unbeknownst to the men, I had an unspoken test for them. Sound therapy was so important to me. I expressed myself through music. If I felt sad, I would play a tear jerking melody. If I wanted to help my heart soar, I would put on beautiful tunes like the Pachobel's 'Canon in D'. I let musicians and their creative works express my feelings and reflect various chapters of my life. *500 Miles, Exodus, Dream the Impossible Dream, Somewhere Over the Rainbow, You've Got a Friend, Knights in White Satin, Leaving on a Jet Plane, Take It Easy,* Rod Stewart's *You are my Friend,* and others eloquently spoke my emotions.

I had lived more lives than necessary this incarnation. I often said that life was like a book. We all have the same chapters, we just choose to step into them at our own rate. Some go through death issues when they are 24 and others wait until they are 42.

I believed we all have a relationship chapter. Some of us married the first man we ever exchanged sex with while another's' chapter of experience didn't stop with the first but went on to sample many flavors of intimate exchanges. At some point in a person's life they would go through the chapter of diversity in relationships and the chapter on monogamous commitment.

Knowing the big book of life is what made us all One. The capacity to not judge the theme of a being's current life chapter was a strength. From the book *Knowing Woman,* an insight resonated through me. We were to look at another and see their highest good. We were not to focus on their weak, sick character flaws but attempt to put our attention to their strongest traits. We do have free will when it comes to mirroring what we see in others.

A sign of a wise person is one who witnesses life, learns from the lessons/chapters of others and discerns appropriateness with exchanges. One can witness violence but does not have to return it. It is important to chose whom one wishes to reflect or associate with in life. If one is repeating the same form of relationship over and over again, it takes the greatest spiritual strength to say to one's self. Stop it. Enough, reflect light, beauty, love right now.

I wished to attract to me this time a healthy, happy and holy companion who walked on the medicine path. I would play music for my male guest and if he did not respond with a similar awareness or feeling with the songs and the tones I would register an 'Ah Hah.' He has not logged the same miles I have. If he exclaimed that this particular music made him remember a time in his life when...I would know we resonated and could possibly walk together.

I journeyed through this watchful time witnessing traits and personalities of those around me. Posted on my wall, I would daily reflect on Elizabeth Haitch's twelve sets of twin characteristics listed in her book, *Initiation.*

TWIN CHARACTERISTICS

KEEPING SILENT	TALKING
RECEPTIVITY	RESISTANCE TO INFLUENCE
OBEYING	RULING
HUMILITY	SELF CONFIDENCE
LIGHTENING LIKE SPEED	CIRCUMSPECTION
TO ACCEPT EVERYTHING	TO BE ABLE TO DIFFERENTIATE
ABILITY TO FIGHT	PEACE
CAUTION	COURAGE
TO POSSESS NOTHING	TO COMMAND EVERYTHING
TO HAVE NO TIES	LOYALTY
CONTEMPT FOR DEATH	REGARD FOR LIFE
INDIFFERENCE	LOVE

Concerning the above twin traits, Elizabeth stressed the importance of balance in a person's life. One deserved to know both sides of the spectrum, but not be stuck only on one end of the range.   If a person had to consistently prove how strong and together they were a silent inner witness would whisper there is a place in that person that must be weak and scattered. In myself I was getting to be better at observing my own unauthentic perceptions.

I so wanted to understand my fellow human beings and myself. The above became a continuum for me to watch my own behaviors. If I hung out on just one side of the balance I was inviting in a life lesson on the other side. I yearned to be victim free.

The time for *The Body of a Warrior Workshop* quickly came. A group of fifty plus peoples met at a local hospital. The entire group was never introduced to each other, just identification tags with only our first names. The focus of this workshop was for our personal use. Brooke Medicine Eagle came in and had us form a circle and then she brought out a candle, smudge stick, feathers, corn, a crystal, whistle and bells and then proceeded to create an altar on a beautiful tapestry cloth. We all watched in silence.

Teaching us through example, the altar represent the Great Spirit or All That Is. Before she began to verbally instruct us, she created a sacred space with symbolic representation of the four direction, the four winds, the mother earth, the father spirit and Maker of all things. As she proceeded to honor our relationship with the sweet earth and expansive heavens, Brooke sang to the four directions calling for help and guidance.

MEDICINE WHEEL
by Kate Wolf

When the morning breaks and the sunlight warms my soul,
In the East the Eagle flies and the Red Tail proudly soars.
I'm on my way to the place of the spirit one.
Grandfather hear me now, I am on fire.
Let the Sundance guide my feet to your desire.
Show me visions for my eyes and words like gold
that glimmer in the sun.

Hi e ya, he e ya, hi e ya

Turn towards the South like water I will run.
In innocence and trust the moon child song is sung,
I'm on my way to the place of the sacred plants.
My emotions and my will at their command.
For the turtle's voice is heard upon the land,
and the wise coyote prowls,
The rattlesnake will call me to the dance.

Hi e ya , He e ya, Hi e ya

When the sun goes down and it grows too dark to see,
I look within to the Shaman's mysteries.
I'm on my way to die and live again.
Grandmother Earth I cry, give me rest.
I take my place with the woman of the West.
Show me the raven and the bear,
The way of herbs and the black obsidian.

Hi e ya, He e ya, Hi e ya

In the deepest night the stars watch over me.
Old woman of the North, my mind seeks clarity.
I'm on my way to the place of the Northern winds,
Let the thunder and the lightening carry me.
Lay my thoughts to rest and send me into sleep.
The hawk and the buffalo,
My dreams white crystal magic medicine."

    She asked us to stand and with hands uplifted we would face literally the South on the wheel, turning to the South, then West, up to the North and back to the East again as she sang the Medicine Wheel song. Then as we listened attentively, Brooke again went through the four directions giving us symbolic references. "Medicine Wheel" is the name given to large circles of stones found on the ground in many places in North America. These circles had been used in ceremonial ways by early Native people, as well as representing the whole Wheel of Life on Earth. They were often aligned with certain other stones or geographic features to indicate solstices and other planetary and astrological events.
    Different tribes and cultures have varied ways of dividing the Wheel of Life into its various symbolic aspects.
    Then Brooke ignited a small tied bundle of cedar and sage and slowly this strong medicine woman circled outside our concentric ring of participants, waving a long majestic Eagle feather fan with tinkling beads, smudging each of us. Native people all over the earth use burning herbs for purifying space and one another. The smoke permeated the room and embraced us with a haunting familiarity.
    As I felt the winds from her fan up my backside and brushing around my heart and then lifting up over my head, a feather fell into my lap. A 'rush' spread through my body. Afterwards I tried to return the feather and she assured me it was a blessing for me from the winged ones.
    After this sensory opening ceremony, she explained that to make the circle a safe container it is essential to call in the powers of the directions. This is done to invite the archetypical qualities of the cardinal points, that they might bear witness, lend support, and impart wisdom to our endeavors.
    This acknowledges that we human beings need assistance to cross the limited boundaries of ego into the essential oneness of self. This aligns us and our intentions with the larger impulses of life. She asked us to consider that every step we take each day of our life is stepping onto the altar of our life. The reverence and

BROOKE MEDICINE EAGLE

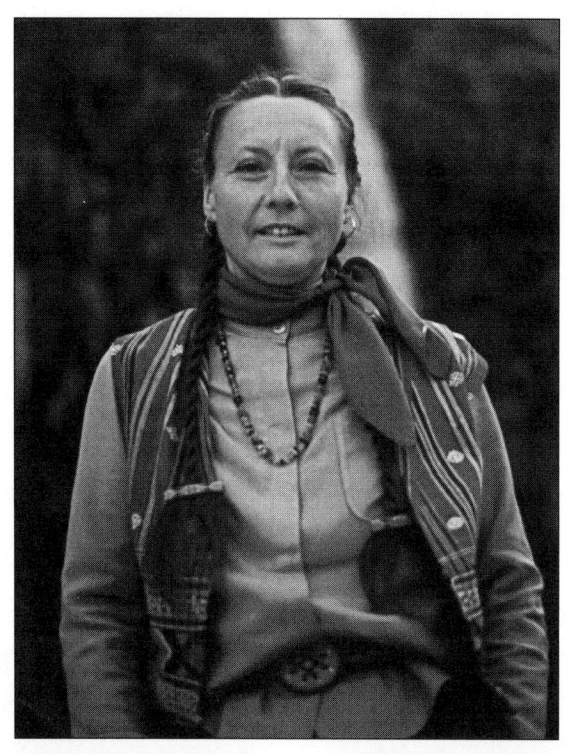

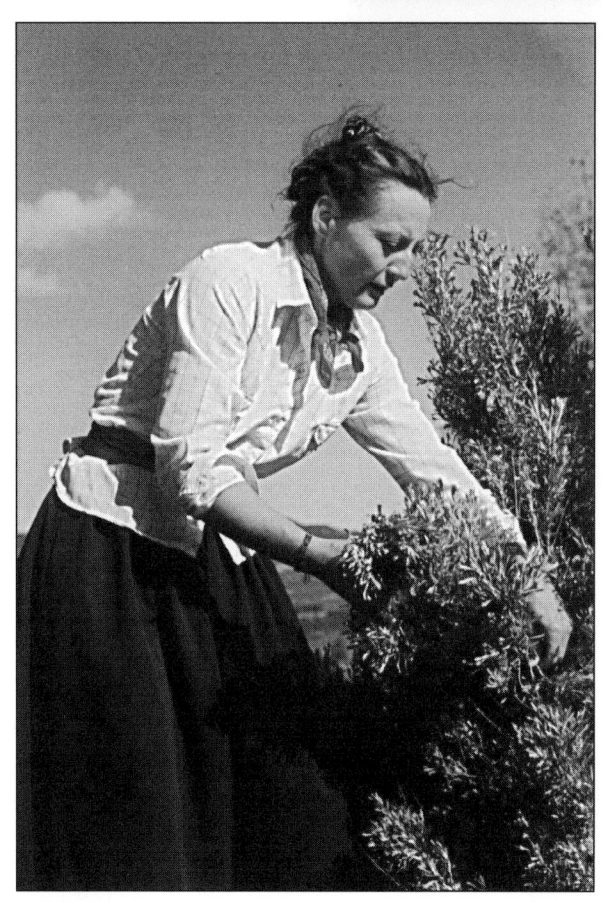

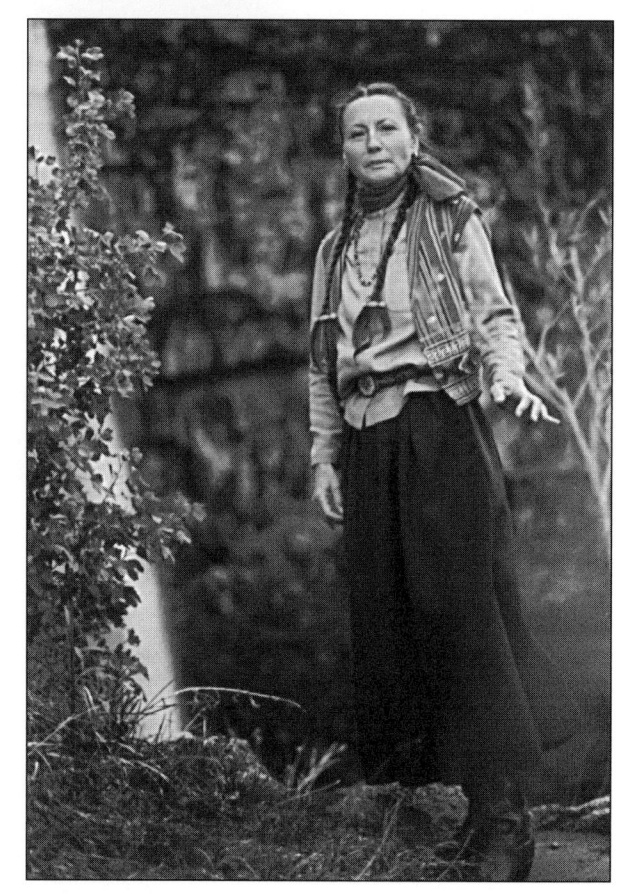

homage observed creates an atmosphere of sacredness. The technology of the sacred involves the ability to invoke, heal, bless, speak, write, dance, symbolically represent and drum and thus be part of the Rainbow bridge.

Brooke asked us to "Walk fittingly where the grass grows. Walk fittingly where the birds sing. Become fully human." She asked us to "wake up and learn quickly so that we didn't hurt ourselves further." "Mother Earth is in trouble, and thus are all of us who are her children. Our earth walk is dangerously unbalanced, and this must be corrected quickly."

The thrusting, aggressive, analytical, intellectual, making-it-happen, and "fixing what Mother Earth didn't do so well" kind of energy has become dominant. It had almost buried the feminine, receptive, accepting, harmonizing, surrendering, and unifying energy. A balancing must take place in which the feminine and masculine energies within each of us, as within all things, can harmonize.

"In our Native way, we are not seen as fully human until we balance these two energies; we cannot make full use of ourselves and our creative gifts until the yin and yang, right and left brain, the active and the receptive are balanced," she related.

"To be fully human is what is being required of us now on Earth. This means that more emphasis needs to be placed on being receptive rather than active; on relationship rather than on separation; on power in flow with great forces rather than on personal dominion over others; on the dark of winter's earthy germination as well as the rapid growth of summer days; on nurturing rather than fighting; on supporting rather than destroying; and on a deep and sacred ecology that deals respectfully and harmoniously with All Our Relations rather than with isolated issues."

She went on to explain that a warrior is:
1) unique
2) fully in service of the people especially the children and
3) in good relationship to all things, people — and
'in-tunement'/atonement—a time of at-one-ment.

Attending the conference alone was typical for me. I was intent on getting well. Brooke Medicine Eagle would be my first truly significant teacher in 'body-mind' therapy. Since I knew no one, I was completely ready to learn to become fully alive. She stressed that "my body is in me not me in my body". I loved her approach to teaching. First, she started out with sacred calling, then some verbal teachings and then we would be directed through activities involving movement with our bodies.

"A new quality of light is coming to the Earth," Brooke related. "A light to find a way into the darkness—our insides. Whatever we think, that very instance, so shall it be. Simplify she impressed, understand that we are at one with all things. We truly have whatever we need right now." She asked us to open up our `dream light' (night space) and let go of what one thinks they are, for the worse the human being can be is light."

There are various possibilities in life. " One, things that we want and have, two, things we want but don't have; three, things we have but don't want and lastly four, things we don't want and don't have."

Brooke took us through a Feldenkrais system of movement called "Functional Integration" in which "the entire process of learning is becoming aware of finer and finer differences, and thus movement was life. Awareness not only hones our perception, it actually improves our functioning." She would make reference to Moshe Feldenkrais's *Awareness Through Movement* and the instructional relearning for our entire nervous system which affects our entire body and its senses.

We mimicked the evolutionary sequence of the brain and behavior as well as the corresponding developmental movements that should have started to occur within the womb and on into our first years of life. Brooke took us stage by stage through the muscular/neurological development of our body. After each movement activity (usually I had my eyes closed so I didn't see others and thus I wouldn't be so embarrassed by some of the actions she asked us to mimic and experience) we would stand and observe any difference in our sense of our self. Using a Feldenkrais language system, to the infinitesimal detail we would first imagine then actually rotate, crawl and lift a portion of our body, form a certain sound with our mouths, and follow through with a developmental stage of our life, hopefully with a lot more grace this time through.

During the course, we listened a lot, but shared little with each other as we experienced the different evolutionary stages of human development. She had us move with a cellular focus, then like a fish, then a like an amphibian, monkey. . . evolutionary integration progression much like Jean Houston described in *The Search for the Beloved* and *The Possible Human*. Brooke explained fully after each animated exercise our reprogramming and renewing journey with ourselves. We analyzed little. We would feel through our body contrasting a before and an after sense.

Towards the end of the workshop, she had our imaginary body lean against the trunk of an tree. We were to remove our shoes and then pretend to put our feet in a nearby stream. We were told the water was very cold. Then with the souls of our feet we were to feel a prickly pine cone rolling through our arches. Her next suggestion was to pick up an imagined stick between our great toe and second toe and roll it successively down pairs of toes until we came to our littlest toe.

By this time my thoughts were stretched way beyond what she was sharing. It wasn't until I was asked to stand and walk and feel any thing different with my two feet- the experiential foot and the passive foot, that I noticed a great pain in the imagined experienced foot. The stick I had thought about had been too big and had sprung my littlest toes too far apart. I literally limped with pain.

A bell of clarity went off in me. I knew through this experience something many fine, past books had suggested was possible. Mind over matter. As the mind perceives so shall it be. I knew the mind could create pain and sickness in the body and it could also create health and peace.

At this stunning moment a light of knowing went off in me. I felt external eyes watching me. Brooke recognized that I had gotten the deeper message and gifting from her teachings.

We were learning how to learn. Our mouth, Brooke contended was the pathway for reorganizing of our nervous system and that was why she had us make the different 'tonals' with each activity. We can only keep so much in the mind, she reiterated. The emotions set patterns in the body and they are the hardest to break.

Most behavior is acquired. There is nothing permanent about it except the belief that it's there. Therefore awareness is first and foremost to waking up. Too many people, Brooke contended were walking around asleep set in habitual patterns. She intended with this Body of a Warrior Workshop to invite us to change, to embody spirit.

At the closing circle, wide-eyed, clear seeing people finally were asked to introduce themselves and their occupations. It was good I did not know initially who was present because I would have been intimidated by the doctors, psychologist, therapists, and counselors who participated. Simple me, how had I come to show up in such a powerful circle?

This circle of peers still influence my life, twelve years later. At the time, it was Brooke who quietly asked if I would be willing to join an 'Elder Sister" Circle she facilitated. I was so pleased. . . of course I would join.

So within days, I was invited to a tall, intense dark haired therapist's home. When I arrived he kindly led me to a den where people sat on the floor circling this huge crystal. I joined the hoop.

Through singing, praying and directed teachings, I began to learn of the teachings of *White Buffalo Woman,* the elder sister.

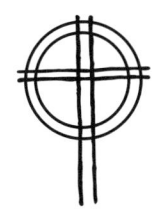

*"THEREFORE BE AT PEACE WITH GOD, WHATEVER YOU CONCEIVE HIM TO BE,
AND WHATEVER YOUR LABORS AND ASPIRATIONS,
IN THE NOISE CONFUSION OF LIFE KEEP PEACE WITH YOUR SOUL."*

WHITE BUFFALO CALF WOMAN TRAINING WITH BROOKE MEDICINE EAGLE

Brooke, a Native teacher, healer, poet; one who was willing to share sacred ritual to assist us to learn or maybe to remember to listen to the earth that is speaking to us. Many signals (earthquakes, pollution, depleted ozone layer, illnesses, drought, forest fires, annihilated medicinal plant species and tribes) are asking us to wake up and pay attention, she reiterated.

This ageless tradition of honoring the Earth by creating a circle which is a powerful metaphor for unity, encourages a healing energy to help mend the land and her peoples. By celebrating with the Earth we are bridging an inner self, outer world reflection of beauty and health.

Through song and ceremony, Brooke honored her ancient lineage that was close to the earth. She shared that the large, multi-faceted crystal in the center of our circle was considered a sacred messenger by the indigenous people. This one she assured would assist us with our intunement this evening. According to the ancient ways, "Every person had the possibility through dreams, prayer and visions to bring through them the life spirit in a form particular and meaningful to them and their time. Spirit lives in all of us presently. We are one family of Mother Earths' children under Father Sky. We are one."

She began the teachings of *White Buffalo Calf Woman,* the elder sister. A messenger that spoke of our oneness. "She taught that whatever we do to one in the great circle of life, we do to ourselves. It's like we've pushed ourselves to the edge and the message is so loud, we can no longer ignore that we are one with all things." Brooke impressed that "the Creator gave only one law at the beginning of time on the Earth, that we are one family and we should be in good relations with each other all things."

Healing, wholeness and holiness all come from the same root woord. To heal the Earth, we must be whole with the Earth. In good relationship with Mother Earth and all that is on her.

"White Buffalo Calf Woman was a mysterious, radiant and beautiful one who came to our land to our Lakota people. A long time ago, the Lakota lived in Minnesota near Saskwash. The buffalo represented the great giveaway as all of it was beneficial for the people to live. The meat fed them, became tools, shelter, clothing and sacred medicine.

A camp of around twenty-four people from the woodlands went to the plains looking for the buffalo. They went to North and South Dakota and the prairies looking for these four legged, great animals. Always at night camping in the cottonwoods as these trees were also seen as good medicine.

Two young scouts went out to make a large circle to see where things were and also to look for buffalo. Their eyes caught a movement in the distance, something unusual, something odd. They also noticed around this figure in the distance was a soft radiant glow.

At this time one of the worst punishments that could happen to a person was to be banned from a tribe and so they saw this person in isolation and they could not believe it. On her back was a bundle and as she came closer this rich, golden soft light reached out to them. The scouts saw not only a lovely, lovely woman, dressed in white buffalo calf leather, but one that was alone. "Not only was her apparel a sign of the supernatural, but as the woman neared, the hunters could see that she walked with a slow, stately gait of the spirits and carried a holy bundle on her back."

Despite strong taboos protecting spirits from worldly lust, the first scout was overcome with desire and walked towards her to take advantage of her. It is said that this beautiful young woman lifted her arms, opening her robes to him to envelop him and a large cloud swirled around them.

The other scout watched and he saw a mist, a soft fog building and swirling and then the two were hidden from his sight. The winds came up and the fog blew away and as the beautiful woman opened up her arms what fell from them were bleached skull and bones. Then the winds came and scattered the bones across the plains.

The other man of pure heart, a warrior, knew that he lived by the creed that he wasn't for himself alone but for the whole of the people, all the Family of Earth. He knew also that when the people forgot why they were on this good Earth often times a messenger would come to remind them. So he approached this beautiful, radiant, mysterious woman and said, "Will you come teach my people?" and the stunning woman said,

"Go before me and have the chief prepare a large tipi for me," and so he did.

This nomadic tribe, efficient at raising tipis rapidly, built the lodge putting several little tipis together and then wrapped their skins around the frames. Then they dressed in ceremonial attire and at sunrise the next day, the woman arrived, carrying her bundle in her hands. Unwrapping it she withdrew the stem of a pipe with her right hand, the bowl with her left. White Buffalo Calf Woman than held the pipe before the chief, saying: "Behold this and always love it! It is very sacred and you must treat it as such. With this you will send your voices to Wakan Tanka, your father and grandfather."

The woman explained that the pipe represented the Earth, and all plants and animals upon it. The stem symbolic of the masculine and the bowl, the feminine. "When you pray with this pipe," she continued, "You pray for everything...all the Earth's family." Then she showed them how to handle the pipe, pointing at the sky and the earth and toward the four winds. She wrapped the object in her bundle and gave it to the elderly chief.

It was to be treated sacredly as a peace pipe. So she taught them through prayers accompanied by pinched tobacco and sacred herbs compressed into the bowl of the pipe to honor all of the Earth's family. Of all the plants known to ancient Indians, tobacco was among the most sacred. Tobacco offered a means of communicating with the spirit world. The smoke shall rise, and one shall speak.

The pipe is a connection for everything through prayer. So they saw how to take pinches of tobacco and then pray for the two legged, no matter which direction they live, the four legged, the winged ones, the green things that grow, the waters, the stars, and on and on. All these great things and more are in the great circle of light. Everything that was here deserved to grow and be healthy, and they also prayed that the answers to who had gone on before them. All earthly, all starry realm seen and unseen, things known and unknown were prayed for in this red catlinite bowl.

Sage was the last thing put in the bowl, which she said represented the mother, the feminine and with this everything not included, not said was asked to be put in completing the filling of the pipe. "When you have that pipe filled, it is a ceremonial representation for everything that is all there is."

The stem, carved from wood represented the green things that grow and also the masculine. An Eagle feather was tied on connecting it to spirit. Then they took fire, the Maker's great gift, the transforming energy to the bowl and she drew in her breath through stem and blew out four times, calling to the four directions.

Literally when one smokes, that smoke going upwards is making with your breath visible that connection and relationship with all that is. The essence of the smoke creates an atmosphere for cleansing and healing. A conscious prayer aligning with the higher power of the Universe, the Maker of All Things, Great Spirit, Heavenly Father, ...God; that I am walking the beauty way. I am making visible what is connected and integrated. Whatever one does to any other thing in the circle of life we do to ourselves.

Each day upon this Earth is a sacred day. We are to respect, love, and treat all things with aliveness and beauty. Everything, every step is sacred and should be treated that way.

Each step is like an embrace, a kiss on the sweet Mother Earth's Cheek. White Buffalo Woman is calling us into account to be in good relations with all things. This special woman gave the Lakota seven sacred rites, which involve the pipe and therefore a portable altar is always with you. She impressed that things have to be empowered.

One, Crying for a Vision, calls for an individual to seek out a place in nature, with prayerful ceremony and request insight to a crucial chapter in their life. A teacher from the community assists the rites of passage.

She impressed that when the visions die, the people die and when people quit seeking visions, life is lost.

The next ceremony she gave was inipi, the sweat lodge. She gave it to us to remember the sacred ceremony of renewal. A symbolic process to return to the Mother and purify and clean out toxicity and be renewed. To get clear down to bare facts. This cleansing lodge was intricately explained. Every step of intention, preparation, prayer and release and renewal was outlined.

The third ceremony was like the rites of passage for the young girls. She called it Her Alone We Sing Over. A young girl comes into her menses and she is like her mother now, she can bring forth life.

For a whole day everything stopped when a woman came into her flow and singing began, deeply honoring of the feminine. Just to touch her was good vitalizing medicine they felt. From that point on in a young woman's life the monthly flow would be honored by allowing a woman to take time out from the community's existence to be quiet to give back to the Earth.

Men would recognize this time as when a woman was most powerful. All the energy of the moon and her cycles flowed through the woman.

The fourth ceremony that she spoke to was concerning sacred life in the four quadrants. She called it Throwing The Ball. Each tribe would pick a young girls of eight or nine who was a paradigm of the Lakota values. She would stand in the center with buffalo hide ball and she would throw the ball to the East. Whoever received the ball in the East was blessed. The young woman would throw to the South and so on around the four directions. Each time the receiver became enhanced with the purity of the cultural's values.

The fifth ceremony that she shared was the Making of Relations. She impressed that any time you take someone as a relation and as a sister, then through that person one remembers every woman as a sister. Brooke impressed that bringing the message to current day was essential. Each one of us at all times were to be in good relations with wholeness in out intent.

This woman was called White Buffalo Calf Woman and she offered the pipe so that every single person could take of the pipe and pray these prayers. She showed them how to take care of the pipe that after a blessing was engaged they would take apart the pipe and cleanse it. She then gave the pipe to the chief as an honor and said, "Hold strongly to this pipe until the end of times and I will meet you there."

When she was done, she left the tipi, walking alone. The people streamed out behind her. The very young would get closer to her because they were very pure of heart. A few followed her way out onto the plateau and they watched as she sat down in a buffalo wallow, where the buffaloes roll and when she came up with a buffalo and when she went down again rolling and dust flying, she came up with another buffalo. She went down two more times and the last time she came up as a white buffalo calf and she ran off and was gone and that is where she got the name White

Buffalo Calf Woman.

    She is calling women to remember that they came forth carrying a beautiful way. They bring forth renewal, future generations and spirituality in their lives. They are called to walk the ways of holiness, to stand for oneness, good relations and aliveness rather than separation and destruction."

    She is still bringing us through visioning ways to remember these messages, Brooke related. She's bringing us holiness, god realization and ecology. She asks us to remember the trees, our waters, the living desert and especially impresses us now about the 'bad waters'.

We are Singing For Our Life. We are to live the beauty way and practice the Giveaway as we are all part of the Circle of Life and Light. As the evening's gathering closed I felt so blessed to be in the circle of the Elder Sister and to be called to do her holy work/whole work. True health comes from our connection with all things. Then we have true power, which is the power of life joined with all of life not separate.

Brooke reminded us that the creator gave only one law at the beginning of time on this earth and that is we should be in good relations with each other and all things. Dawn star the energy of Christ in the Americas spoke the same message of light, love and unity. He healed the sick and raised the dead and walked on the waters, stopped the winds and talked to people of a way of love and light. Asking us to let love's light shine unrestricted through our hearts and connect with all things around us.

"He loved the Mother Earth." He walked upon her and used metaphors as teaching examples. One of the things he did was walking among the tribes/communities teaching the people that the earth is our mother, sky, spirit is our father and lives in all of us as mother lives in all of us. So we are the children of Mother and Father of Earth and Sky. So, in fact, we certainly are related to everything else that lives between Earth and sky.

    "Dawn Star spoke of the same family metaphor the White Buffalo Calf taught of. Love one another and cooperate with each other. He went amongst the people teaching that and they began to follow his ways. So several thousand years ago we had an opportunity to live together with a sense of oneness as he modeled. Today life held the same teachings on relationships.

    When he left the people he said, "If in fact you can keep together this light, this loving family, remembering the Father and the Mother; you will come to golden time where amazing things will be known. If you don't, things will shatter and be blown apart." Warrior like behavior with much fighting and destruction will occur and it did.

Through the teachings of White Buffalo Calf Woman we have the tools to reunite in wholeness, oneness. It felt true to not only acknowledge an elder brother, Dawn Star; but an elder sister, White Buffalo Calf Woman.

Throughout my youth I had sought a comprehension of God, his son, Jesus; and the ways of living a spiritual existence. Seldom, with the exception of the current Mother Theresa, had I heard of a female in the role of spiritual leader, especially not in the great Holy Bible.

India currently had two fine women, Ghandi's mother and the Mother Theresa. I was distraught spiritually and wanted a formula for living and loving in my own backyard, not in a third world country across the great oceans. Learning of the prophetic teachings of White Buffalo Calf Woman encouraged my heart to be okay as a strong, sensitive, nature honoring, spiritual woman who could revere the Elder Brother as well as the Elder Sister. This felt so good.

I heard Brooke's interpretation that women to women had important 'codes of good relations' to uphold. She inferred that White Buffalo Woman was asking us to honor another's commitments and not interfere with another woman's family. She also insinuated that men had much to improve in the area of respect and honoring of woman.

> "Be kind to the weak
> the children and women
> be kind to all men
> and all living things...
> If you see a girl or woman alone
> do her no harm
> nor have any bad thoughts about her
> but protect her
> For she is a sacred being
> And this is the teaching
> of the Above One
> Women are sacred
> because they are the givers of life
> and their purpose is to raise that Life
> in harmony with all creation..."

(by Crazy Horse, Legendary Mystic and Warrior)

As I rose to leave, the man to my left finally spoke. He told me that he had been watching me at the Pain Clinic workshop and he was a Barefoot Physician who announced he had strong, healing hands. He felt we would be working together some time for recognized in me my sensitivity. He also sensed he could help me with the pain he saw in me. He made me nervous. I did not commit to connect to meet him again.

I cautiously watched the other tall dark haired man, who sat to my right in this powerful Elder Sister Circle. I would name him Gentle Heart in the days to come and the touch healer who sat to my left would become Iron Fingers. Gentle Heart's sensitive strength and fervent spiritual dedication interwove through his gay nature. This marked the beginning of long term association with a 'safe' male. In time we would share our recognition of also being Living Disciples this lifetime. With Gentle Heart, I have been able to deepen my understanding of the masculine and the feminine aspects of spirituality and discover the combined oneness.

I was unsure when this respectful Elder Sister family would come together. I was told that there was an invisible telegraph system that one could tap into and receive the message or quite literally a call would be put out to reconvene. Brooke would continue her way home to Montana. In the meantime, each of us was asked to do our work for the highest good of the Earth's family.

An old Chinese Proverb sums this up:

"If there is righteousness in the heart,
    there will be harmony in the home.
If there is harmony in the home,
    there will be order in the nation.
When there is order in the nation,
    there will be peace in the world."

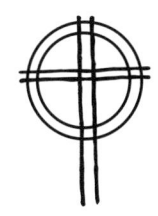

"MANY FEARS ARE BORN OF FATIGUE AND LONELINESS"

THE FUTURIST — SETTING ONE'S INTENTIONS

Offers to help me regain my health were coming from other body therapists. One, the facilitator of the *New American Medicine Show,* was a yoga teacher who did integrated deep body tissue release work. This therapist proceeded to introduce me to his good friend who was a Futurist hired by the local university.

My first exchange with the Futurist was like meeting a 'blood brother'. With strong Indian facial features, sharp dark eyes and eagle nose, this tall, dark haired 'wise' man reached out through conversation to meet the spiritual searcher of faith in me.

Highlights of our conversations were the statements of our political involvements of the Viet Nam Error. He shared memories of Kent State and work with Martin Luther King. He knew the feel of police batons, social scorn and death of heroes.

The Futurist invited me to participate in a workshop he taught on *Abundance at Hand.* I saw money as an evil. In my view, it corrupted people. For years I prayed for a peer/tribe that was beyond the fixation of 'needing something to be happy' and the "If only I had . . ." or "I would be content if. . ." So if I heard someone whom I was wanting to share deeper with say what it was they wanted, I went about helping them get it. I gave my monies away. . .trying to get people to focus on a spiritual life to return to knowing Heaven was on Earth right now.

I wanted to live in the Garden with companions as soon as possible. As long as I had access to money, I refused to let some material 'need' get in the way of a spiritual companionship.

The closure of the bookstore and the continual consumption of funds from the farm, had brought me to the end my savings. Just six years earlier I had thought that I would never have to work for others again, and now I was broke.

It was clear that I needed to look at money and prosperity another way. Bureaucracy and materialism was a heavy weight to carry, and I judged them harshly.

Early in 1982, I began the reframing of my anger towards money. Prosperity - Well Being and Growth taught by the Futurist addressed one's spiritual, mental, emotional, physical and financial aspects. I needed to learn how to be 'hard as nails. . .sensitive as a nerve.' It is always said that during hard times, hindsight finds one has experienced some of the most meaningful times. When times get easier, it's just not as thrilling.

The Futurist asked us to look at what belief around prosperity blocked our ability to experience more. . .one's own self-doubt (denial of deserving abundance) or money is an evil and love is golden. He suggested that we see money as love and include a better understanding of being responsible for everything and everyone else.

This mandate to put one's self first, called for trust and faith. Indulgence comes with lack of purpose and direction, the Futurist emphatically espoused. The closet fear that there is not enough trust reflects back to one's prosperity. One who is looking for abundance rather than accepting it insinuates that they are looking at lack rather than abundance.

He shared four affirmations:
' God Am I.
I am a living statement of God.
God is with me! and God is abundant.'

The Futurist asked us to look at the ease with which we walked our lives. He, too, contended that the only difference in the old and the young is stiffness. By believing or not believing, we were able to respond or be blocked. Money is God in action.

It is important to consistently program, on and on, with trusting. Attune and attain, he declared. Envision and allow stuff in. Next, he share a guided visualization to assist us to discover our blueprint, our original connected with the one source, God. After the imagery activity we were asked to write our goals. I wrote "by allowing myself to be in harmony, to be cognizant of an inner `rush' of connection with the electrical current of life that I interpreted to be God, trust would be rebuilt and then I would be able to rejoice that I am now living exactly as I should be."

Creative Visioning as the Futurist explained entailed:
(1) Visualization (steps given) to aim for one's goal
(2) Energize with emotion love/gratitude/acceptance
(3) Affirm—decree/command 'speak to your work'
(4) Allow/receive act with acceptance.
(5) Be thankful

"God's gifts puts man's highest dreams to shame." The teacher appealed for us to not spread the energy by talk. He referred to a book called *Super Beings* by John Wesley and the gifts the author shares relating to one's ability to be awake in the present moment on this Earth.

TWELVE STAGES OF A SUPERBEING

<u>Phase One</u>

A Phase One person may or may not have an awareness of his true identity—and if he does, it is only an assumption; there is no comprehension of the real meaning of this revelation. However, a person in this category may have a strong self-image as a human being, and even though his overall belief system may be faulty, he can on occasion "pull himself up by his bootstraps" and overcome handicaps and achieve a degree of success through sheer sweat,strain and personal will power. At the present time, the majority of people are in a Phase One onsciousness — regardless of how "religious" they may profess to be.

<u>Phase Two</u>

In Phase Two, the understanding faculty is beginning to develop on an intellectual level. You perceive and approve of the idea that there is a Power within you, another Self on a higher vibrational level, a pattern of Perfection that is the potential You, a Higher Nature that can be brought forth is much enthusiasm for reading, studying and exploring of new ideas. There is interest in the techniques of self actualization, mind dynamics, meditation, visualization and affirmations. Your mind is beginning to open and you are fascinated by your new discoveries.

Phase Three

The Phase Three person begins to feel subjectively that "Man's not all included between his hat and his boots" as Walt Whitman put it. But the primary emphasis is on what can be done with "mind power"—basically a mental approach with little superconscious or spiritual foundation. The individual on the third rung usually tries to give the impression of being a bit mystical—the "I know something you don't" attitude, resulting in an exaggerated ego and much false pride. And when a Phase Three man or woman demonstrates a particular good, heaven help every one within shouting distance because the experience is going to be told over and over again. If you can identify with this level, you know that you spend too much time trying to convert others to your "New" way of thinking with philosophical jargon that does nothing but turn people away. And you are retarding your own progress in the process. The key to moving past this stage is to keep your lips sealed and let the Power grow and develop.

Phase Four

The Fourth Phase must be entered into with great caution because it is in this stage of consciousness that most Superbeings-in-training experience the greatest difficulty. In Phase Four, the Truth or spiritual faculty has been partially developed in your deeper mind, but is not ready for full expression. But because the consciousness tunes in at times to this illumined awareness, so-called miracles will occur, and there will be opportunities for magnificent demonstrations of the Power at work. At the same time, you may also find that your optimism is ahead of our understanding and errors in judgment will result, plunging you into a "how could this possibly happen" state of mind. It is not until the Truth Idea is fully manifested in consciousness that "miracle follows miracle and wonders never cease."

Phase Five

In Phase Five, an individual's consciousness is directed toward the good at lease fifty-one percent of the time, i.e. the positive thoughts and feelings outweigh the negative. Now the clouds seem to part and more sunshine than ever comes into your life. There is more harmony, money is more plentiful, those old aches and pains are not as frequent, and things seem to be "right" in your life. The exceptional heights of sudden miracles and the deep valleys of futility experienced in Phase Four have passed and there is more stability and order in life. The marvels and wonders indeed continue, but they are now recognized as the natural out-picturing of an uplifted consciousness rather than as supernormal. But there is a caution light on this level too. People on the path say that Phase five is straight and narrow, and if the shield of protection from the race mind is not strong enough to ward off concentrated negative influences, the scales of your mental atmosphere may be tipped and you'll find yourself backsliding into the roller coaster side of Phase Four again. It is during the Fifth stage that a firm and definite commitment must be made, a covenant with your Higher Self, an unwavering dedication to principle. In essence, you now take your vows to achieve mastery.

Phase Six

Phase Six is the beginning of mastery, a dying to the old consciousness and a rebirth into a new understanding of the cosmic power within. This consciousness knows only spiritual man, and is content to simply experience this joyful communion. Very little outer work is done during this stage, and is thus referred to as the "Sabbath" by the evolving souls. When you reach this level, you know you are the Power, but being a time of rest, the knowing is sufficient. By the Law of Consciousness, you experience harmony, but there is no strong desire to reach out and demonstrate your realization. The next six phases, Seven through Twelve, signify the evolving consciousness culminating in total Mastery.

Phase Seven

As a Seven, you understand that you now have the power to establish a life of heaven on earth in this incarnation—and you begin to use the power accordingly. Creative imagination becomes a major factor in this stage and through it, you find the world shaping to your thoughts. You are quickly "Placed" in work that is best suited for your talents and where you can experience the greatest fulfillment. There is financial security because you "see" all the money needed to achieve your purposes being attracted to you in abundant measure—and so it is. Your health is excellent, and your relationships with others loving and caring. The basic thinking of a Seven is to get his life up to the standard of his highest vision, and to achieve the maximum degree of livingness. And while it sounds as though a Seven is completely self-oriented, it must be pointed out that this stage represents a greater degree of givingness than the others before it. Reason: A Seven knows that he cannot use the power for himself without decreeing the same good for all others within the range of his consciousness and beyond. So he sees himself as whole standard. This is "loving thy neighbor as thyself."

Phase Eight

In Phase Eight, you know that your life is now in a more advanced stage—you are reaching wholeness in mind and body and your spiritual nature is in a higher degree or radiation. Your desires are fulfilled, so your attention begins to focus outwardly almost exclusively, and as if "by chance" people are attracted to you for guidance and counseling. In this phase you have remarkable healing powers for another's body and affairs, but your effectiveness depends to a great extent on the receptivity of the individual being treated. For that reason, you usually will not attract those who knew you when you were living out of a lower-vibration consciousness. It is during this stage that you will find a new light on the ancient Truth teachings. This Gift of wisdom and understanding will enable you to develop a new way of thinking and teaching based on the extension of this sacred body of Knowledge, and you will spend much time absorbing these new concepts and preparing the message" for the people of the world.

Phase Nine

A Phase Nine person tends to "go public" with his Message. Here, your tendency is to attract a following for your particular teaching and miracle works. Where an Eight is more individual oriented, the Nine Man is committed to service on a much broader scale. The founders of Unity Religious Science, the Infinite Way, and other New Thought groups were most likely men and women in this state of consciousness, along with many other spiritual teachers and writers of the past and present who are making significant contributions to the uplifting of the race mind.

Phase Ten

An individual in Phase Ten is an Earth Master, with dominion over matter and the forces of nature. He has the ability to project his spirit body and be seen at two places at the same time, and clairvoyance, clairaudience, telepathy and precognition are a part of his nature. Translating pure energy into visible form is another characteristic of a Ten. But it is interesting that as a soul passes from Phase Nine to Ten, he begins to separate himself from the masses and goes apart for a more solitary life of meditation and contemplation. Even so, the Power of a Ten radiates throughout the earth plane, enveloping the world with a light of an illumined consciousness. Others on the path frequently "tune-in" to the consciousness of a Ten with spectacular changes occurring in mind, body and affairs. Thus the evolution through the various phases is helped considerably by these Earth Masters.

Phase Eleven

Phase Eleven is the stage for Universal work, not only on earth but in other dimensions as well. A Master in this stage of evolution is able to move from the earth place to the realms beyond and return at will. While a master Ten is concerned primarily with earth life, the Master Eleven is more universal in scope, working on both sides of the "curtain" — helping in the evolution of all souls. The Masters frequently referred to in occult literature and in the ancient writings are in this stage of soul development.

Phase Twelve

A Soul in Phase Twelve is a Master of Heaven and Earth and as far as we know, the last Twelve on Planet Earth was Jesus Christ. More about this Master Superbeing later.

The great majority of the advanced trainees and the Superbeings themselves (Phases Six through Nine) are living lives that appear to be ordinary from all appearances. They raise families, pursue meaningful careers, watch television, enjoy vacations, engage in social activities, and participate in civic and community affairs. But the more advanced they are, the less they talk about their abilities—so you can enjoy a friendship with one and possibly not realize that he or she is actively working the Power in this life experience. But don't be too curious about that strange neighbor down the street, or the friend who seems to suddenly have it all together. Even with a close watch, you probably won't see either one practicing psychic tricks or flying around the backyard. The only truly recognizable feature of an advanced soul is the feeling you pick up when you are around one. Intuitively you know that you are in the presence of a higher consciousness; you sense a love vibration, a deep sense of peace, a radiance not usually expressed by ordinary mortals.

Just be content to know that in every community you will find individuals who are daily tapping the Supermind and releasing a healing, prospering, guiding, protecting Power that does not understand the meaning of the word impossible. These men and women are not running around playing God. They are God—in expression, and they know that the human or earthly side of their nature is but a channel through which the Power works."

A BASIC OUTLINE FOR THE EXPANSION OF CONSCIOUSNESS:

1. What do you desire in life? You must focus your thoughts on what you really want.

2. You must make a definite decision to accept the fulfillment of your desires.

3. Your desires cannot be fulfilled in the outer world of experience and form unless you have the consciousness or mental equivalent for them.

4. The first step in building the mental equivalent is to recognizethat the Divine Idea corresponding to your desire already exists in your Superconsciousness. This is the intellectual awareness.

5. But an intellectual awareness alone does not have sufficient power to shape the outer picture. Your feeling nature must also be brought into play. When the two are combined, a powerful reaction takes place in the subjective phase of mind, setting up a vibration that corresponds to the spiritual equivalent of fulfillment in your Superconsciousness.

6. This fusion of mind and heart along the lines of a particular desire-fulfillment—if protected from thoughts to the contrary—will develop into a conviction. The conviction of mental equivalent becomes the pattern

through which the Creative Energy of Mind flows or radiates. As this Energy, Light, Power, Substance passes through the pattern it takes on all the attributes of the pattern and goes forth into the outer world to manifest corresponding circumstances, experiences and form.

7. Do not outline the way your desire is to be fulfilled—do not be concerned with how your good is to come forth. You must trust the wisdom and ingenuity of the Power, which is God.

8. You develop your subjective convictions through a dedicated program of contemplative meditation, affirmations, and the proper use of our power of imagination.

9. Be filled with a sense of thankfulness and gratitude that your desires are already fulfilled (they are in Mind), and that they will come forth into visibility at the right time and in the right way.

10. Be active! If you just sit around and wait for your good to fall into your lap, your lap may be far removed from the point of contact and channel that the Power has selected specifically for the outpouring of your good.

(John Price. *Super Beings.* 1981.)

HOW THE BODY REFLECTS THE MIND

Subconscious patterns	Possible physical manifestations
ANGER-HOSTILITY	Appendicitis, arthritis, boils, constipation, heart problems, high blood pressure, indigestion, inflammation
CONFUSION-FRUSTRATION	Colds, flu, headache
CRITICISM	Arthritis, liver problems, ulcers, high blood pressure
FEAR	Accidents, asthma, flu, headache, heart problems, indigestion
GRIEF-DEPRESSION	Cancer, colds, gallstones
GUILT-SELF CONDEMNATION	Back trouble, cancer, hay fever

LACK-LIMITATION	Anemia, asthma, Kidney trouble
OLD AGE CONCERN	Hardening of arteries, (afraid of growing old) Kidney trouble
RESENTMENT-UNFORGIVENESS	Arthritis, cancer, heart problems
TENSION-STRESS	Colds, constipation, headache, high blood pressure

Prosperity is your willingness to express your own aliveness. "You can experience anything you are willing to become," the Futurist impressed. "Prosperity is a state of mind. God is now meeting all my needs in time in full." The Futurist also restated that evil turned around became live. He encouraged us not to postpone our knowing that all that we were was God. Tithing five percent of your net is very important, the Futurist went on to attest. Tithe for the deep sense of thanksgiving given you and your willingness to participate in the greater circle of life. The *Prospering Power of Love,* by C. Ponder, expands upon God, Money and Love. "If you raise your prosperity consciousness, everyone benefits."

"In order for the flower to bloom,
The bud must cease to exist.'

That which must be lightning
Must for sometime be a cloud."

As the Futurist summed up, abundance simply is "We can have what we can behold — or what we can hold in our minds. There is enough for all of us to live full, happy and prosperous lives. We don't have to fear lack of clean air, water, food, energy or any of the other things of a `good life.' We can make ends meet and have plenty more, for there is a power at work within us that can achieve all this if only we believe. Matter is simply mind slowed down to visibility."

He quoted Paraculsus as saying "Could we rightly comprehend the mind of man, nothing would be impossible to us upon the Earth." So he ended the workshop by asking each of us to make a list of what we wanted in life, claiming it as our own, visualizing the experience of having the fulfillment of our desires, affirming that it is done and giving thanks, and then, to stand by for a miracle."

"PEACE, BE STILL, AND NOW I AM ONE WITH THEE, GOD." *(The Impersonal Life: A channeled book)*

A handout a dear friend had given me by Louise Hay called *How to Love Yourself* reappeared in my journal. It seemed to tie into the abundance and love wisdom that was coming through. It had ten steps that I would read and reread. They are:

HOW TO LOVE YOURSELF

1) **STOP ALL CRITICISM**! Criticism never changes a thing. Refuse to criticize yourself. Accept yourself exactly as you are. Everybody changes. When you criticize yourself, your changes are negative. When you approve of yourself, your changes are positive.

2) **DON'T SCARE YOURSELF!** Stop terrorizing yourself with your thoughts. It's a dreadful way to live. Find a mental image that gives you pleasure (Mine is a rose in full bloom) and immediately switch scary thought to a pleasure thought.

3) **BE GENTLE AND KIND AND PATIENT!** Be gentle with yourself. Be kind to yourself. Treat yourself as you would someone you really loved.

4) **BE KIND TO YOUR MIND!** Self hatred is only hating your own thoughts. Don't hate yourself for having the thoughts. Gently change your thoughts.

5) **PRAISE YOURSELF!** Criticism breaks down the inner spirit. Praise builds it up. Tell yourself how well you are doing with every little thing.

6) **SUPPORT YOURSELF!** Find ways to support yourself. Reach out to friends and allow them to help you. It is being strong to ask for help when you need it.

7) **BE LOVING TO YOUR NEGATIVES!** Acknowledge that you created them to fill a need. Now you are finding new, positive ways to fulfill these needs. So lovingly release the 'old', negative patterns.

8) **TAKE CARE OF YOUR BODY!** Learn about nutrition. What kind of fuel does your body need to have optimum energy and vitality. Learn about exercise. What kind of exercise can you enjoy? Cherish and revere the temple you live in.

9) **MIRROR WORK!** Look into your eyes often. Express this growing sense of love you have for yourself. Forgive yourself looking into the mirror. Talk to your parents looking into the mirror. Forgive them too. At least once a day say, "I love you, I really love you."

10) **DO IT NOW!** Don't wait until you get well, or lose the weight or get the new job, or the new relationship. Begin now. Do the best you can.

1982 TEEN SURVIVAL SCHOOL IN THE HIGH COUNTRY

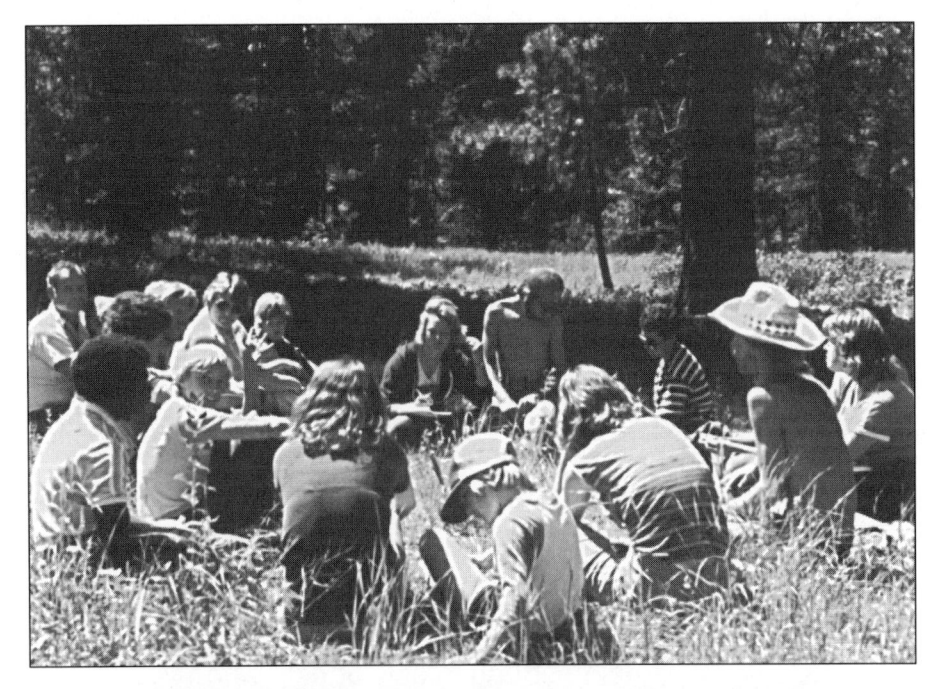

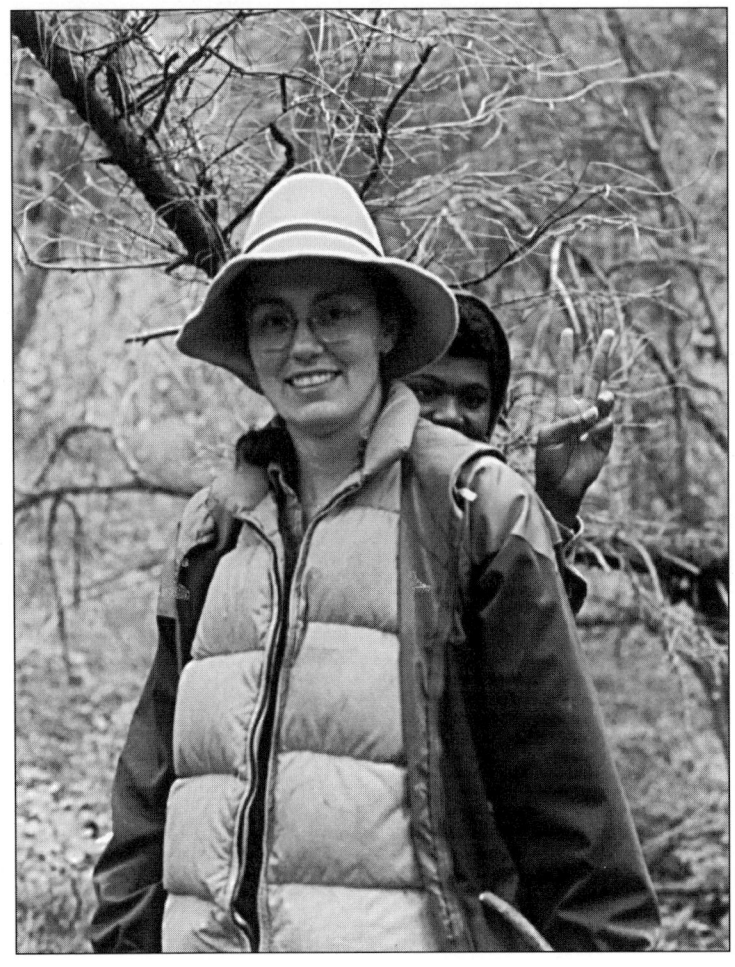

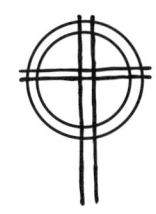

THEREFORE BE AT PEACE WITH GOD, WHATEVER YOU CONCEIVE HIM TO BE, AND WHATEVER YOUR LABORS & ASPIRATIONS, IN THE NOISY CONFUSION OF LIFE KEEP PEACE WITH YOUR SOUL. WITH ALL ITS SHAM DRUDGERY & BROKEN DREAMS IT IS STILL A BEAUTIFUL WORLD.
BE CAREFUL. STRIVE TO BE HAPPY."

WHOLE PERSON—WHOLE PLANET

The spring and summer of 1982 were intense. While pain and death were constant threatening companions, I was surrounded by intense passionate warrior-like men.

The week before the Two Raven's Festival, my friends facilitated a Wilderness School for a local Foundation. We focused on troubled teenagers who were no longer safe to reside in their homes. Because I was simultaneously assisting with the promotion of a *Local to Global Peace Conference* at the university featuring a Hopi spiritual messenger, Thomas Banyaca and an international peacemaker, Gordon Feller, I would only attend the first week of this teen survival school in the high country of Idaho.

Out of doors I supplemented the curriculum by teaching self health and esteem. Letting this setting in the wilderness assist youth to regain or recognize a nurturing connection with the Earth was part of my heart work. After being a teacher of mathematics under fluorescent lights and darkened windows, this provided my dream classroom, nature.

I could not put my total attention to the survival school, though, because of my obligations back in the city.

When it came time for the teens to set out on a four day trek, I left to return to the city. This long hike would afford them enough time away to be quiet, to listen, and ask for visioning help in their goal setting. They didn't know that yet.

I ached as I felt some of the teens shudder and watched as some cried when they heard I would not be on the walking part of the journey. There was another woman guide who did go. She was the friend who had helped fund me to go North to the Healing Camp and had also given me the important moral document, *How to Love Yourself.* I recognized that I was like their mother figure, one who really liked them.

Not until the moment when they walked up the trail turning, oozing pain did I understand how much I represented security and safety to them. I was saddened by the realization, but part of me knew it was a critical life lesson, reliance on self not others. We are often called to journey alone in life with just our relationship to spirit and nature to keep us peaceful. In this case I would return and be there for their homecoming.

Quickly I shifted into a facilitator for our elder Hopi spiritual messenger, a round, jovial twinkling eyed grandfather, and a saucy, mid-twenties, outspoken, planetary peacekeeper. From the moment I picked up Thomas Banyaca from the airport, I knew this stout, withered, elder held keys to my spiritual pursuit. That night as he delivered his message from ancient Hopi tabloids, I clung to each concept. I heard him share the prophecies:

> ***Until people from all races, all colors and spiritual pursuits can stand in circle and be heard...we would not know peace on this good land.
> ***He called us to watch the mountains, especially the sacred Mother's original mountains on his lands. If the mountains were destroyed, pillaged by man for the material mineral worth, cataclysm would come to the Earth.
> ***He spoke of his call to go the United Nation and ask to be heard. As a planetary peacemaker, he was charged to go four times and request an audience. If after the fourth visit, he was still not heard, his assignment as spiritual messenger was complete and he would then return to his lands and await the time when the earth would shake and crack, and the volcanoes would spew. At this time he had gone twice and was soon to journey a third time.
> ***He again explained the concept that all of nature is interrelated. What one part does or receives affects all others. We cannot get away with being unconscious.

I knew his truth was my truth. Oh, another family member that knew of my innate natural spirituality. It also helped to explain the part of me driven to heal and to make changes. I felt deeply connected to the Earth. I had constantly felt the threats from the nuclear plants to those living towards the Southeast part of Idaho and 'wind over' debris up from Nevada darkened our atmosphere and mutated our waters.

I felt this but had not known how to speak about it and be heard. Throughout my years as a fifth generation Idahoan, I had heard friends relate nightmare dreams about big mushroom explosions in the sky, death of communities because the well waters were poisoned and on and on. I knew our intuitive nature was screaming for attention, but our government's military regime commanded more power than the average citizen.

His truths settled in my heart. I responded to his call for assistance in speaking the word. I announced myself to be a Planetary Peacemaker. I would be outspoken when it came to speaking for the Earth and her family. I would watch the mountain, seeing the storm beings and feeling the waters. I would take action. I was not alone. My Sioux Medicine man teacher had referred to we rebels for the Earth as 'dog soldiers'. We were people out on the fringe of society, assuring safe passage for the tribe/family to travel.

Now my sense of family had greatly expanded. I was part of a global family. I returned with Thomas and Gordan to the high mountain festival sight. I reconnected to the Youth Wilderness Camp ready to welcome them back. Simultaneously, I was going to share the festival time with my playful Irish friend I had met at an earlier Red Cross training. Some say God is a comedian performing for an audience that has forgotten how to laugh. This particular 'production' was huge. I prayed to stay well enough to get through this hectic demanding major sequence of events.

Here we all were, many different participants at the crossroads of life; on the majestic Two Ravens at Tall Pine camp sight, inhabited by grand tipis and a crowning glory view; a welcoming back celebration occurred with the dozen teenagers; a Hopi Elder returned to the round lodge to rest and city funding officials scrutinized the training. Meanwhile, the funny Irishman brought chuckles and stories to the young.

A few of the youth met me with warm smiles and hearts while some of the others were instantly mad at me. After the feast, the storytelling and the rewarding of their accomplishments, the dancing began. I joined in and soon the teasing began that I looked like a chicken. Laughter and acceptance of each other occurred and I prayed that they would see the pattern that it is great to be able to be in community with another being aware that at some point one or the other may have to walk alone. It is possible to have a reunion in time and not experience abandonment. I knew with my own healing journey, that I was healing with the Earth, her feelings and responsiveness, her aliveness and consistency.

As the youth departed a part of me was desperately wanting to be 'just a participant' and not a responsible leader at the high country earth festival. I wanted to play and be in loving company. Every direction I turned, out popped another intense man. These were men who appeared to really want to know me. Whatever the vibration or attracting senses I was emitting, it was felt by many.

As the magic of the Two Raven Festival intensified, a powerful electrical storm dumped pounding rains. The torrential rains seemed to mirror the intensity of the men who were "hitting" on me, from young teens to the elders. I was attracting men and I could not believe it.

The grand dance performance was scheduled to occur on Saturday night down in a green grassy meadow surrounded by tall pine. All day it rained, poured. Late in the afternoon our prayers were answered as the waters let up. The decision to go on with the performance was intense as our power source was a generator with thick wrapped wires running a quarter of a mile that would have to be dried as well as the stage.

What occurred next was close to a miracle. A rainbow appeared as well as the calling of birds, so the go ahead occurred with nature. Young and old began mopping up the waters to provide safety for our evening performance.

As I stood in line for our evening dinner a frantic person ran by me, turned and came back and asked if I could assist one of our star performers. A flutist from California whose two year old daughter had accidentally poked her finger in his eye. He was in great pain. Eye injuries are one of the most painful things the body is called to endure. So off I went to lay on of hands to his eye hours before the performance. I had watched this sensitive man interact with his daughter from a distance this weekend. I had been impressed that a single father would bring a child here.

While administering to the flutist I would hear that he and his wife were getting a divorce and this was his first time alone with his lovely, emotional child. The evening beauty included a glowing full moon that journeyed behind dark, water drenched clouds to beam luminous specialness. I am sure all who attended this Earth Celebration still can revision this spectacular work of Earth Art. I was so impressed when the flutist shared with us a musical video impression of Heaven on Earth; he set his pain aside and transformed all of us with his artistic expression.

The next morning my photographer, river runner friend departed early.

Within minutes another magnetic man bounded from the hillside demanding me to give him some time. He was from San Francisco and aspired to run for president of the United States. He sparkled with enthusiasm concerning his knowledge of the Iroquois confederation and their influence on our young government. He prophesied a

1982 TWO RAVENS FESTIVAL

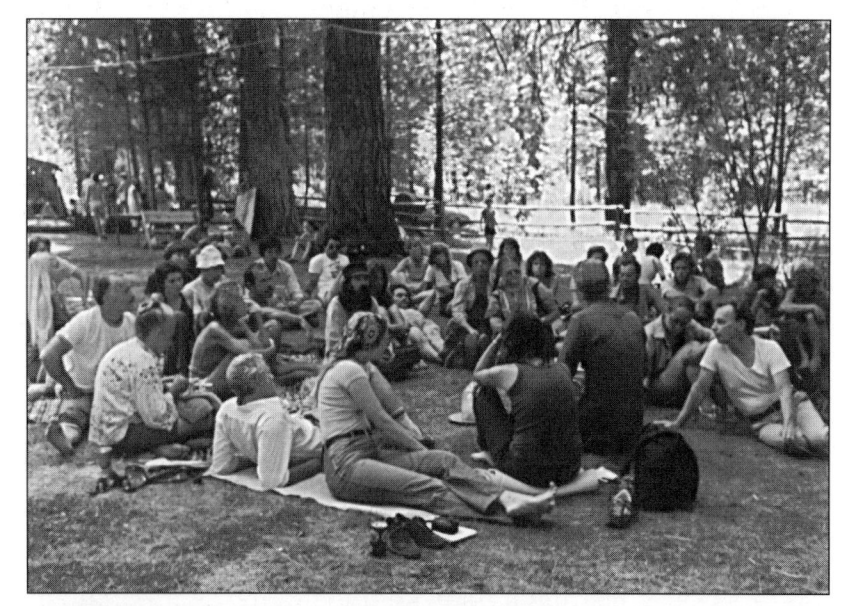

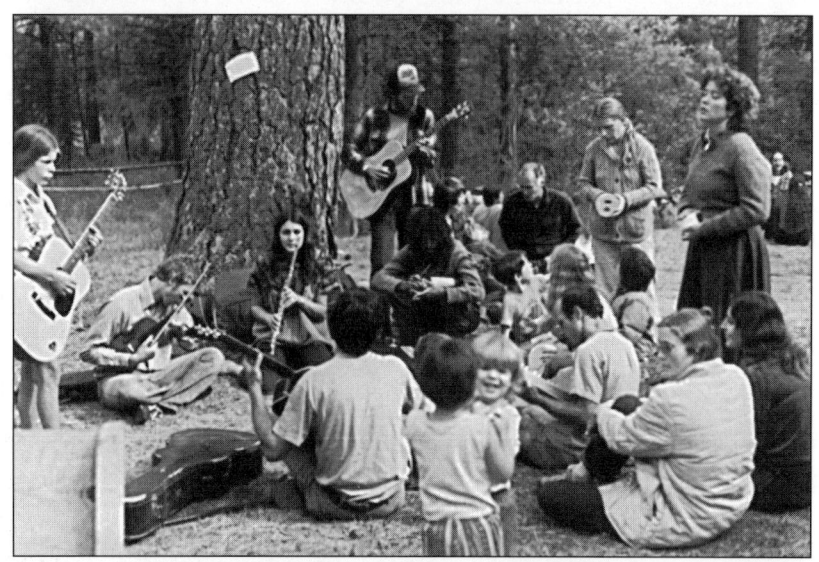

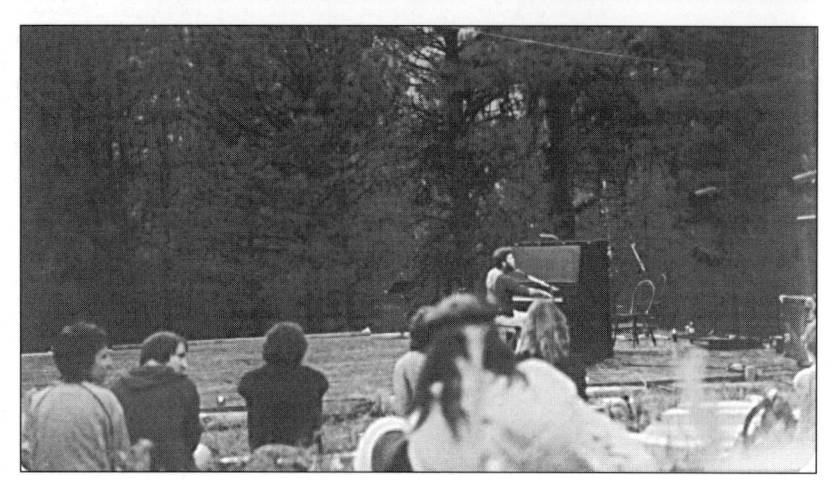

1982 TWO RAVENS FESTIVAL

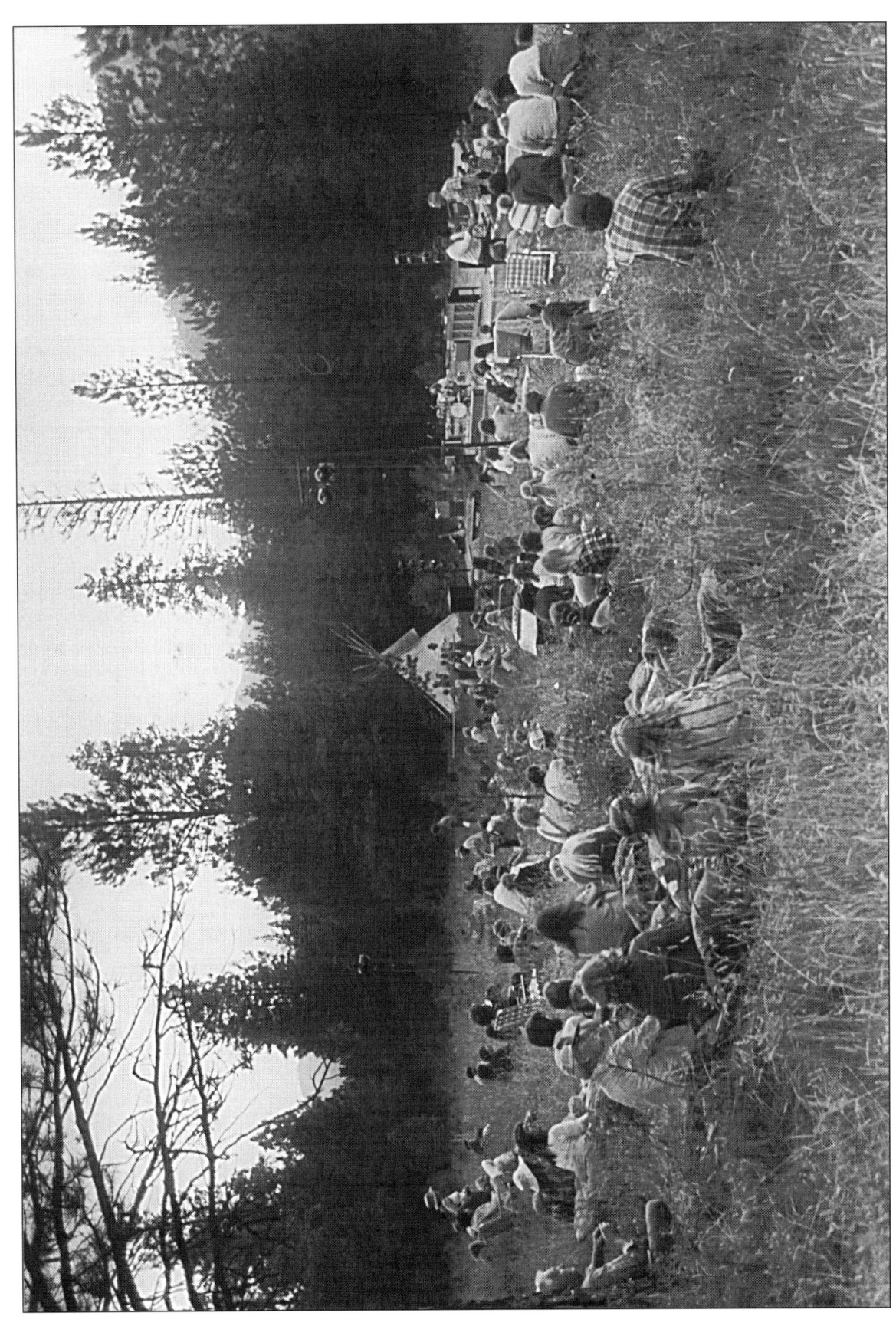

telephone computer hookup to communicate with the nation. He saw my organizational skills and wanted me to come to California and help with this major project.

This had never happened before in my life. Perhaps I was on the edge of aliveness and death and felt I had nothing to lose that was attractive. I was courageously giving my all to know and live spirit-filled. Days felt like lifetimes and I was learning a lot about life very quickly.

After all the crowds left this magical, musical, dance-filled, self-health, earth communing festival, the facilitator conducted a closing sweat. I had been eager to sweat with the couple who were planning to share this deep renewal, cleansing process. The sweat leader openly proclaimed the value he put to having his wife help with this deeply reverent process. The two ran outdoor youth programs out of the high country in California and Oregon.

'Nana', the medicine person's wife, had fallen and injured her knee the week before the festival. Because of the remoteness of the festival site, she had no access to medical help and day by day she was becoming more lame and infected. Because of my observation of other 'medicine women', I was extremely cautious to offer my services, although my hands and heart were pressuring me to announce my capacity to be of service to her. Finally I approached her husband, and then her and soon I was assisting with comfrey compacts, Reiki, and treatments to her brain. By this time, I was convinced that until the brain could balance and allow the healing presence to come through, illness would stay in the body.

The time for the sweat arrived, and the only other woman was wounded and could not participate. There I was again, in close quarters, dominated by intense men. Through prayer, the spirit of the hawk came into the lodge. A small Merlin-like bird hopped to my shoulder and demanded that I leave the lodge and attend to the ailing, elder woman. I responded and left.

I had committed to following my intuition, the second nature that truly caretakes our every move. I was learning that when I ignored the inner voice, often painful consequences unfolded.

When I went to the woman, her face lit up and love spewed forth from her center towards me. She said she had been praying for some help. The pain was great in her. Together we worked with natural earth medicines, prayers and intentions to remove the fire that was consuming her leg.

Later, I learned second hand that after I left the sweat, my Sioux medicine teacher was hurt in the lodge. He left the 'inipi', and gave away his pipe and his tools of medicine. Somehow he had misused his gifts, and only he knew how.

Meanwhile, the San Francisco leader continued to teach me of the Iroquois Federation system for healthy communication in a community, in a nation. It was so interesting. Anytime a decision was needed, the elder women's circle was consulted. The concern was aired, their input asked for.

Next the elders would examine the effect a decision would have on seven generation to come. Decision were not made lightly. Then the recommendations were given to the tribal legal chief system and a dictum would be emitted. Our own constitution is copied much from the Iroquois treaties. For more information read *Basic Call to Consciousnes.* Wow. This was a culture that honored women's wisdom, something totally unfamiliar to the male hierarchial family, religious and government systems practiced in the U.S.A.

Now I was being shown a way to assist in re-establishing of creditability regarding woman's knowing to honor family, community and the raising of children. When asked why Native Americans were so structurally weak today, a wise elder responded that our missionary process imposed upon them removed the native children from their blood family and community and the social training necessary for personal pride, esteem and closeness with all of nature.

In the church schools and in the legal system it was a crime for Native Americans to practice or speak to their ancient natural spirituality. My politician friend stated that the elder women he knew in various tribes asked the white men to give them back the Native American children so that they could be trained in the earth respected ways, to be reminded of who they truly are. We had shamed their race and abused their people for a 100 years. It must stop.

We sparked conversations that I had only heard murmured inside myself or read in idealistic books. Now there was a potential American leader who wanted my help. He offered to bring me to San Francisco to work on his campaign. Quickly I said yes.

The farm had continued to be a retreat place for me. The people on the land were distant since the closing of Book Magic. I wanted my life to be meaningful and expansive. I had nothing to lose and everything to give.

My 'ol' sunshine' man was living in my farm house and I did not feel like disrupting him, so after the festival I moved in with my 'spiritual soul sister, Synthony' and prepared to leave for San Francisco and the world.

My newly acquired California politician changed his mind two days before I was to depart. All my repeated internal messages about men shouted inside me. I didn't demand enough respect for myself. I was confused about what it meant to love, to know loyalty and sincerity.

The fall and early winter of 1982 were cold in the ancient Victorian, three story old hotel my friend owned. Knowing only that we are to do our 'heart work', 'heart art', my friend and I opened an art gallery on the ground floor of this wondrous historic home. She was recently divorced with four children and together, with my own energetic son, we lived as family, scraping along on hopes and dreams and little physical money.

The mystery surrounding men deepened as my Irishman friend just disappeared. We were to meet around Thanksgiving to see how each of us were doing. He never showed up.

Hauntingly in my dreams, I was visited by a woman dressed in white leather, with long dark hair. She whispered knowings to me and called on me to let go of the 'living dead' parts of myself and feel the rebirthing that was growing stronger in me. My artist friend, not knowning of my dream guide woman, painted an original oil Indian piece that looked just like my dream image.

It has hung on the North wall of my Sacred Space Office. Anytime I meet with someone who is pushed up against the wall deeply needing 'wholing', I share the picture. Without words we can nod our heads, seeing the promise of new growth in front of the dead of winter. If we will take a risk and step out, with great trust, life does begin again.

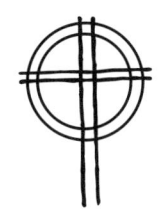

"GO PLACIDLY AMID THE NOISE AND HASTE & REMEMBER WHAT PEACE THERE MAY BE IN SILENCE"

THE LOST YEAR - 1983

From mid November through December, the ground floor of this giant Victorian home became the business known as *Idaho Christmas.* In years gone by we had this sale in the bookstore. We brought in the community's wonderful artisans and gave them a place to market their artistic expressions.

My son and I lived in one of the rooms and shared a makeshift kitchen as the main one downstairs was a display room. I appreciated the warmth and kindness of my friend to invite us in her home, but living in a storefront seven days a week stretched my wounded soul.

With the new year, my attitude shifted concerning my farm home. No longer did I feel like my 'ol sunshine man' deserved to stay in my comfortable farm home. He was no longer my ward to protect. Enough with this Earth Mothering of everyone else but me. I asserted myself and asked my ex-soul lover and yogi guru to leave and allow me to live alone just with my son. The attitude that had me give every thing to the man and that I would make it somehow with less than I deserved broke. A single man had lots more opportunity for self maintenance than a mother and child. I returned to the farm.

This was the first time in my life that there was no other man present overseeing and criticizing me. I pledged to seek solace and return to my health vigil. What was once my sanctuary became my lost paradise.

I call 1983 the lost year. One of the rules of my right conduct was love thy neighbor as thyself. On the farm lived the man who initially was one of my ex-husband's best friends in the BIFC Boy's Club, a 'jock' hero, and a woman user. This Big Man was also the male I intentionally set out to prove my worth to and gain his respect. At the time of finalizing my divorce, Big Man walked beside me supporting my process, affirming my worth as an individual.

Big Man became my second lover in my life. We co-owned Book Magic together and soon after the demise of our relationship; the book store structure began to crumble.

Big Man's new family became his priority. The years of training to become the Farm's farmer had strengthened his conviction that he by himself should tend the land. He no longer wanted to share with us the trials and gains of this eighty acre parcel of hopes and dreams. He broke the rules of our farm's communication process.

For years our group had hired Mennonites to farm the land as the Big Man learned to work with nature, its' seasons and its cultivating, rejuvenation, planting, harvesting and marketing. Now that he was doing well and still ripe with anger over the 'con' man at our now defunct store, he and his lady wanted me off the farm. Daily I felt bombarded by their anger about my return to 'their' home. I was judged harshly. I was worse than the plague to them.

Life did not get better as my Medicine man, True Creed, who had relinquished his tools, communicating with me anymore. Only upon pressure from me to determine if our teen survival school was scheduled for the next summer was I finally told that I was not to be hired back on the team. Both women from the first school were rejected, although all the men were back on line to teach. The betrayal of our common dream of reaching teenagers, plus the strength of the expanded community system collapsed. My brain was shattering; nothing made sense.

We had always teased that the farm was the 'crazy farm'. The most interesting of peoples frequently found their way to this God graced land. I often felt like I lived in a glass bubble that many longed for but chose not to commit to and help grow with.

My mind hesitates to remember this last year on the land. I used to dream of rocking in chairs, telling stories with friends and children and making sure there was tea available when someone was weak. The land had a personality that soothed the aches. The fruit orchard was ready to finally produce fruit, the acres of grapes were budding, the rose and herb garden had matured and I was being bombarded by the people who were to be my extended family.

This year of final retreat with the land gave me the opportunity to write repeated political letters, quizzing on the inappropriate consumption of waters, swayed views of politicians, treatment of youth and to report on a system that judged people as guilty before even being tried by their peers. My fury over various areas of the culture that I viewed as out of integrity raged in my journal writings.

One of my original valley friends married a wealthy woman who subsequently bought an adjoining farm. Even though he was now a neighbor I seldom saw him since his union. His wife was best friends with the Big Man's wife.

In the fall I noticed he started visiting at different times of the day. It occurred to me he was sneaking over to see me while watering the back acres. This blunt outspoken side of me challenged him to get honest with his mate. I clarified that if she did not know he was visiting me, then he could not come over. With eyes cast down, he simply stated it would be devastating if his wife knew he was here.

I was striving for integrity and honesty. Outside the winds picked up and the atmospheric pressure was changing. I climbed up into my loft bedroom for a better view of the South where big, dark storm clouds were building and I saw the distant bolts of lightning flash. My friend climbed upstairs to look. Immediately I heard that inner voice say get down from here. I commented, 'It would be just my luck to get hit by lightning and be found crispy with you in my bedroom.' All the rumoring about me would be substantiated.

I demanded that we get downstairs immediately. Within minutes my farm home was hit by a giant cosmic, glowing red charge. All the lights went out and there was distinct smell of smoke. I felt like I was inside a bell that had just been struck. I was vibrating and fuzzy. Visibly shaken, my old friend left immediately and we never had another conversation.

The phone lines were down, and the pump was blown, but my house was not on fire. I sat through the night praying. As the sun rose in the morning, a knocking on the door below awoke me. My friends brought a hot air balloonist to the farm and we were off to an open field to lift off into the blue sky.

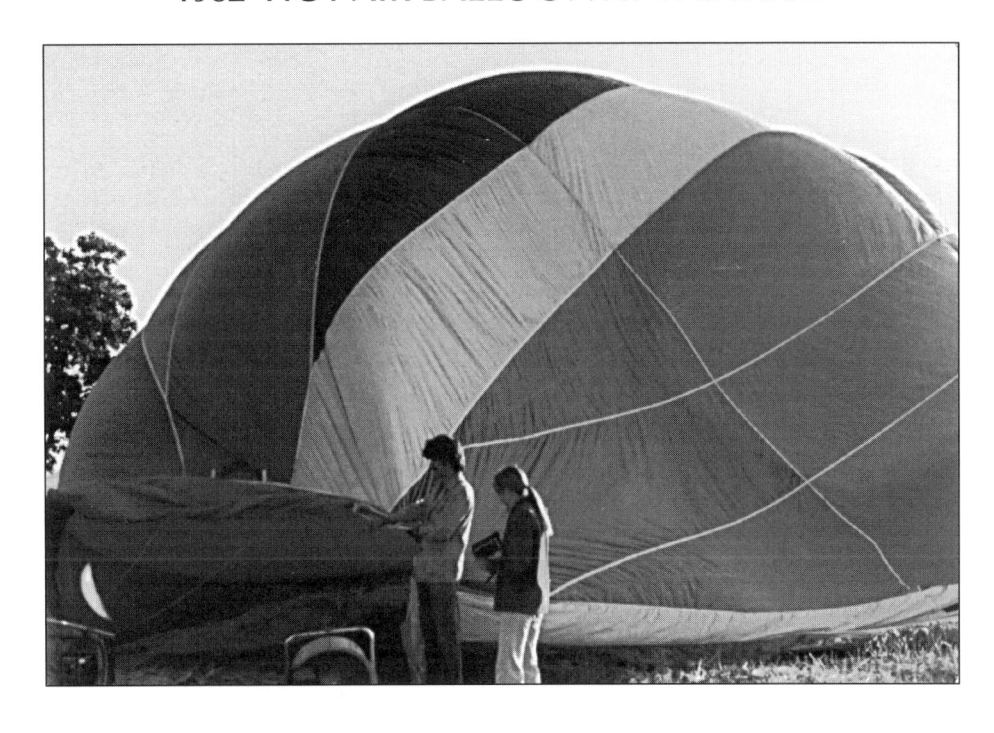

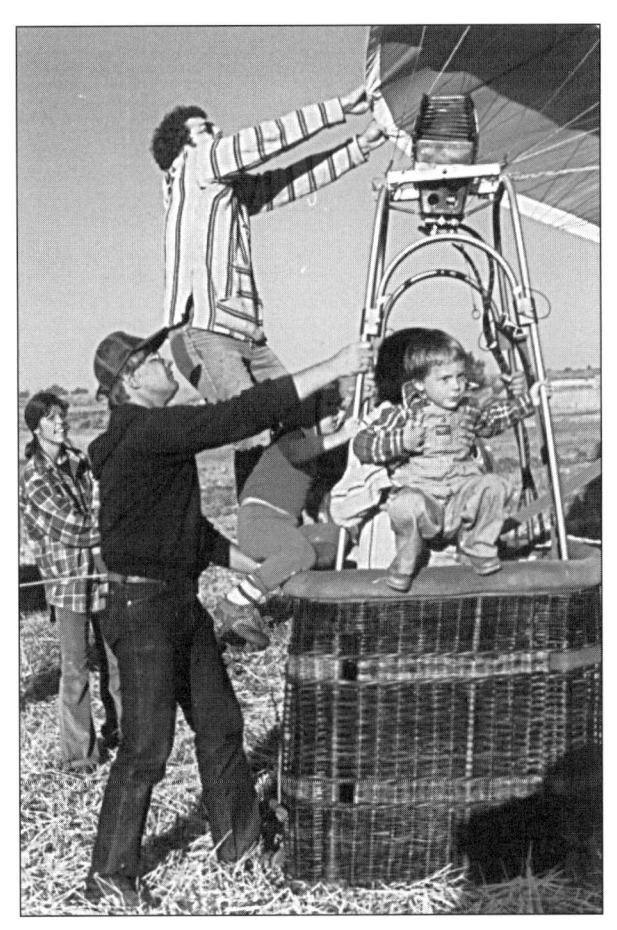

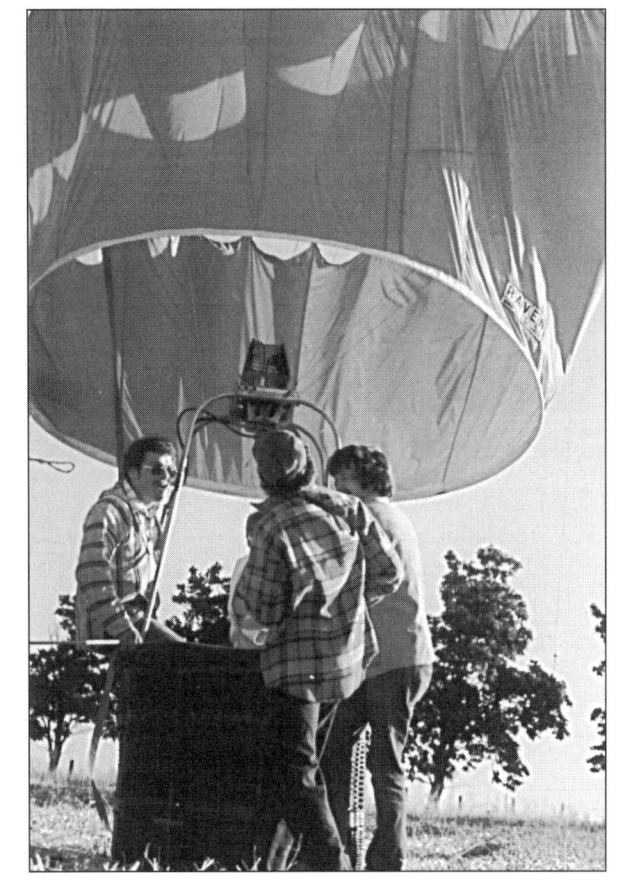

1982 HOT AIR BALLOON AT THE FARM

Out in the field I watched as neighbors and passerby congregated to see what was happening at this crazy farm. Repair people arriving to reconnect my home to the outside world. Life was truly a circus that morning. The winds blew and we were unable to take the balloon ride. Oh, such was the story of life. Great potential, almost making it, but not yet.

An old friend who had introduced me to the Georgian lawyer who had, a year or so earlier, returned to our valley. This family therapist/psycho-therapist chose me as his free client. In the stillness of a long, dark, cold winter he shared hours of questioning and examining my mental and emotional decay. He asked me a million 'whys', especially around relationship decisions. My brain screamed for silence. He asked hard questions.

He shared his deep envy of my spiritual beliefs. There was something just of me that oozed a belief in God, in Jesus, in being a Living Disciple that was broken in him. As a young man he had entered a monastery to become a priest but disillusionment drove him away. He came from a matriarchal system where his mother was a powerful medicine women in her own ranks. He seemed to have a similar pattern to mine, attracting powerful partnerships that could not sustain their idealism.

Proud of his roots and his blood, somewhere this sweet Chicano had broken and now was filled with disillusionment for a God that would create such prejudice, hunger and grief. We commiserated on the plight of women, minorities, children and the health of the good Earth. Regularly he would leave his family practice, secure income, comfortable middle class existence and journey to South America to do missionary work to help his people.

Winter was a hard one plagued by several feet of snow early on and deathly cold spells which kept us close to the wood heater in the farm home. For a few days we were snow bound. A neighbor was able to plow out my driveway and lane so I could journey to town for supplies.

I picked up a broken beer bottle on the sidewalk and accidentally cut my finger. In the middle of the night, the storms returned dumping more snow. In the early morning hours, I sat sipping tea looking out at the sea of white when I noticed a stream of water flowing towards my back greenhouse door. Then my mind screamed. "River of Water!" unbeknownst to us the plowing to release us the day before had pushed down the frozen layer of snow into the stream in my backyard, plugging the necessary underground culvert, thus damning the flow of the stream. The bottleneck caused this tiny trickle to flow an alternative route right towards my back door.

Immediately I stepped into action. I put on a new pair of leather gloves and raced out to unplug the culvert. Where are the cameras when heroic deeds occur? Hours later the flood averted, I collapsed back in the farm house. My hands were thoroughly soaked and stained by the dye from the leather gloves.

In the dark of the night the hand and arm that had been cut by the broken glass began to throb. In my loft, I felt the fire run up my arm, my head ached. No healing treatment, touch, massage, or ointment helped. My life energy was diminishing and by early dawn the haunts of death danced with me again. I didn't have enough energy to get mad at God, for again finding myself in this pervading grey limbo. I had blood poisoning and it was up to my shoulder, inches from my heart. I was in big trouble.

Dazed, all but unconscious, I called a friend in the nearby community. I knew the roads were all blocked. After I diverted the floods at my home, the waters unleashed, rushed to the major road a half miles away and filled the low point on the highway, stopping all passage. I could not drive out.

My friend connected with an EMT friend and within an hour I was rescued by a snow mobile and was taken to the local physician. The community pharmacy gave me medication and the stores supplied me all I needed on good faith for I had no monies on me.

Faith in this tough, tight rural farm community was sparked. Even with the starting of a book store, opening a food co-op, being a teacher, participating in local fund raising, I had still felt like an outsider, judged and not accepted. Now I knew I was. It moved me. Even though the feelings of the farm community were tense and the man who walked beside me had challenged my brain to the hilt, I quit thinking. "Delete the need to understand, Delete the need to judge and Delete the need to compare," ran through my thoughts.

After this scary situation I prayed for what I was to do with my life. Should I stay on the farm and continue the fight for respect or leave and join a more accepting community. If I was to leave, where would this wholistic community be? Over and over I heard, "Simplify, Unify and Purify."

The book *2001* which addressed micro-macro consciousness by Thea Alexander came to me. It could have been my story. Through the world of meditation and sometimes pain, I could alter my view of reality. I, like the hero in the book, found myself in an idyllic Garden of Eden with beautiful golden human beings. All the codes for how I wished to live were practiced there but not here in the physical Earthly reality, only in the dream world-non-ordinary reality. I longed to live in that garden.

I dreamed of dancing in a circle with a group of kindred souls. In the dream, we were in harmony with each other and this Earth world that we lifted up off the ground and slowly became transparent and went to this other realm of pure energetic being. Much to my dismay and that of the hero in the story, I, too, was told I must live out those codes of integrity, right livelihood, boundaries, Earth wisdom, and loving in the here and now, on this physical Earth. The internal directions went on to say to me 'put your books away and be it.'

Until I lived it out here, it being that place of peace, health, relationship, and spiritual wholeness, I would not get to there to stay.

I started actively journaling my ongoing process of living spirit fully. Each time I would get distracted on my weak male/female knowledge, I would tell myself to 'stop it.' and put my attention to living as the elder brother Christ spoke of. My mind was told to be still and listen. I was willing.

Synchronistically, that spring Brooke Medicine Eagle was returning to Idaho to do a course called the *Warrior's Leap.* I knew I would attend. The whole reason I chose to live on the land initially was to heal with the Earth, to know God and be in a caring community. After the divorce, I vowed to never marry again. I felt broken and unable to believe in that institution. I put a lot into friendship. I never wanted to focus all my attention towards just one person again. I vowed to be a good friend, to show up, to work together, to care. To my senses, The Farm had failed to be that community.

My psychotherapist friend warned me repeatedly, "You really are being called to do bigger things. It looks like your time at the farm is ending." I was ready to leap into a new way of living and loving.

Brooke's *Warrior's Leap* class occurred again in a distant town. Upon arriving I could tell that the amazing telegraph system in the Planetary Peace Movement had reached many special people. The room was full of wonderful teachers, counselors, ministers and ordinary folk. Before Brooke began her sharing we watched her again create her altar with a candle, bells, sweet grass, sage, corn, fire and *intention*. She prayed to the directions and then proceeded to call in the animal protectors, elements, elders, ancestors and teachers. I wondered as she sang if I would ever learn the medicine wheel.

Her emphasis was in integrating our whole body, remembering that the deeper part of one's self loved metaphors. She was calling us to embody spirit. Learning how to learn was the key to awareness.

She impressed upon us to be 'Rainbow Warriors', bridging Heaven with Earth, knowing we have a calling and that we are all family on this Earth. Each of us must get on with our heart work. She helped deepen our knowledge of nuerolinguistic movements through deliberate exercises. By engaging our active imagination she taught a hand exercise to be used any time we came to a situation in life which was an 'either - or' response. We learned how to weigh our options and then turn it over to grace for a mediated divine intervention.

To deepen our trust, we found a partner and designed a process for surrendering to trust. It might have been walking on a plank suspended above the ground to represent a fear of heights or falling backwards into embracing arms that would reflect healing a distrust in relationships. Whatever or wherever we felt stuck in life, she had us set up a challenge that mirrored or was a metaphor for that situation and then with great trust move through it.

The partner I had was Gentle Heart from the Elder Sister circle . He was a safe male for me as he was gay and thus some part of me felt trusting to share how broken my male-female connection was. We created a bond that represented human beings, regardless of sex, who are willing to reflect the highest good in each other. Today our relationship is still strong; we know we are living disciples this lifetime.

Brooke's closing exercise had us affirm what it was that we truly wanted in our life, our right livelihood, and then announce to the group who we were and what our intention was and do a running leap into the linked arms of our group as they chanted our name and our intention. These exercises blended all our senses touch, smell, sight, hearing, and knowing with outside positive responses. A true warrioress leapt calling herself Suzanne and affirming sacred healing work with her hands.

When I returned to the farm, an amazing offer came from an established city grandfather to manage a sophisticated clothing store. I allowed myself to say yes, knowing that the life I had dreamt of at the farm was completed. This elder gentleman had observed me through the book store chapter and then as I was a manager substitute for my friends who owned businesses downtown. He said I was respected and powerful and he wanted those qualities to help manage his forty year old clothing store. I sensed that this would be a temporary position where I could be trained by a wise man to manage and to increase my monetary notions.

I was moving on. My son was thrilled, for the last few years he had repeatedly expressed wishes of living in a city where he could play soccer and be with more action. I was glad he had his preschool years in nature and I was amazed at the intensity of his wishes to get out in the world and in time prosper. He wanted to be very rich. My therapist friend with tears in his eyes said 'I told you so.' Our intimate relationship ended and I left the farm to never return again.

One Saturday evening at a local pub, I was celebrating the end of the work week when a man across the way kept staring at me. This tall, angular man came over and introduced himself as the gentleman who had sat beside me at the Elder Sister circle. I was stunned because I scarcely recognized him.

This Barefoot Physician was regularly doing treatments in our Magic Valley. He noticed how difficult it was for me to stand straight. My head was on crooked and on many days it felt by mid-afternoon that I could not even keep it up. He asked if I was ready to start working with him and his type of therapy.

I had to admit all the spiritual and mental exercises I had been practicing had not removed felt pain. He said my facial bones were out of symmetry and my jaw reeked of tautness. He sensed the tremendous pain in my head and knew of resulting Endocrine glandular imbalances in my spleen and ovaries. He knew my body better than anyone I had ever met just by looking at me. Few people knew the intensity of my illness as I kept it private and stayed away from others when in the height of pain.

I began an ongoing, restructuring of my out-of-align, out of balance, frayed person. I was receiving deep body tissue and Oriental meridian acupressure from this talented touch physician I called Iron Fingers. My health regime consisted of daily administering a personal Reiki treatment, Zen with the land, soaks in geothermal water, lap swimming, eating vegetarian, locally grown meals, and meditation.

The barefoot physician, being trained in ancient oriental ways also addressed my mental and emotional states of mind. He saw the fear and disbelief in living I carried. The sadness oozed from me covering deep anger at the painful repeated relationships I created. He would shift into what the Native American's might call shaman role or spiritual journeyer and helped mend my lost soul parts.

Iron Fingers facilitated medicinal sweats. Even though I had been participating in the sweat lodge ceremony for a decade, I could not in the beginning sit through one round of his intense, soul purging experiences.

He felt that by facing fears, we gain freedom and vitality. Since I had an intense dislike of heights, he and I would go out to the canyon's edge and knowing how terrified I was, he would suggest I walk on the edge and find peace and safety because I was connected to the Earth through my feet. I'd like to report that it was easy. It was not. Every cell of my body and nervous system would fire. I did not trust enough, and I would fall over the edge and get hurt some more.

One time a group of us had prepared for months to do a long dance on the solstice in June at a magical natural waters overlooking the Snake River Canyon. By the time the evening fell dark, there was no one able to dance. Each in our own way were lame or too exhausted.

What was curious, is that for years I had prayed to see, and while training with Iron Fingers, he knew that I saw non-ordinary reality through my senses. No one had ever known about the flashes of light, the dancing of sparkle that fluttered in my periphery, the sound the trees murmured, the communication with the birds, the language of the waters. He knew I saw and repeatedly he would check into what I was sensing.

With hindsight I know this was an extremely important chapter in my life, facing my fears, including death. I learned that my physical eyesight may never get back to perfect vision, but that I could see through my hands and other senses. A crack of light was finally filtering in where endless years of prayers had seemed unreachable.

An opportunity came to buy an inexpensive home in the town where the clothing store was. My son was in the second grade now and I was displeased with the teaching techniques in our small rural town. My worst fear was to have his innate

NATURE HEALING SOJOURN

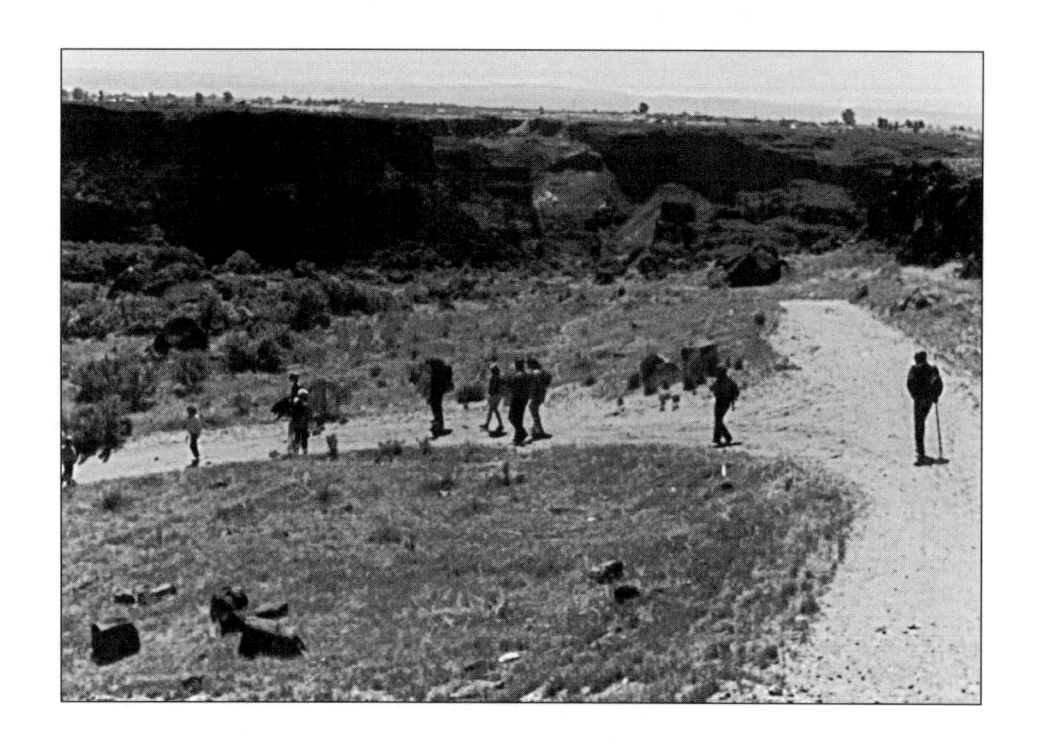

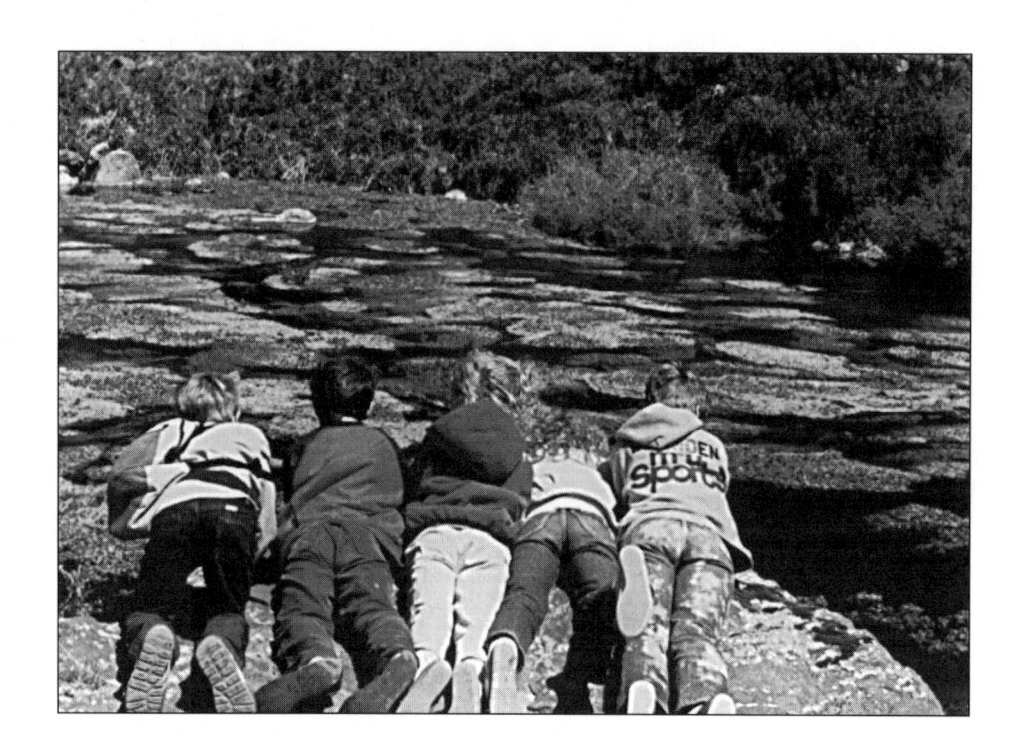

wisdom and expansive creative nature stifled. As a teacher and active parent I was prepared to do home schooling but my son was outspoken about wanting to be part of peer group. He was very social as I was very remote. In the fall I chose to buy a second home, moving quickly, not knowing I would never return to the farm and my dream community.

    I knew that my career as clothing merchant and manager was a temporary step.. I felt I would not be in the position more than a year. I wished to glean the skills of the patriarch of merchants. He was an elder grandfather figure, who admired my honesty, character and intelligence. He was willing to groom me. In the past, I had made many mistakes trying to let someone else be responsible and while doing service for others. I truly needed to make decisions wisely and then stand firm. I did not know of the embedded problems with this almost 100% female staff of clerks, bookkeepers and 'hench woman.'

    The world of beauty, texture, and design was rich. My duties extended to assisting others to express themselves with comfort in the world of clothing. The time was ripe for me to explore and express my own personal beauty through attire and stature. Being a flower child in exotic flowing skirts and braless underwear was inappropriate.

    An old crone I called the 'She Wolf of the West' was the bad guy on this elder's staff. She was the disciplinarian. Her techniques were verbal abuse, defaming character and an evil eye. Constantly I went nose to nose with this tyrant. I did not condone her treatment of the staff who worked with me or me, period. She had an underlying distrust of me.

    With a degree in mathematics I had a knack for budgets, figures, percentages and after watching the books for several months, I knew the figures were inaccurate. I learned the clothing mark-up world, which was much more lucrative than that of the bookstore markup system, but I just could not get the same results as this matriarch.

    I was soon to learn that the elder owner would rather be known as roaring success, his net results were always in the black. All it took was erasing the red. He played with the numbers and added more dollars when necessary. So, the community truly did have a Santa Claus like merchant. I pondered the duality that he wanted to train me to be a wise merchant, but he himself was distorting truth for his own self imposed successful image.

    The sales were phenomenal. He gave merchandise away at below cost. It stunned me. I found I actually took minimal earnings home, but my wardrobe was outrageous.

    The She Wolf criticized me from day one to cut my long dark brown hair with it's white rosette of grey. "A mature woman in her thirties would not sport long hair and truly be considered sophisticated," she scorned.

    I let the clothing boutique become an extension of my healing practice. When the fluorescent lights and stress of life would find someone hurting, with permission we would slip into a dressing room. I would lay on of hands or I would practice a headache release acupressure technique.

    On weekends I would continue to train with Iron Fingers. Not only was Iron Fingers in my life to assist me to wellness but he considered me a talented touch therapist. I too, had a healing presence in my touch. I was being taught through observation as he requested that I put my "hands" away for a year and learn the ways of a Barefoot Physician. He was willing to discuss any thing I observed while he was administering to others. If I did not see a technique, he would not present it.

A hidden part of my quiet inner female was leaping for joy. Finally I had attracted a medicine person who worked with his hands. A recurring dream of mine had me and another pair of hands doing team heart, mind and body work with a recipient. This was my right livelihood. Here was this teacher who was courageously out there practicing a healing art that was pretty much unheard of. I would call it 'therapeutic touch or touch therapy'. It was definitely not the massage work I had learned in the late seventies.

Iron Fingers not only had an intense feeling for the Mother Earth, being part Native American himself, but he spoke with familiarity of the Chinese five element wellness process. Most of all, he saw the pain in my head and could feel the irregularity of my heart. He understood the spiritual emergence that had consumed my last years. He felt he could help me regain wellness in my life.

He had a special affinity to the red tail hawk as Brooke did to the Eagle. I loved the chance hearing of the Red Tail's searching screech. I was getting more excited about getting well, though the episodes of intense pressure in my brain were more frequent. It was difficult to always believe I was getting better. Quite honestly I felt worse before I felt any relief. Was I fooling myself with my brain and ego again?

As clear as this man was that I was a 'healer', he was also sure that we were family and not to be soul lovers. At this point my heart was so overwhelmed, my blood pressure constantly being blocked by improper circulation and posture and my mind had faced and felt death so often—something had to change. Life was not a pleasure, it was a strain and that was nothing new, just a recurring script of broken heart, flooded feelings, and vulnerability because of betrayals.

Iron Fingers knew too that my life cord was very frazzled. Part of Iron Fingers standards were that if he could not assist someone to better health he would aide them to find someone who could. He insisted that I travel to his teacher, Dr. Timothy Binder a homeopathic, chiropractic, osteopathic naturopathic physician in Montana. He felt that if anyone could help me it would be this talented herbalist and registered healer. He was willing to make the connections and literally drove me there to begin treatments.

The drive to Montana was done in the dark of night, after a full week of work. Hours before the appointed meeting, my Barefoot Physician would take my son and I to a sacred grove of cedar on a high mountain pass. Just walking in the thick circular grove was like entering the most immense cathedral. I prayed for health and vitality. I prayed to be an instrument of the maker's purpose. I prayed for a quality to my life that I knew I deserved.

Walking into Dr. Binder's solar heated office was unnerving. I would bare my whole health history to this short, dark eyed, very unique looking physician. After the verbal exam, he proceeded to do an over view, using electrical probes, gentle and then complicated structural balancing. (I had been trained in his aligning program called Postural Integration.) This physician would not see people unless they had done a bunch of prerequisite treatments.

He stood looking at me with those direct, piercing eyes. He was in deep scrutiny of my facial bone structure and he asked "Have you ever been hit or received an injury to your face?" Tears sprung out without permission. Which time, I responded! He asked my history of facial abuse. Quickly, I related the knock-out blow my ex-husband had delivered in 1977, but my memory simultaneously recalled the punch my father had delivered when I was a teenager, that had also knocked me flat.

It was almost a family power point to strike about the face. I knew my mother had been hit in her youth and it was second nature for her to strike us especially on the face. I had thought I had healed those impacts because my involuntary response no longer had me flinch anytime a hand or a motion came towards my face.

Here was a trusted physician explaining the structural damage done and the resultant pressure on my Pituitary gland. This accounted for excruciating pain behind my left eye, and the secondary influences of stress and imbalance to my hormones through the endocrine system and especially the inter-relatedness to my menstrual cycle, or rather lack of menses.

He began the complicated unwinding of my neck vertebrae, and the intricate work within my mouth and ear region to start releasing and balancing my battered jaws. Jaws that had responded to childhood messages. . . "You are to be seen, but not heard." "Open your mouth and I'll knock your head off." "Smile pretty but say nothing." Painful, painful work, searing pain. . .I did not like the jaw work but I knew I had to have it.

Next he educated me on the effects of the life threatening 'quinsy—rheumatic fever' I had as a teenager that had weakened my heart. Finally someone put into words why my heart felt breaking and unsteady. Iron Fingers had brought it to my attention that I literally pounded my heart to keep it going. I also hit my heart region when I felt angry at myself and my actions. My pulse was extremely irregular and my breath often difficult to get.

There were many treatments he needed to do with me, Dr. Binder related. Would I commit to continue coming north and working with him on an extended basis? If so, he would start me on a homeopathic, natural cleanse. He also recommended I go through a complete restructuring of my whole skeletal/muscular body to accompany his work so my structure would maintain my health and not continue to collapse forward.

He did some initial cranial adjustments, including inserting balloons up my nasal passages. By inflating the balloons, muscles and bones in my face moved. As this first release occurred at the most inner part of brain, I heard a crack of inner release that set tears flowing again. I flashed through my life history of my 'to date unnamed abusive facial blows' and knew the mysterious dark unattainable reason for continued illness was finally reached and I was going to heal.

The immenseness of that moment of breath into my brain initiated the promise within me to tell my story so that others who might be on a long road of pain and recovery surrounding battering and accidents in their youth might believe they too could heal and regain a vitality to life.

At the end of the session, he recommended some homeopathic and herbal concoctions to assist my liver, kidneys and endocrine system. During the weeks that followed, as I was cleansing out the toxins in my brain and nervous system. I was again visited by the thoughts that this stuff is killing me. I felt bad, but I was committed for my brain was breathing, and the stagnation was leaving. I was hopeful.

After the treatment, I received apothecary concoctions that Dr. Binder created. With instructions to keep up with specific exercises and promised healthy diet, I left to go soak in some Montana sacred waters.

We went to this hidden away, geothermal lodge called 'Sleeping Child Lodge and Therapy Spa' to rest and release in the geothermal waters. Sleeping Child was named after an old Indian Spiritual story of rebirth and healing. I was so exhausted I slept and soaked for the next few days. I was healing.

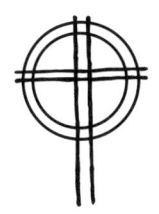

"IF YOU COMPARE YOURSELF WITH OTHERS,
YOU MAY BECOME VAIN & BITTER;
FOR ALWAYS THERE WILL BE GREATER & LESSER PERSONS THAN YOURSELF. ENJOY
YOUR ACHIEVEMENTS AS WELL AS YOUR PLANS."

TRANSITIONS - 1984

My health regime and therapeutic training became the most significant aspect of my life in the Magic Valley. While I knew my days were numbered at the Clothing Store, my attention focused on treatment of myself and others who were asking me to share touch therapy with them. I did not charge for my touch sharings but I strongly contemplated how was I going to get on with my 'right livelihood'.

A strong Buddhist influence filled my yearnings to be healthy, happy and holy. I desired to integrate my heart values, inborn talents and the lifelong quest for self realization with my work and daily life. Right livelihood seeks a mindful, focused approach to all work, especially the jobs we loathe (Housecleaning). Perseverance, self-mastery and the attitudes of service and selflessness were calling to my very way of being with constant practice of non-judgement to any script that life was giving.

All these good thoughts scrambled during the end of 1983. My Grandfather had fallen at the nursing home and was being sent to the hospital. My service and love script demanded that I go see him immediately. The reality of being a single mother, manager of a major store and the peak of the holiday season would not allow me to journey the seven hours to get to him. I felt miserable, part of me wanted to be there to help him, to see if I might even touch him and ease his pain. Though I knew the family would never condone my therapeutic touch, I felt the need to be there. I whipped my mind and heart with self judgement and criticism at my failure to show up for my dear grandfather.

During my last visit with him a few months earlier, he spoke for the first time in my life of his knowing that I carried the spirit of our family and our ways of believing. He encouraged me to keep doing what had heart to me and stated he was proud of me. No one in my family had ever spoken of understanding that sensitive, connected to the earth spiritually. I was thrilled and yet, now when my Grandfather truly 'needed' me as his worse fear became real of dying in a foreign hospital away from his beloved high mountain valley home, I could do nothing but fret.

My personal health was immersed in the intensity of cleansing and I felt like I was healing, but the renewed stress over my grandfather had me scrutinizing my path to enlightenment. I knew money did not own my soul. I knew that to be spiritually and physically well was important to me and that I wanted right livelihood. The Buddha said we become enlightened by sticking with mundane tasks. We use tiresome, repetitive work as a life mirror.

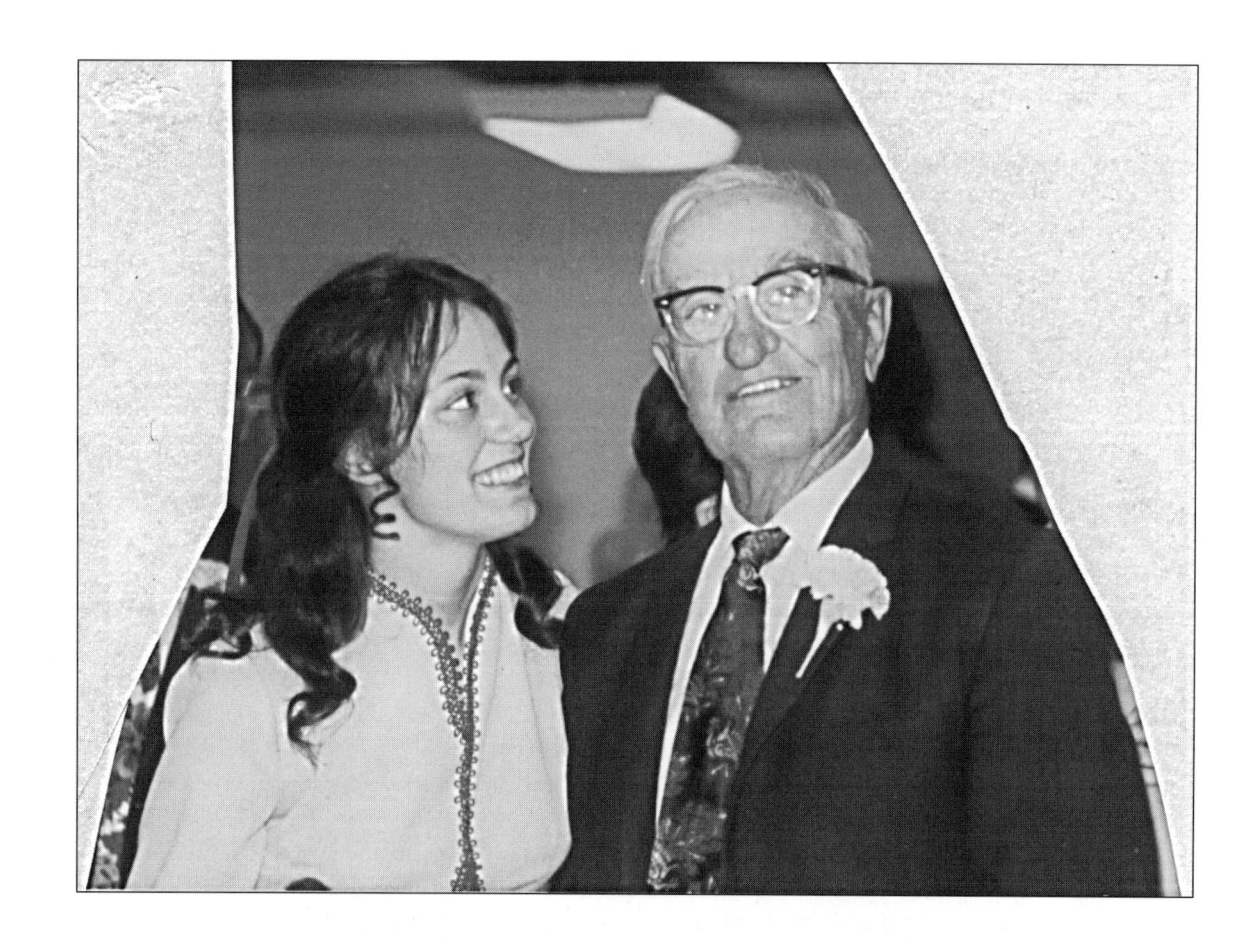

GRANDFATHER

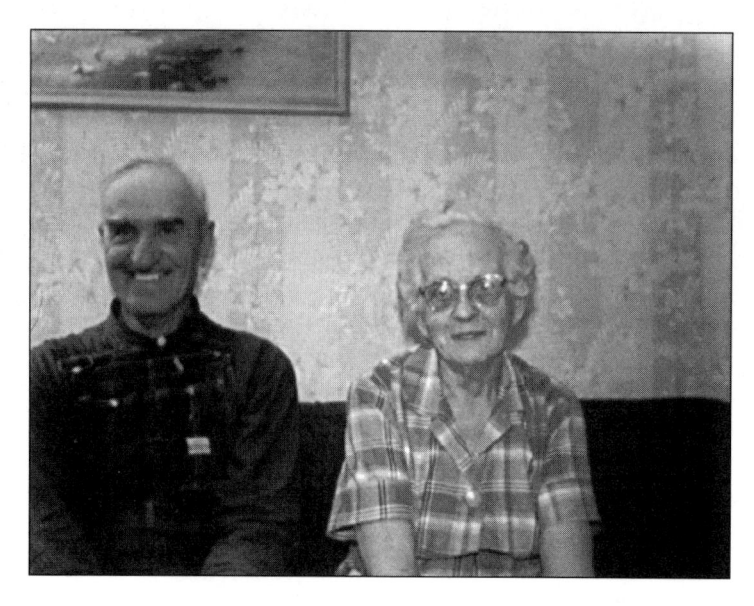

GRANDFATHER

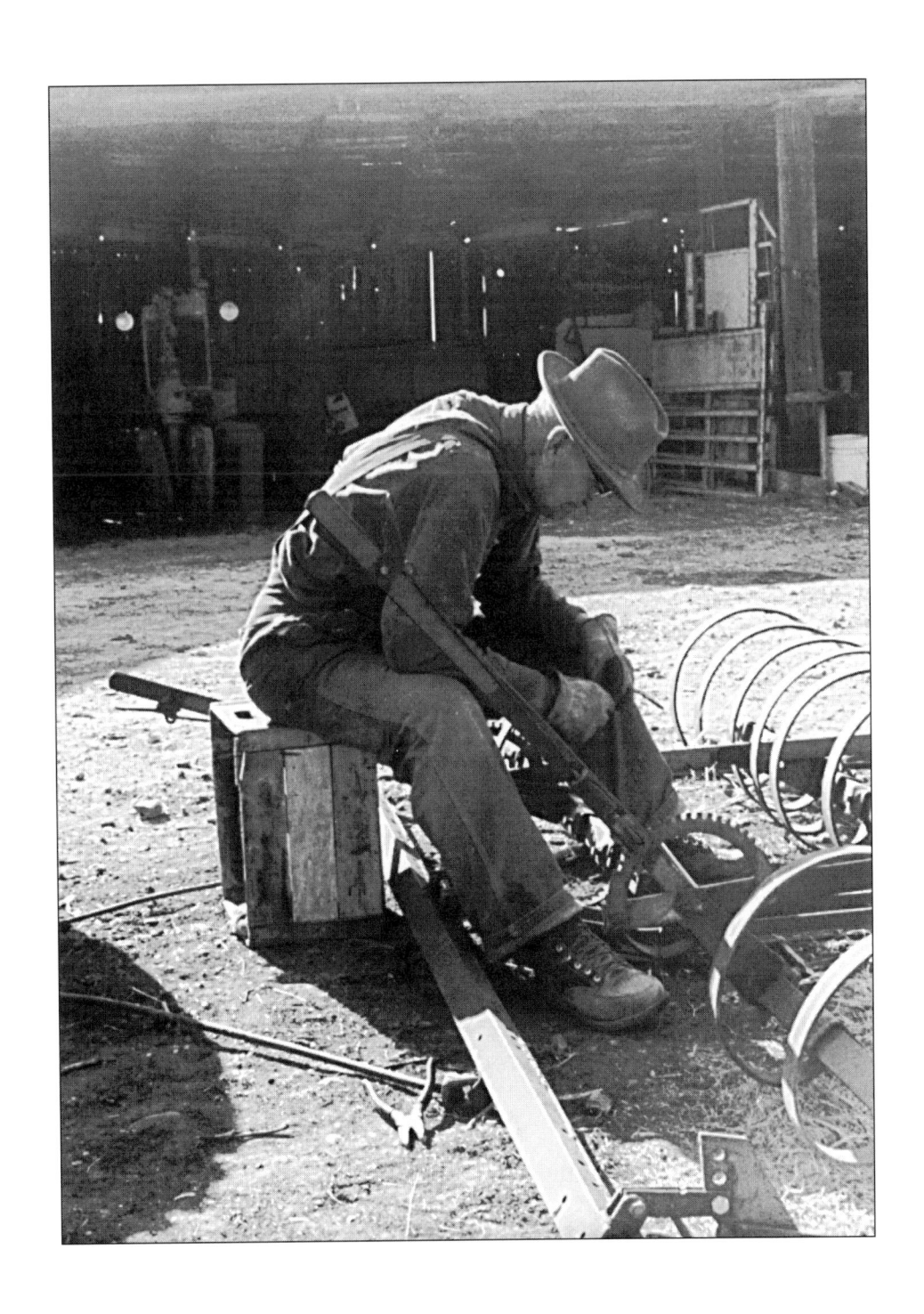

For myself, it was clear my 'work' this lifetime dealt with relationships. As each day is fully the Sabbath, and I was walking on the altar of my belief system. Learning to walk peacefully with longevity beside a man was my life work along with the sense of health and wellness. Christmas came with all its work responsibilities and my son journeyed to another town to be with his father. I spent the holidays alone, just working. I could not be with my grandfather for a multitude of reasons and I was alone.

Just after Christmas, I received a call that my grandfather had died. Because of the after Christmas sale, my elder boss would only allow me to be gone the day of the funeral. Out of the lack of kindness from this boss, I drove in the dead of winter five hours each way having time to only attend to this sad passage for just a few hours.

My improved jaw was tense as I drove the winter roads of Southeast Idaho to return to the land my ancestors had settled in the mid-1800's. I moaned and raged that the only man beside my son that I truly loved had died and that I had failed to be present for him. I tried to assault myself for not knowing how to get to that loved state with another that I so hungered for. All my life I had wanted to be special. I pushed, stretched, challenged, and surrendered trying to get some male to say "You are special."

I heard myself challenge my ability to love, and as I breathed in, I knew I did know how to love, it just wasn't with a grown male. I knew of my love for my artist friend, a woman. I could sense her there shining her love and acceptance and I decided that I would rewrite my old script of having to be special and in love with some outside male. I also gained clarity on how much I felt love with the Earth and her trees, waters, animals, birds, rocks, winds and fruitful soils.

By the time I arrived at the funeral, love had returned to my heart and I could say goodbye to my last male saint. As I sat with my thirty cousins, and dozen aunts and uncles, I could share my tears and disconnect from the critical attitudes I had felt judged by all my life. Maybe they would never know my specialness. I did not have to be vulnerable with them anymore. I knew I was okay, just different.

The next day I returned to work, tired but ready for grueling sales and expectations. Shortly before lunch, my elder male boss asked me to go for coffee. Something was up, I thought, he had not made that request for months.

Within the first few sips of coffee, he delivered what I call the 'blind left swing,' an impactful situation that I don't see coming. Ms. Lewis, he stated with his deep, gruff voice, "I am letting you go. You have lots more to get on with in your life. You have a lot of special talents that don't match the clothing business." The old she wolf's influence was more important than mine. He needed someone to do the dirty work around the business. I was too kind and honest. He said I could work for two more weeks and then it would be time to go. Symbolically another grandfather was marking a huge passage that I did not consciously chose.

I knew I was relieved not to have to enter that phony existence much longer and I decided it was time for me to get on with my heart work. It was time. For the first time in my life, I qualified for unemployment compensations and I was going to seek out a community that lived a wholistic approach to life.

Much to my dismay, within days a neighboring community approached me asking me to teach what I called my 'dream teaching' position. I was hired on a grant to write an individualized program for what I called the 'dead lightbulbs' in the back of classroom. I was integrating reading and mathematics for these special teens, the ones that take extra time, attention and communication.

Simultaneously that Spring, Big Man, the farmer and shareholder of the farm approached the remaining stockholders to buy us out. He had a new stepmother with money. They did not want us on the farm anymore. It was humorous, here I had thought the Earth was ending in 1984. All the last decade we had gone out of our way to be a healthy example of community and organic integrity with the Earth and economy and now it was The Farm that was ending.

It was clear that if I chose to resist the sale of the eighty acre farm, several other dear farm members would support my vote. I knew that, but none of my owner allies lived on the farm land to be good neighbors with. The energies of those surrounding my home and life at least had to be neutral, loving was aimed for, but dislike and hate was to be avoided. My son knew clearer than I, it was time to let go of the safe retreat center the farm had offered me since the mid-seventies.

I was teaching the educational program in an ideal setting with a 1-4 ratio with students. My test scores were showing that my concept around teaching the unteachable was real and worked, but deep in my soul I felt like a caged bird under fluorescent lights. I did not want to teach in a structured system.

Prayerfully I continued to journey north to work with my doctor. Since he was also the teacher of my close friend, Iron Fingers, whom I was training with in integrated deep touch therapy, I asked if he would teach another Barefoot Physicians course based on the Oriental five elements and meridian bodymapping and balancing one's nutritional system. He said soon, but not quite yet.

During the spring of 1984 I chose to facilitate Iron Fingers and a Feldenkrais trainee who had originally brought Brooke Medicine Eagle to Idaho, in a weekend course called *Path With Heart* at the local junior college. Our objective was to allow people to discover their own internal compass. To assist individuals to get in touch with their inner connectedness with life in the present, past and future. The past few years worth of guidance I had journeyed was worthy of sharing in this sleepy, agricultural based community.

At this well attended event, Iron Fingers met a professional children's advocate that would capture his heart and eventually influence him to move from Boise.

A few weekends later I would again facilitate this talented duo in the Magic Valley. This time we shared a weekend themed around *Reunion With The Sacredness of Self.* A tribe of people were coalesing in Southern Idaho. We were a diverse group who were willing to explore the illusion of limitation placed culturally upon us. We were knocking down the fences, walls or unconscious places in the American soul that was learned. 1984 was about responding to a healing call that required us to integrate the body and the soul and not be dominated by the brain between the ears.

It was a cold, wet and dark early spring weekend. We chose to meet at our dear friend Synthony's mansion home. The first night we congregated this ancient home's electrical system blew out. It was as if Nature took a hand in mandating our closeness. Warmth was derived only by her fire place, so we all cuddled close.

Iron Fingers and the NLP trainee directed us through sensory and guided journeys. We allowed ourselves to know each other as if we had known each other from old. We would write, draw, touch, dance and sing our way into harmony. The words I don't know or I can't do were eliminated and encouragement was given to trusting, prayer, asking and listening to allow co-creativity with the Maker of all Things, God and union with the sweetness of the Mother Earth.

1984 HEALING SUZANNE

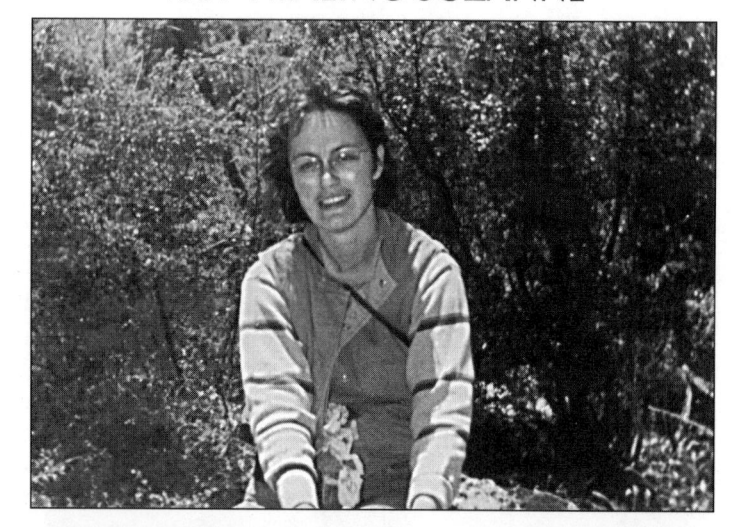

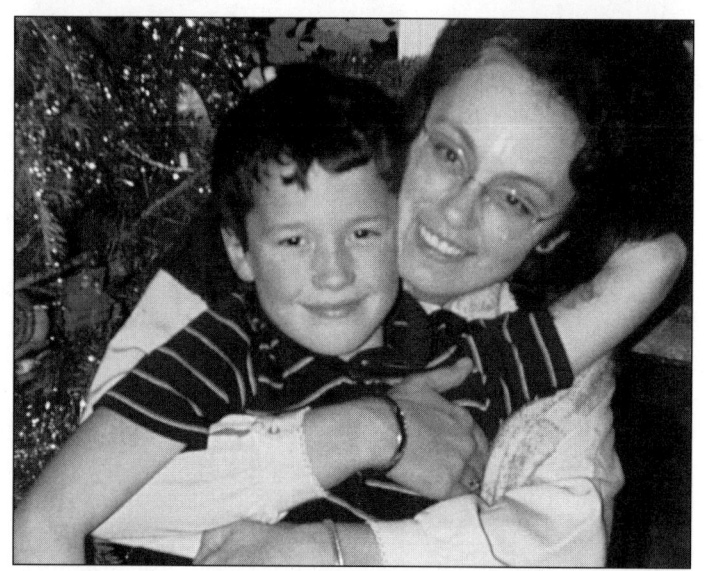

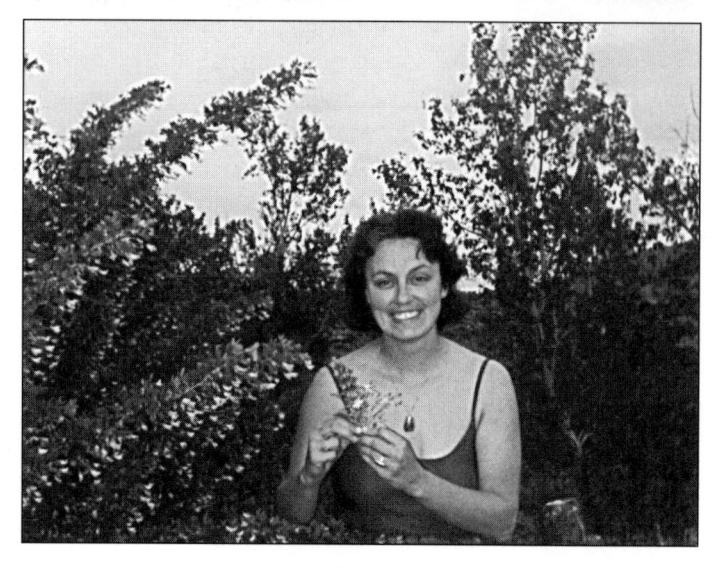

It was during this creative spontaneous process that I learned about Haiku, an Oriental, short prose process with measured beats that always has a nature metaphor built into the three lined verse. It was so liberating to playfully and briefly sum up what was currently a theme in my reality.

We ended the weekend with a longer prose writing exercise that to this day exhilerates me. In a circular group process we wrote a collective poem for each other. It was an allowing and conducive way to show that with trust and willingness we can do anything including expressing ourself symbolically.

Within days after this weekend event the 'human telegraph system' that exists on this Earth, sent word that Brooke Medicine Eagle had issued a plea for peoples all over the world to do a sacred sweat ceremony for the wetlands and the plants and trees of South America. A time to synchronize our efforts was given. Up to this point in my history, I had never facilitated or rather been in charge of this sacred cleansing, prayer full process. I was really 'up creek without a paddle'. There were no men around to do the sweat at the appointed time.

The East of the Medicine Wheel is often represented symbolically by the Eagle and Red Tail Hawk. Both birds are recognized by their clear sightedness and ability to see great distances. The last few months I had been gifted twice by the Red Tail Hawk. It is extremely rare to come upon the hawk or eagle. When one finds a bird that has passed over, one is called to honoringly take care of its bodily remains. I knew that I was being gifted. At this time in my studies with Brooke Medicine Eagle, I received it as a spiritual message.

My life was filled with prayers at this time in my life. I courageously agreed to be responsible for a sweat in our valley, even if I was not sanctioned by a medicine person. The receiving of the Red Tail Hawks helped in making this big decision. The Earth deserved our prayers. Before I could announce the ceremony, I received permission to come back to the farm and use the lodge.

Ten women met as the moon rose the spring of 1985 and I would be in charge with what was a monumental leap of faith for me as in the last sweats my body had been so stressed I had felt death whisper through my body. Now, I was committing to be responsible for the whole process, could my body be well enough to do it? I prayed to be an instrument for the evolvement of consciousness and healing, pleading for the two-legged to get connected with the consequences of their unconscious consumption of the trees, the waters, the air, the sweet Earth.

During the sweat process, I became aware of oversouls, winged spirits surrounding us, praying with us. My hands were miniaturized by giant felt hands moving through my intentions and fingers. With each round of added rock, more waters, and intense prayers, strength and integrity coursed through my energy channels and spirit. The knowledge that thousands of others were praying with common intent was astounding. The words, the feelings were magnified. I was so thankful I was willing to respond to the invite. I wanted to be of service to the bigger Self, to the whole Earth and all her family.

When the final prayer ended, honoring our ancestors and willing to do good actions for seven generation to come, the flaps opened. Individuals crawled out, birthing into a newness, an awareness that would be felt by all the world (Emerald Forest is an excellent film the depicted this sacredness loss.) My hands were so alive, they felt four times their regular size. I felt blessed and validated. I was the Teacher of Heart and my hands would do body/mind/heart work. I could see through my hands and with pure heart and intentions assist myself and others to health and vitality. I knew I was to write my book, *TEACHER OF THE HEART: A Self Health Journey.* I was aware how closely I was in contact with Brooke because Red Tail Hawk and Field Hawks continued to soar and dive towards me.

Meanwhile people from Boise were driving to my area for touch treatments and workshops that I was facilitating. Different folks were asking me to come to Boise and do therapeutic touch.

I had mixed feelings about Boise. When I left it ten years earlier, my broken spirit and health had me sever all connections. Rarely had I visited the city and now the thoughts of returning challenged me. Having my son around his blood father was attractive.

In May, my friend Synthony and I were invited to journey to Boise to attend a four day *Peaceful Settlements* conference. My Futurist friend insisted we be present for this innovative event that focused on ways to promote peace rather than litigations and lawsuits. The theme also encouraged inner peace making as well as community.

My artist friend would create two spectacular pieces to display at this event. One was called *They Brought Us Christianity* and the other, *The Peacemaker.* For myself, I was reintroduced to a wonderful mediative, conflict resolution oriented peer group. I would learn of an effort in San Francisco called *The Sounding Board* where neighborhoods had people trained to mediate conflict through an intricate system of communication and listening. I was so impressed that progress was being made to help us be better neighbors that I vowed to become a trained in this program.

I began to feel welcomed by sectors of this Boise Valley. By late summer, I was driving to Boise and had a half dozen committed recipients of my therapeutic touch. I had worked on a logo for over a year and my new business card had to have three roses with a circle surrounding them. The rose is my connection with Christ and the Circle my understanding of the interconnectedness of all life.

Still not certain about the move to my old hometown, I chose to go to the ocean to pray and seek clarity on my birthday in September. Time by the waters is always high in my books for self healing. But the journey to the grandmother waters was troublesome/unsettling this time. On the return journey, a friend and I traveled a different route through the high, lava filled mountains of Oregon.

At one stop, we decided to take a walk on the volcanic bubbles and blisters. Behind me I heard a grandmother shuttle her four grandchildren onto the hard rocks. The next thing I heard was that terrible sound of flesh and bones crunching against rock. I turned and saw blood gushing from the face of this elder woman. I knew I had to get involved. So I went to her, the grandchildren crying, "She's a bleeder, she's a bleeder." With little thought, but great prayers, I asked if I could help, explaining my talents to have healing touch. She said please do, so I `layed on my hands'. The light of day intensified brightly. I prayed. My friend stared in disbelief. I heard and felt God's healing presence, handily come through my hands. Do you still question your heart work it asked?

The bleeding ceased, the gash above her eye sealed, she was almost as good as new. The fragile part of me wanted to run away. It is always difficult to acknowledge the miraculous. But a miracle had just occurred, once again, and I saw it and confirmed, that yes I did have hands that were gifts from God, and my human self did deserve to live healthily and well. Allowing my hands to do my lifework did not mean I had to live as a pauper.

SUZANNE AT THE OCEAN PRAYING FOR DIVINE GUIDANCE

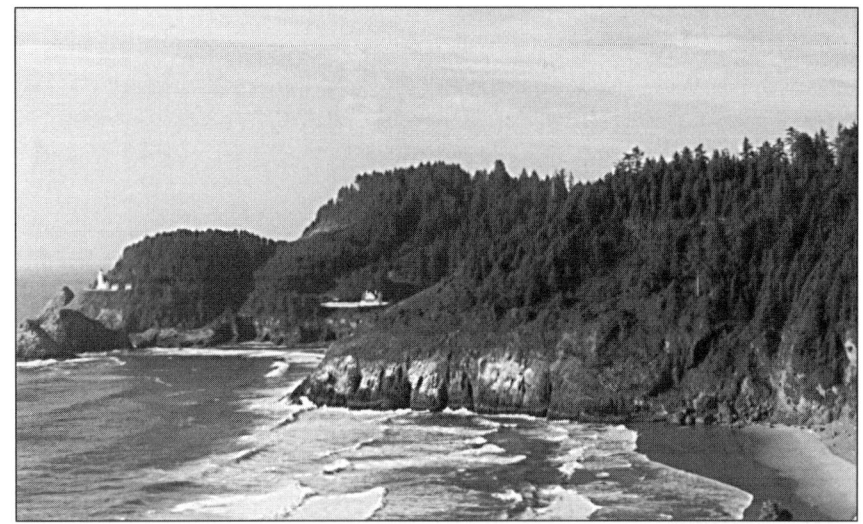

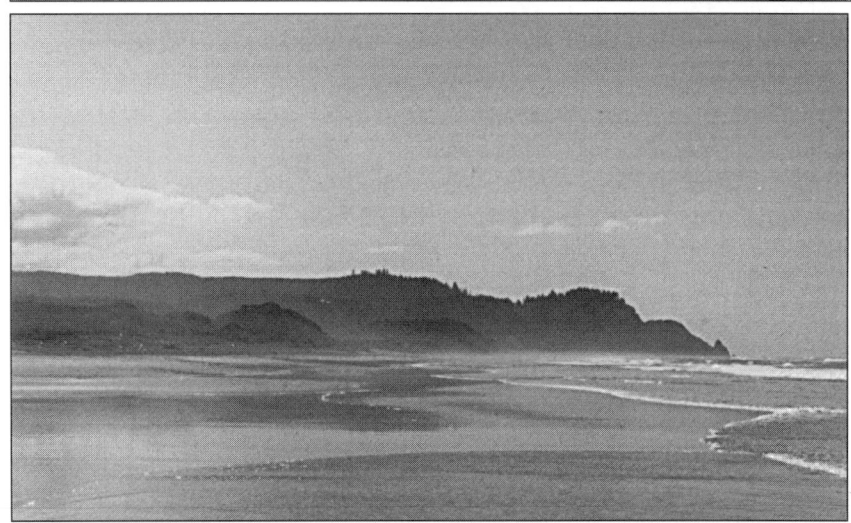

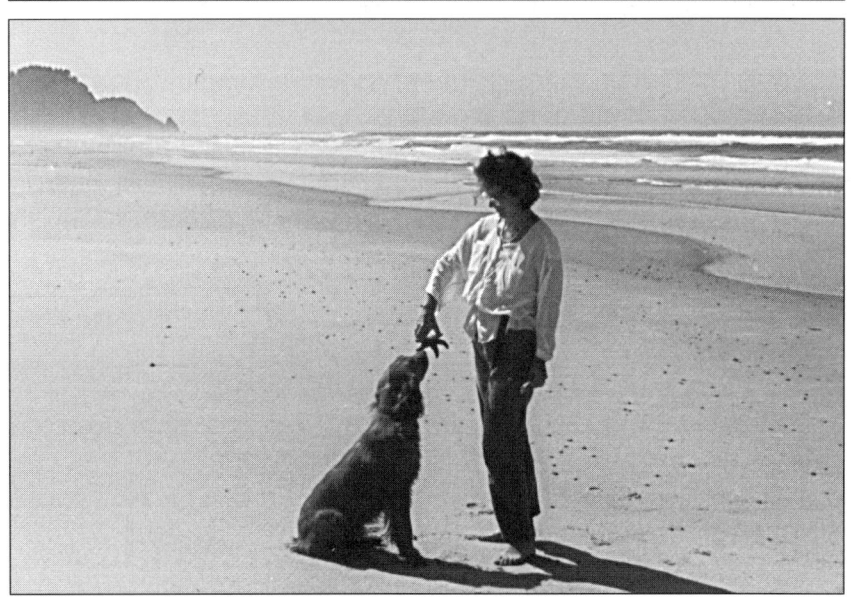

I had an appointment to meet back in Boise. Iron Fingers had arranged for me to meet and touch someone with lupus, an immune related, joint congested confusing disorder. When I arrived I met a gentle man, with lots of personal spirit and commitment to his wellness. After working with him, he announced he was a Psychologist and he would welcome me to Boise with referrals if I would come there.

I announced if I could easily relocate in this city of the trees I would do so. Within weeks, friends located a completely furnished home. I drove to Boise with my son and what my small car could hold.

A surprise came my way as I journeyed to Boise. Iron Fingers and I were to work together in this capitol city, but his heart was smitten and as I drove West, he drove East to be closer to his loved one. I definitely was doing a move of faith, that demanded that I stand on my own two feet. No leaning on the established clientele of Iron Fingers, though he did bequeath me his phone number in Boise.

In the fall of 1985, I returned to the town that I grew up in and graduated from college. I came back not as a teacher of secondary mathematics, but as a Wholistic Touch Therapist. I called myself the "Professionals' professional touch therapist." My blood family lived within fifteen minutes of my home and my son could easily access his father. In addition, he could finally play his long yearned for soccer.

I was in close communication with Brooke and had committed to follow through with her four year healing vision. The next cycle was called *BREAKING THE CHAINS - Healing Dysfunctional Family Patterns* and it was going to be facilitated in Oregon. I was back amongst some of most harmful, hurtful and confusing co-creators of such patterns. I wondered how long I would be able to stay 'out in the world'. I already was missing my farm retreat.

I knew I was the Teacher of the Heart. All that I had to share was gained through authentic experience. If by telling my stories, others would be helped to mend frayed hearts and nerves, it was worth the decade plus effort of completing and editing the chapters of my life from 1974-1984.

I basically believe we are born whole, whether abuse, trauma, confusion sets in while in the womb or shortly thereafter. We start out graced. Once illness, a dis-ease patterns set in, we proceed with greater sickness, confusion and disorder until we get to the point that we will not allow ourselves to get any worse. Death haunts us.

My path to recovering that natural God given grace was just shared. I contend that life is like a book. We all have the same chapters, we just choose to live them out at our own rate and order. Some of us get critically ill in our twenties, others in their forties. Some of us go through relationship fallout in our teens others in their thirties and so on. I believe we all have the same chapters. So, onward to wellness within ourselves, with our families, with the Earth and with the relationship with the Maker of All Things, God.

POSTSCRIPT:

It is now 1997 and I intend to have a second book available covering the first ten years of being a wholistic therapist and educator in Boise, Idaho. It is a curiosity that in our culture one does not call oneself a healer, but is known for it. The success of those of us in this therapeutic touch world reflects the results one's clientelle recognize. Not only will this next book, called *WATER MEDICINE WOMAN: Healing is the Revealing of Feelings* elaborate on the four-year healing cycle with Brooke, it will also expand on the integration of the Indigenous People's Medicine Wheel as it interweaves with the Oriental five element theory and meridian flows.

    I pray this next book takes only a few years to write and edit instead of a decade plus. Peace, joy and health to each of you, right now.

1985 SUZANNE HAPPY WITH CHILDREN AND SUPPORTIVE FRIEND

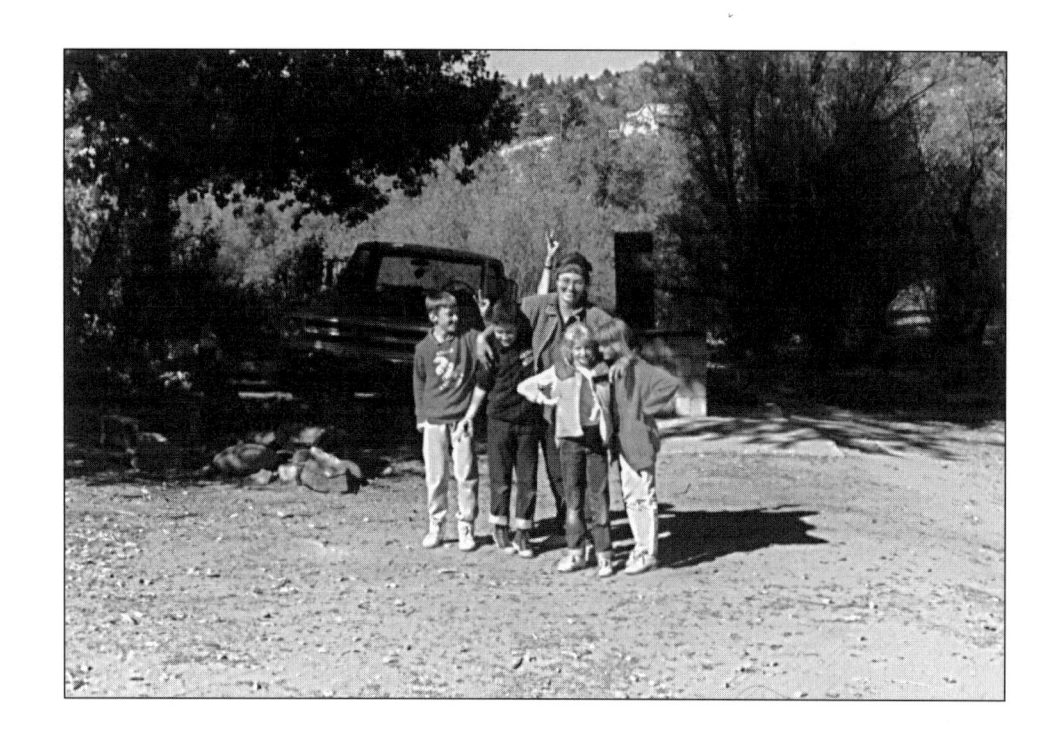

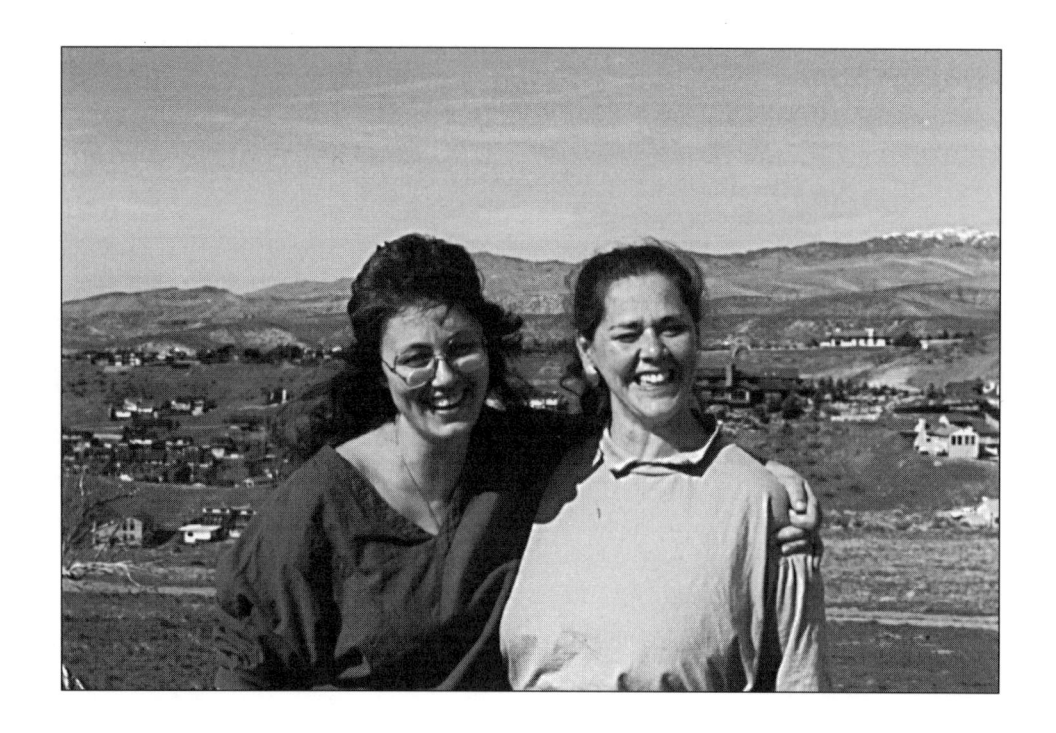

LIFE SONG

I DREAMED A DREAM
Words and Music by Patti Weber Lightstone

1. I dreamed a dream a long time a go
   'Bout a land where the rivers run wild.
   Where flowers grow wherever they choose.
   And the breezes blow gentle and mild;
   Where the trees stand in silence yet singing their song.
   In natural harmony:
   Where the earth freely gives to nurture all life
   And creation is boundless and free.

2. I dreamed a dream a long time ago
   About people who know how to live.
   Their words and their deeds are simple and pure.
   And their love they most willingly give.
   Each day of their lives is a reverent prayer.
   Their joy fills each moment with Light:
   And the peace found within is reflected without,
   Like a day softly echoed by night.

3. My dream slowly fades with the passing of time,
   Yet my vision grows clearer each day.
   I know what a wonderful world it will be
    When we each learn the part that we play.
   But each one of us must find the Truth for ourselves
   And live it the best that we can,
   And I'll sing my song just as you will sing yours.
   What a beautiful vision for man.

MY SON, NATHAN'S "WISH FOR THE WORLD" AT AGE NINE

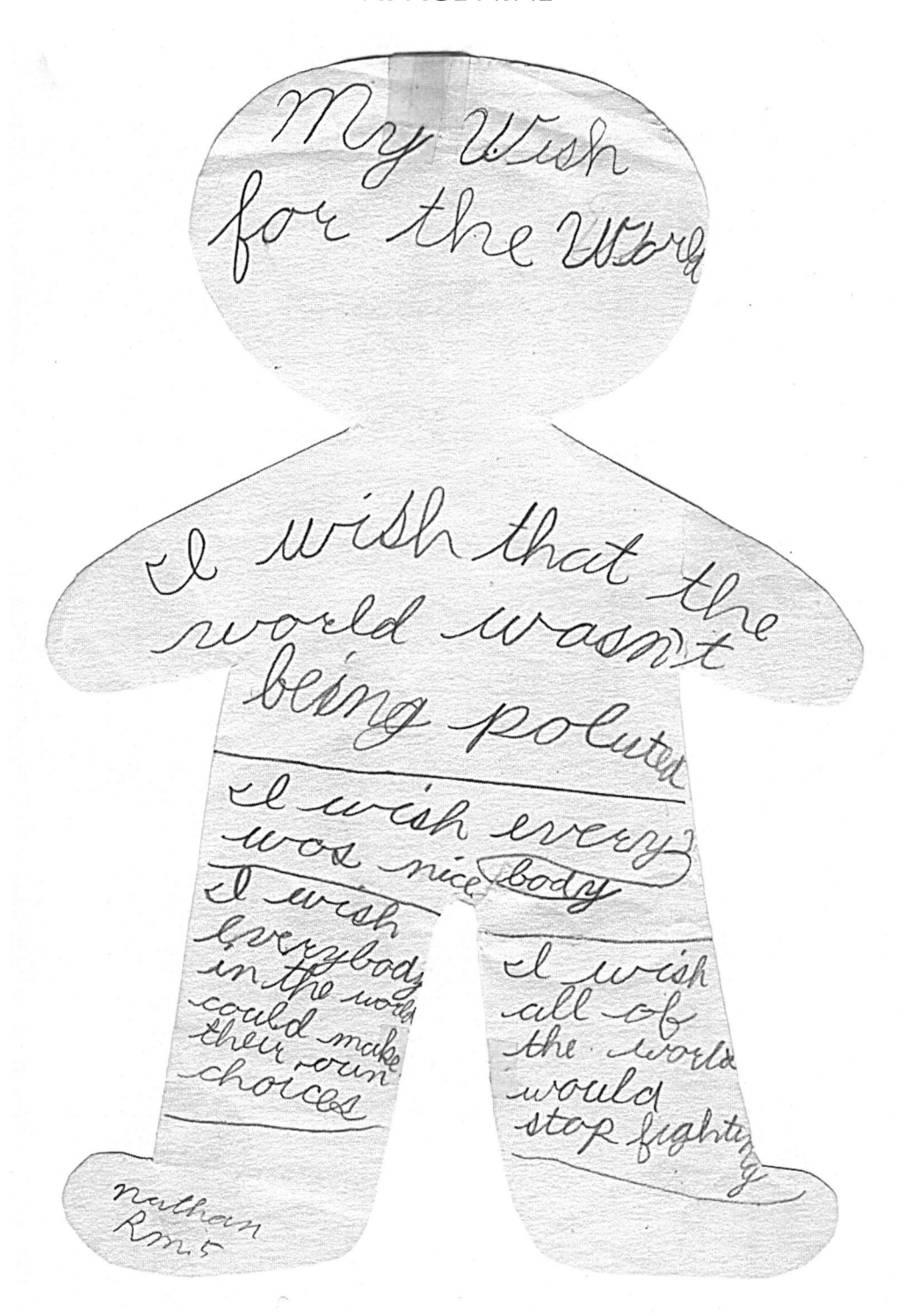

My wish for the world

I wish that the world wasn't being poluted

I wish every body was nice

I wish everybody in the world could make their own choices

I wish all of the world would stop fighting

Nathan Rm 5

SO BE IT!

REFERENCES

Abbey, Edward. 1975. *The Monkey Wrench Gang.* Holt Rinehart Winston.
_____. **1966.** *FIRE ON THE MOUNTAIN.* Holt Rinehart Winston
_____. **1968.** *DESERT SOLITAIRE.* Holt Rinehart Winston
_____. **1971.** *BEYOND THE WALL.* Holt Rinehart Winston

Bach, Edward, M.B., B.S., D.P.H. 1931. HEAL THYSELF *An Explanation of the Real Cause and Cure of Disease.* The C.W. Daniel Company Limited. London.
_____. **1933.** *THE TWELVE HEALERS and Other Remedies.* The C. W. Daniel Company Ltd.

Bach, Richard. 1977 . *ILLUSIONS The Adventures of a Reluctant Messiah.* Delacorte Press.
_____, **1975.** *Jonathan Livingston Seagull.* Delacorte Press.

Bandler, Richard. 1979. *FROGS INTO PRINCES.* Real Peoples Press.
_____. **1985.** *Using Your Brain — for a CHANGE Neuro-Linguistic Programming.* Real People Press.

Bayly, Doreen E. 1984. *REFLEXOLOGY TODAY The Stimulation of the Body's Healing Forces Through Foot Massage.* Thorsons Publishers, Inc.

Bean, Roy E, N.D. 1975. *Helping Your Health With Pointed Finger Pressure.* Parker Publishing Company, Inc.

Binder, Dr. Timothy. 1977. *POSITION TECNIC The Science of Centering.* Dr. Tim & Sharon Binder.

Brown, Dee. 1971. *BURY MY HEART AT WOUNDED KNEE An Indian History of the American West.* Holt, Rinehart & Winston, Inc.

Buck, Pearl S. 1961. *THE GOOD EARTH.* Pan Books Ltd: London.
_____. **1965.** *THE MOTHER.* Pan Books Ltd: London.

Bunker and Javane, Dusty and Faith. 1979. *NUMEROLOGY and The Divine Triangle.* Para Research, Inc.

Castaneda, Carlos. 1968. *The Teachings of Don Juan: A Yaqui way of knowledge.* Ballantine Books.
_____. **1971.** *A Separate Reality Further Conversations With Don Juan.* Pocket Books New York.

Dass, Baba Hari. 1974. *THE YELLOW BOOK.* Lama Foundation.

Dass, Ram (Alpert, Dr. Richard). 1971. *BE HERE NOW.* Lama Foundation.
_____. **1974.** *THE ONLY DANCE THERE IS.* Bantam Books.
_____. **1976.** *JOURNEY OF AWAKENING: A Meditator's Guidebook.* Bantam Books.
_____. **1977.** *GRIST FOR THE MILL.* Bantam Books.
_____. **1979.** *Miracle of Love Stories About Neem Karoli Baba.* A Dutton Paperback.

de Castillejo, Irene Claremont. 1973. *KNOWING WOMAN A Feminine Psychology.* Harper Colophon Books.

Deer amd Erdoes, John Lame and Richard. 1972. *Lame Deer Seeker of Visions.* Washington Square Press Publication of POCKET BOOKS.

Dillard, Annie. 1977. *Holy the Firm.* Harper and Row.
_____. **1982.** *TEACHING A STONE TO TALK.* Harper & Row.
_____. **1984.** *PILGRIM AT TINKER CREEK.* Harper & Row.

Downing, George. 1972. *THE MASSAGE BOOK.* Random House — The Bookworks.

Dreikurs, Dr. Rudolf. 1964. *CHILDREN THE CHALLENGE.* Hawthorn Books, Inc.

Dukas and Hoffman, Helen and Banesh. 1979. *Albert Einstein The Human Side.* Princeton University Press.

Dychtwald, Ken. 1977. *BODYMIND.* Jeremy P. Tarcher.

Eagle, Brooke Medicine. 1991. *BUFFALO WOMAN COMES SINGING.* Ballantine Books.

Feldenkrais, Moshe. 1972. *AWARENESS THROUGH MOVEMENT Easy- to-do Health Exercises to Improve Your Posture, Vision, Imagination and, Personal Awareness.* Harper & Row, Publishers, Inc.

Ferguson, Marilyn. 1980. *THE AQUARIAN CONSPIRACY Personal and Social Transformation in the 1980s.* Tarcher Houghton Mifflin Company.

Findhorn Community. 1975. *THE FINDHORN GARDEN: Pioneering a New Vision of Man and Nature in Cooperation.* Harper Colophon Books.

Fromm, Erich. 1956. *THE ART OF LOVING.* Harper & Row.

Gibran, Kahil. 1928. *JESUS The Son of Man: His words and his deeds as told and recorded by those who knew him.* New York - Alfred A. Knopf.
_____. **1923.** *THE PROPHET.* Alfred A. Knopf. New York.
_____. **1960.** *thoughts and meditations.* Citadel Press, Inc.
_____. **1962.** *Spiritual Sayings of Kahil Gibran.* Citadel Press, Inc.

Haich, Elisabeth. 1965. *INITIATION.* Seed Center

Hashimoto, Keizo M.D. 1977. *SOTAI Natural Exercise.* George Ohsawa Macrobiotic Foundation.

Heinlein, Robert. 1961. *Strangers in a Strange Land.* New English Library.

Hesse, Hermann. 1951. *SIDDHARTHA.* New Directions Publishing Co.
_____. 1930. *NARCISSUS AND GOLDMUND.* Farrar, Straus and Giroux, Inc.
_____. 1956. *THE JOURNEY TO THE EAST.* The Noonday Press a Division of Farrar, Straus & Giroux New York.

Hodgson, Joan. 1974. *ANGELS and INDIANS.* The White Eagle Publishing Trust.

Huxley, Aldous. 1942. *The Art of Seeing.* Montana Books, Publishers, Inc.

Joy, Dr. Brugh. 1977. *JOY'S WAY: A Map for the Transformational Journey.* Ballantine Books.

Jung, C. G. 1961. *MEMORIES, DREAMS, REFLECTIONS.* Random House, Inc.

Kazantzakis, Nikos. 1962. *SAINT FRANCIS.* Touchstone.
_____. 1960. *THE LAST TEMPTATION OF CHRIST.* Simon & Schuster.
_____. 1963. *The Saviors of God—Spiritual Exercises.* Simon & Schuster.

Kapleau, Philip. 1965. *THE THREE PILLARS OF ZEN: Teaching Practice Enlightenment.* Beacon Press.

Keyes, Ken, Jr. 1982. *the hundredth monkey.* Vision Books
_____. 1975. *HANDBOOK TO HIGHER CONSCIOUSNESS.* the Living Love Center.
_____. 1979. *a conscious person's guide to relationships.* Living Love Publications.

Khan, Hazrat Inayat. 1978. *THE COMPLETE SAYINGS OF HAZRAT INAYAT KHAN.* Sufi Order Publications.

Kriyananda, Swami. 1973. *EASTERN THOUGHTS WESTERN THOUGHTS.* Ananda Publications.

Kushi, Michio. 1980. *See Your Health Book of Oriental Diagnosis.* Japan Publication.

Laubin, Reginald & Gladys. 1957. *THE INDIAN TIPI: Its History, Construction, and use.* The University of Oklahoma Press.

Mabbutt, Richard. 1982. "Abundance at Hand". New Realities Magazine.

McLuhan, T.C. 1971. *TOUCH THE EARTH: A Self-Portrait of Indian Existence.* Outerbridge and Dienstryfrey.

Montagu, Ashley. 1971. *TOUCHING: THE HUMAN SIGNIFICANCE OF THE SKIN.* Columbia University Press.

Montgomery, Ruth. 1974. *COMPANIONS ALONG THE WAY.* Popular Library.
_____. **1973.** *BORN TO HEAL.* Popular Library.
_____. **1971.** *A WORLD BEYOND.* Coward.
_____. **1979.** *STRANGERS AMONG US.* Coward.

Moody, Dr. Raymond A. Jr. 1976. *LIFE AFTER LIFE.* Mockingbird Books, Inc.

Moss, Dr. Richard. 1981. *THE I THAT IS WE: Awakening to Higher Energies Through Unconditional Love.* Celestial Arts.

Muramoto, Naboru. 1973. *HEALING OURSELVES.* A Swan House Book published by Avon.

Nuernberger, Phil Ph.D. 1981. *Freedom From Stress: A Holistic Approach.* Himalayan International Institute of Yoga Science & Philosophy Publishers.

Orwell, George. 1949. *1984.* Harcourt Brace Jovanovich, Inc.

Pelletier, Kenneth R. 1977. *Mind as Healer Mind as Slayer: A Holistic Approach to Preventing Stress Disorders.* Dell Publishing Co., Inc.

Price, John Randolph. 1981. *THE SUPERBEINGS.* Fawcett Crest.

Rajneesh, Bhagwan Shree. 1975. *The Mustard Seed: A living explanation of the sayings of Jesus from the Gospel According to Thomas.* Harper and Row.
_____. **1975.** *ONLY ONE SKY: On the Tantric Way of Tilopa's Song of Mahamudra.* A Dutton Paperback.
_____. *Tantra Spirituality & Sex.* 1983. Ma Anand Sheela, M.M., D. Phil. D. Litt., Acharya.

Rimmer, Robert H. 1961. *THE HARRAD EXPERIMENT,* New England Library.

Roberts, Jane. 1971. *SETH SPEAKS: The Eternal Validity of the Soul.* Prentice-Hall, Inc.
_____. **1974.** *THE NATURE OF PERSONAL REALITY: A Seth Book.* Prentice-Hall, Inc.

Robbins, Tom. 1976. *EVEN COWGIRLS GET BLUES.* Bantam Books.

Roffman, Roger A. 1982. *MARIJUANA as MEDICINE.* Madrona Publishers.

Salinger, J.D. 1961. *FRANNY and ZOOEY.* Bantam Books.

Sandars, N. K. 1960. *EPIC OF GILGAMESH.* Penguin Classics.

Snyder, Gary. 1969. *THE REAL WORK: Interviews & Talks.* A New Directions Books.
_____. **1974.** *TURTLE ISLAND.* New Directions.

Stewart, Mary. 1970. *THE CRYSTAL CAVE.* A Fawcett Crest Book.
_____. **1973.** *THE HOLLOW HILLS.* A Fawcett Crest Book.
_____. **1976.** *THE LAST ENCHANTMENT Merlin Trilogy.* A Fawcett Crest Book.

Storm, Hyemeyohsts. 1972. *SEVEN ARROWS.* Harper & Row.

Suzuki, Fromm and DeMartino; D.T., Erich and Richard. 1960. *Zen Buddhism and Psychoanalysis.* Grove Press.

_____. **1948.** *THEORY AND PRACTICE OF BODY MASSAGE.* Milady Publishing Corporation.

Williams, Paul. 1973. *DAS ENERGY.* Warner Communications Company.

Watts, Alan W. 1966. *THE BOOK: On the Taboo Against Knowing Who You Are.* Collier Books, New York.

Werner, David. 1977. *WHERE THERE IS NO DOCTOR: a village care handbook.* The Hesperian Foundation.

Whitman, Walt. 1855. *LEAVES OF GRASS.* Penguin Books.

Yogananda, Paramahansa. 1977. *AUTOBIOGRAPHY of a YOGI.* SELF-REALIZATION FELLOWSHIP Publishers.
_____. **1976.** *MAN'S ETERNAL QUEST and other talks.* SELF-REALIZATION FELLOWSHIP Publishers.

ORDER FORM

IF INTERESTED IN PURCHASING ADDITIONAL COPIES OF THIS BOOK OR MORE INFORMATION ON SUZANNE'S WORKSHOPS AND FUTURE WORKS, FILL IN SPECIFICALLY BELOW:

Name _____

Address _____

City _____

State _____ Zip Code _____

_____ copies of **TEACHER OF THE HEART A Self Health Journey**
@ $24 ea. $_____

Idaho Residence add 5% sales tax $_____

Send 10% for shipping $_____

TOTAL $_____

include check for total amount, or use credit card as indicated below:

___ Visa   ___ MasterCard   Credit Card No. _____

Signature _____ Expiration Date _____

_____ Please put me on future workshop and mailers.

I am especially interested in _____ topics.

To order by phone call:
1-800-358-1929
Quantity orders invited — Call for bulk pricing

To order by Mail:
Make checks payable to:

STAR ROSE PUBLISHING COMPANY
SUZANNE LEWIS
623 West Hays Street
Boise, Idaho 83702
U.S.A.